Second Edition

ENDODONTICS

E. NICHOLLS
M.D.S., L.D.S. R.C.S.

Consultant Dental Surgeon, University College Hospital, Dental Hospital

Senior Lecturer, The London Hospital Medical College Dental School (University of London)

JOHN WRIGHT & SONS LTD.
BRISTOL 1977

First Edition, 1967
Second Edition, 1977

CIP Data:
Nicholls, Edward
  Endodontics. 2nd ed.
  1. Endodontics
  I. Title
  617.6′34   RK351

ISBN 0 7236 0427 4

Printed in Great Britain by John Wright & Sons Ltd., at the Stonebridge Press, Bristol

TO
MY WIFE AND CHILDREN

Preface to Second Edition

In the 10 years since the first edition of this book there have been considerable changes in the scientific basis for endodontic treatment and in the pattern of endodontic practice. The maintenance of pulpal vitality by direct and indirect pulp capping has received considerable study, and there is a growing awareness of the interrelationship which sometimes exists between pulpal and periodontal disease. Root canal treatment of molar teeth is now performed far more often, especially in Great Britain, whilst various forms of endodontic treatment rarely employed a few years ago, such as the use in suitable cases of endodontic stabilizers and the so-called 'apexification' treatment of immature pulpless teeth, are now commonly practised.

These and other changes have necessitated not only substantial alterations in the text but also some enlargement, and in consequence this second edition is rather more than an updated first edition. Although the chapter titles and order of presentation have for the most part been retained, many chapters have been partly or completely rewritten and many new illustrations have been used.

A further alteration concerns the references cited in the text. These have not only been updated but also, in response to requests following the first edition, they have been increased in number. It is hoped that the text has not become unduly burdened as a result of this change. Although the book is intended primarily for undergraduate students and general practitioners, it is hoped that postgraduate students with a special interest in endodontics will find it of use.

As in the first edition, a distinction has been drawn between the terms 'endodontic treatment' and 'root canal treatment'. Endodontics is that branch of dental science dealing with diseases of the pulp and periapical region. Thus, by endodontic treatment is meant any procedure which is designed to maintain the health of the pulp or the periapical region of a tooth when either is in imminent danger of disease, or which, when disease is present, is used to treat them in such a way that the tooth can safely be retained. Root canal treatment is one such procedure.

My sincere thanks are due to Mr D. Derrick for his encouragement during the writing of this second edition, and indeed for first suggesting the need for this book, and to my publishers John Wright & Sons, for the considerable patience and forbearance they have shown to a week-end writer such as myself.

I am most grateful to Mr G. Walters for preparation of the new illustrations, to Miss C. Symondson for typing the altered manuscript, and to Mr C. Mercer for his diligent reading of both the manuscript and proofs. Finally, I would like to record my thanks to Surgical Equipment Supplies Ltd., to J. and S. Davis Ltd, and to Mr P. Kurer, of Kurer Developments, for kindly supplying the photographs illustrated in *Figs.* 80, 84 and 132*a*, and 132*b* respectively.

July, 1977   E. NICHOLLS

From the preface to the First Edition

Since the end of World War 2 there has been a growing awareness of the important role that endodontic treatment—and in particular root canal treatment—can play in the dental care of patients. However, in Great Britain alone, as the figures of the Ministry of Health indicate, millions of teeth are still extracted each year, and there is little doubt that many of these could be retained as useful functioning units with the aid of root canal treatment. Although the teeth are sometimes replaced by a denture, or more often by a succession of dentures, and occasionally by bridges, neither substitute is as effective as a tooth which has been properly root treated and restored, and in the long run both are often less economical. When root canal treatment is carried out, it is too often of a standard that would be unacceptable in other branches of clinical dentistry, particularly conservative dentistry in general. Dentists capable of making a fine crown or bridge can be completely at sea when faced with the prospect of root treating other than a simple anterior tooth, nor is it a rarity to see a well-made crown or bridge supported by a poorly filled root.

Root canal treatment is all too often a hit-or-miss procedure, and the approach to it commonly one of apprehension. In few other branches of clinical dentistry is there such a marked tendency to use methods and short cuts which the operator himself knows are unlikely, in the long term, to result in success. And yet there is no doubt that root canal treatment, when it is properly performed, has a high rate of success, especially in comparison with other dental procedures, or at least with those for which the rates of success have received detailed study.

There are a number of reasons for this unsatisfactory state, but one of the major ones is undoubtedly the lack of a clear concept of what should be done and why, and not an actual inability to do it. Like crown and bridge work, the bulk of endodontic treatment is definitely within the capabilities of most operators. This book has been written with this belief, and tries in a rational way to present to undergraduate students and general practitioners the essentials of endodontic treatment. Whilst it is hoped that the inquiring reader will find the large majority of his questions answered in its pages, it does not claim to be encyclopaedic. The treatment of primary teeth has not been included, and the bacteriological and histopathological aspects of endodontics have been described only to the extent considered necessary for understanding the rationale of clinical procedures. Inevitably, some of the generalizations made will be shown by future research to be in need of modification.

Contents

Chapter 1

Diagnosis of pulpal and periapical states: causes of pulpal injury

Correct diagnosis is of obvious importance. If a patient has signs or symptoms suggesting pulpal or periapical disease, it is necessary first to confirm that they are in fact due to such disease, and to identify the causative tooth, or teeth. If, when this has been done, it is planned to retain the tooth, the general state of the pulp and the periapical region beyond has to be assessed in order that appropriate treatment may be instituted.

CAUSES OF PULPAL INJURY

A knowledge of the causes of pulpal injury is important in the diagnosis as well as in the prevention of pulpal and periapical disease. In the account which follows it must be remembered that the reaction of the pulp to injury is variable, so that the result of such injury is difficult to forecast. Although some of the causes listed usually result in only slight irritation with reparative dentine formation, in some teeth they may lead to pulpitis. Conversely, a severe injury which would normally cause pulpal necrosis may sometimes be followed by recovery.

The causes of pulpal injury may be divided into two groups, according to whether or not they are associated with dental procedures.

1. Causes unassociated with dental procedures

a. Bacterial

Caries, leading to irritation of the pulp by micro-organisms and their products, is undoubtedly the commonest cause. Although Langeland and Langeland (1968) have shown that pulpal reaction can occur even with early lesions of dentine, the work of Reeves and Stanley (1966) and of Shovelton (1968) suggests that there is no significant pulpal change so long as the remaining dentine is at least 1·0 mm thick. With progression of caries beyond this level, and before exposure occurs, inflammatory cells start to accumulate in the pulp in the vicinity of the involved dentinal tubules, so that by the time the pulp is exposed it is already chronically inflamed (Seltzer et al., 1963).

Periodontal disease may also lead sometimes to pulpal irritation by micro-organisms. Thus, the presence of a deep periodontal pocket extending to the vicinity of the root apex will eventually result in pulpal inflammation. The latter

1

may also result from less extensive pocketing if the orifice of a lateral branch of the root canal becomes exposed by the destruction and loss of periodontal fibres. Furthermore, if the pulp has died previously from some other cause, then the bacteraemia associated with movements of a tooth with periodontal disease may possibly result in invasion of the necrotic pulpal tissue by micro-organisms.

The studies of Seltzer et al. (1963) and others have shown that regions of pulpal atrophy and necrosis may sometimes be associated with periodontal pocketing. This interrelationship between pulpal and periodontal disease is discussed further in Chapter 14.

There is one further route by which micro-organisms may reach the dental pulp, namely the bloodstream. There is evidence from studies on experimental animals that, during a bacteraemia, organisms may be attracted to damaged tissue, such as an inflamed dental pulp or periapical lesion (Gier and Mitchell, 1968). This phenomenon is known as *anachoresis*. However, whether it is responsible for pulpal infection in humans, and if so how often, is uncertain.

b. Mechanical

Injury to the pulp may result from wear of the teeth by attrition or abrasion, or from trauma.

Trauma may occur in a number of ways. Commonly it takes the form of a fall or blow on the face, with or without fracture of one or more teeth. If the pulp of a tooth is exposed it not only becomes inflamed in the region of the exposure but is also contaminated superficially by micro-organisms. The treatment of teeth involved in such accidents is dealt with in Chapter 16.

Pulpal injury may also result from a traumatic occlusal relationship between maxillary and mandibular teeth.

Longitudinal fracture of the crown of a tooth, sometimes extending into the root, may occur without any evidence of trauma. This condition is usually seen in posterior teeth, especially molars, and is dealt with in Chapter 12.

c. Chemical

Erosion of the substance of a tooth by acidic liquids may also lead to pulpal damage if it is not checked.

2. Causes associated with dental procedures

a. Mechanical

The mere act of cutting dentine during cavity preparation leads to pulpal injury in the vicinity of the involved tubules. Rotary instruments at speeds of 3000–30 000 rev/min seem to be the most harmful in this respect. However, provided adequate coolant is used and the tooth is satisfactorily restored, recovery of the pulp may be expected.

Both friction-grip and self-tapping dentine pins have been shown to produce stresses within dentine, and even cracks extending to the pulp chamber. Suzuki et al. (1973) found that pulpal inflammation, albeit of a minor nature, occurred in association with such cracks.

Sometimes during cavity preparation the pulp is exposed not by the removal of caries but by the injudicious use of instruments. Such an accident is followed by acute inflammation of the pulp in the region of the exposure. Moreover, unless treatment was being performed under strictly aseptic conditions, the exposed pulpal surface will have become contaminated by micro-organisms.

Micro-organisms may also be forced into the pulp through dentinal tubules by rotary cutting instruments, and by such restorative procedures as the taking of impressions and the cementation or condensation of restorations (Bender et al., 1959). Normally the pulp seems to survive these insults, but in deep cavities, where some degree of pulpal inflammation probably already exists, care should be taken not to cause further irritation. Rotary cutting instruments should therefore be used with minimal pressure, and the cavity floor adequately lined before taking impressions or inserting restorations.

Other mechanical causes of pulpal injury associated with dental procedures are excessively rapid movement of teeth during orthodontic treatment and the use of undue force during the insertion of restorations, as may occur during the malleting of gold-foil fillings.

b. Thermal

Besides the mechanical injury inflicted on a pulp from cutting dentine, thermal injury from the use of rotary cutting instruments may also result unless the dentine is adequately cooled. With high-speed instruments, water is normally used to prevent overheating. With low speeds a jet of air is sometimes advocated, but care must be taken to avoid excessive drying of the dentine, since this also leads to pulpal injury.

The transmission of excessive heat to the pulp may also occur when polishing metallic restorations and during the lining of a cavity with a cement having an exothermic setting reaction, especially if the cavity is deep. An inadequate lining beneath a metallic restoration will allow the transmission of heat and cold to the pulp.

c. Chemical

Most of the materials used in restoring teeth act on the pulp when applied directly to the dentinal floor of a cavity. The pulpal reaction depends not only on the material but also on other factors, including the depth of the cavity. Where the cavity is shallow a productive reaction, with the formation of reparative dentine, may occur; with deeper cavities an inflammatory reaction is likely.

Outstanding in their irritant effect on the pulp are silicate cements. Although one possible reason for the toxicity of these materials is their high degree of acidity when first inserted into a cavity, cases of pulpal necrosis following their use without linings are seen frequently enough to indicate that some other mechanism of pulpal injury, perhaps associated with marginal leakage (Hansen and Bruun, 1971; Qvist, 1975), most probably also exists.

The autopolymerizing acrylic resins constitute yet another group which is capable of causing severe pulpal injury unless used in conjunction with a lining. Their toxic action is considered to result from free monomer in the materials.

Phosphate cements also have a pronounced irritant effect on the pulp when applied directly to the dentinal base of a cavity, especially if the cavity is deep. With these materials the effect is attributable to their pronounced acidic reaction at the time of insertion.

Various studies have shown that unlined composite fillings produce pulpal inflammation. Although this generally seems to be mild in degree, Dickey et al. (1974) found that a severe response, comparable to that produced by silicate cements, could result, particularly in deep cavities. Brannstrom and Nyborg (1972) have drawn attention to the frequency with which micro-organisms are found beneath unlined composite fillings, due to marginal leakage, and consider that this probably represents a more serious threat to the pulp than the material itself; from the former aspect alone, therefore, lining of the cavity floor is desirable. Acid pre-treatment to clean the cavity and etch the dentine preparatory to the insertion of composite fillings has been shown by Eriksen (1974) and Stanley et al. (1975) to be followed by significant pulpal inflammation.

Polycarboxylate cements may lead to pulpal inflammation in deep cavities, although the effect is apparently only transient and mild (Plant, 1970, 1973).

Drugs used in an attempt to sterilize or dehydrate a cavity preparatory to filling —such as phenol, chloroform and alcohol—may also lead to pulpal injury, particularly if the dentinal floor of the cavity is thin.

d. Electrical

The presence in a person's mouth of dissimilar metallic fillings—typically gold and amalgam—may lead to pulpal injury due to the flow of electric currents arising from galvanic action. The dissimilar fillings may touch only during mastication, so that contact is intermittent, or they may be adjacent and make continuous contact. Alternatively, since saliva acts as an electrolyte in the flow of current, pulpal irritation may occur even though the fillings make no contact at all.

Although the presence of dissimilar fillings in the mouth is usually without clinical manifestations of pulpal disease, discomfort does occasionally occur.

PATHOGENESIS OF PULPAL NECROSIS

By the time the pulp is exposed by caries, part or all of its coronal part already shows chronic inflammation. Exposure with resultant infection of the pulp is followed by the accumulation of acute inflammatory cells and necrosis in the vicinity of the exposure, so that the chronic pulpitis becomes acute in this region. Despite this acute inflammatory reaction, however, the tissue defences of the pulp are unable to eliminate the organisms in the carious dentine, so that as more of the pulp becomes exposed by caries pulpitis becomes more widespread. The inflammatory exudate which is formed is largely confined within the pulp cavity, unable to escape because of the surrounding wall of dentine. It was formerly believed that the resultant increase in pressure caused strangulation of the veins passing through the apical foramen, so leading rapidly to necrosis of the entire pulp. However, recent work suggests that the accumulation of exudate causes an increase in tissue pressure locally; this leads to venous collapse followed by stasis and ischaemia with resultant tissue necrosis in the area (Brown, 1968; Van Hassel, 1971). The subsequent release of intracellular inflammatory agents, together with the growth of micro-organisms into the necrotic tissue, leads to further irritation and repetition of the process. Thus necrosis followed by invasion by micro-organisms gradually spreads to affect the entire pulp. By the time the apical part of the canal is reached, the irritation caused by breakdown of the pulp and the diffusion of bacterial toxins has led to extension of the inflammatory process into the apical part of the periodontal membrane and the periapical bone (*Fig.* 1).

Amongst the factors affecting the spread of necrosis in the pulp is the possibility of drainage into the cavity in the crown of the tooth. If the pulp maintains a free communication with the coronal cavity and thence with the mouth, inflammatory exudate may escape, with the result that the pulp may remain in a state of chronic inflammation for a comparatively long time before it becomes totally necrotic. Occasionally, especially where root formation is incomplete and there is a good blood supply, the pulp is gradually replaced by granulation tissue. This may grow into the coronal cavity, forming what is sometimes called a 'pulp polyp' or a

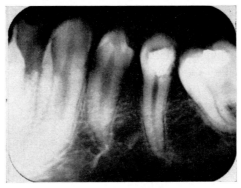

Fig. 1. ⌐5. Early periapical change with inflamed pulp.

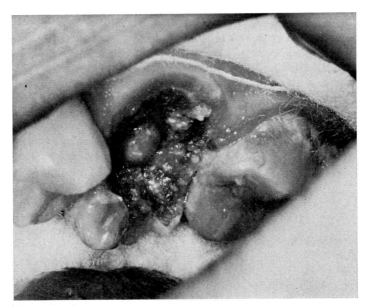

Fig. 2. ⌐6. A pulp polyp.

'chronic hyperplastic pulpitis' (*Fig.* 2). More often, however, the opening into the pulp cavity becomes suddenly occluded by food impaction, resulting in an acute exacerbation with a rapid spread of inflammation and necrosis.

Another important factor affecting the spread of necrosis is the stage of formation of the root apex. Where this is complete, and the apical foramen is narrow, venous collapse and ischaemia with resultant necrosis are likely to occur sooner than in an incompletely formed root with a wide apical foramen.

Following operative procedures, such as cavity preparation, an acute inflammation of part of the pulp may develop. Provided that further irritation does not occur, resolution generally takes place. Even where the pulp is exposed during cavity preparation—by instruments, that is, and not by caries—with adequate treatment it may still recover, provided it was only superficially contaminated by organisms and was only slightly injured by the exposure. However, where the pulp has been lacerated and severely injured, or where it has been heavily contaminated from the penetration of instruments, recovery is highly unlikely. Under these circumstances, inflammation and finally necrosis of the pulp take place in the same way as following carious exposure.

DIAGNOSTIC METHODS

Diagnostic methods include both history taking and examination. Often the cause of a patient's complaint may be determined from the symptoms described and a visual examination of the mouth, with perhaps one or two simple diagnostic tests. In other cases a diagnosis can only be reached after obtaining a detailed history and making an exhaustive examination.

1. History

a. General medical history
The patient's medical history, if not already available, should always be obtained, since it may be relevant not only to diagnosis but also to treatment. For example, sensitivity to a particular drug, especially penicillin, will preclude its use. If the patient has a history of endocardial damage, systemic administration of an antibiotic, typically penicillin, is needed when treatment is performed within the root canal and for the immediate treatment of acute periapical conditions.

b. History of present complaint: pain
A complaint of pain or discomfort is usually the reason for initially suspecting pulpal or periapical disease. History taking is therefore largely concerned with this symptom. The patient is questioned on the location and nature of the pain, on how long it has lasted, and on the factors which excite and relieve it.

Some of the descriptive details included in the following account are largely without direct significance in diagnosing the state of the pulp and periapex, or in locating an offending tooth. They are given, however, not only because the patient's pain may not be pulpal or periapical in origin, but also because they illustrate the variability of the pain experienced.

i. LOCATION
When the disease is still confined to the pulp and has not involved the supporting tissues, it may not be possible for the patient to localize the pain more precisely than to the right or the left side, to the mandible or the maxilla, and to the front or the back of the mouth. Often the patient says that both upper and lower jaws, or both the front and back of the mouth, are affected. If this is so, the questioning should be directed to determining where the pain actually starts. Sometimes pain due to pulpal disease is felt in the opposite jaw to that in which the offending tooth is located. Pain may even be experienced on the side opposite to the causative tooth (Logan, 1964; Friend and Glenwright, 1968; Harris, 1973), although this is rare.

Later, when the periodontal membrane becomes inflamed and its proprioceptive nerve endings stimulated, the patient can localize pain to a small region of the mouth, and can usually identify the causative tooth.

ii. NATURE

The pain may range from slight to severe; it may be dull or sharp; it may throb or it may seem to bore into the jaw; it may take the form of intermittent spasms lasting a few seconds or minutes, or it may continue for hours on end; it may occur frequently or only very occasionally; and it may be experienced at any time or only at certain times, such as in the evenings after work.

iii. DURATION

The onset of pain may have been relatively recent, or it may have occurred weeks or months previously.

iv. EXCITING AND RELIEVING FACTORS

The pain may be initiated, or aggravated, by such things as hot or cold foods, sweet or sour foods, toothbrushing, pressure on the tooth during mastication, and bending or lying down.

A lower atmospheric pressure than normal, resulting from an increase in altitude during air travel or induced experimentally in a decompression chamber, may lead to toothache. This is known as 'aerodontalgia'. Its occurrence is associated with pre-existing pulpal damage, which may be symptomless until a decrease in pressure takes place. High altitude *per se* does not cause pain in a tooth with a normal pulp. Aerodontalgia is said not to occur when the pulp of the tooth communicates with the mouth.

The patient may have found that, besides analgesics, certain things relieve the pain, for example holding cold water in the mouth or sucking on the tooth.

Pain of non-pulpal origin

Sometimes the pain described by a patient as 'toothache' arises from a source within the mouth other than the pulp of a tooth. For example, it may be associated with ulceration of the oral mucosa, or with a restoration which makes premature contact on closure of the teeth. It may also arise from periodontal disease, commonly following on food impaction between two teeth which do not make firm contact. Cases such as these are generally easy to recognize by visual examination of the painful region and, where appropriate, examination with mirror and probe of the periodontal condition. Where any doubt remains, the tests used to diagnose the pulpal status, described presently, will settle the matter.

REFERRED PAIN

The referral of pain to teeth other than the causative one has already been described. Occasionally, pain of dental origin, including that arising from a diseased pulp or periapical region, is experienced in some other region of the head (*Fig.* 3). Conversely, pain from other regions is sometimes felt in the teeth or jaws.

For example, pain in or around the eye may be associated with disease involving the maxillary anterior teeth; pain in the cheek with diseased maxillary posterior teeth; and pain in the ear with diseased mandibular posterior teeth. Conversely, maxillary sinusitis may lead to pain in the maxillary posterior teeth, and infections of the ear may cause pain in the mandibular posterior teeth. Ischaemic heart disease may lead to referred pain in the mandible.

The differentiation of referred pain from pain of pulpal or periapical origin depends partly on confirming the absence of pulpal and periapical disease, and partly on obtaining evidence of disease in the 'referring' region. Thus, in maxillary sinusitis there is tenderness of the cheek on the affected side, sometimes with alteration in the sound of the patient's voice and a history of a recent cold. Several teeth, rather than just one tooth, are painful; they may be sensitive to both temperature change and percussion. Radiographic examination will show evidence of sinusitis.

Occasionally, a dental opinion is asked for in cases of suspected trigeminal neuralgia, where pain may be felt in oral and dental tissues as well as in other regions. The duty of the dentist in these cases is to ensure that there is no oral or dental cause for the pain.

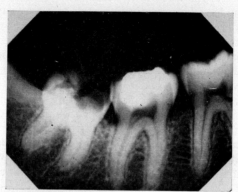

Fig. 3. 8̄]. Diseased pulp which was associated with referred pain in right ear.

c. Other aspects of history taking

Sometimes, especially when it is uncertain that pulpal or periapical disease is actually present, or when it is difficult to identify the tooth involved, many other questions may be asked, for example if there has been trauma to the face, such as a blow or fall. If there has, the patient is asked when it happened, if any particular tooth was loosened, if there was pain or swelling afterwards and if treatment was sought at the time. Again, questions about individual restorations in the teeth are often indicated; for example, if local anaesthesia was used for certain fillings, if a water spray was used for a cavity prepared with an air turbine drill, if the onset of pain was related to the insertion of a particular restoration, and if a warning was given that a certain cavity was deep or might cause after-pain.

2. Examination

a. Visual examination

Useful information may sometimes be gained from the patient's facial appearance. For example, localized puckering or indentation of the skin surface may be associated with a long-standing sinus from a periapical lesion (*Fig.* 4). Oedema of the face from an acute periapical abscess is usually easy to see, especially where it is away from the midline and has led to asymmetry. Such a patient may have had little sleep the night before, and often looks pale and tired, if not actually ill. Occasionally the appearance is one of exhaustion and near-collapse, and in such cases it is advisable to take the temperature and pulse.

Before attention is concentrated on a particular region, the entire mouth is examined with a view to obtaining a general idea of the oral and dental condition. In this preliminary examination, particular attention is paid to the occlusion, to the general periodontal condition and to the evidence of previous dental care and caries susceptibility. From the findings that result it may be decided that the offending tooth, when found, should be extracted rather than conserved.

In examining visually a particular region, any external swelling is first noted. The intraoral soft tissues, particularly in the buccal sulcus, are inspected for swelling, inflammation and evidence of a sinus. The teeth are examined for their

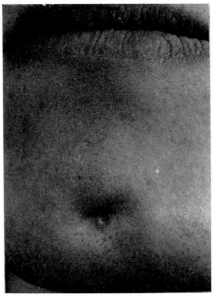

Fig. 4. Indentation of skin over chin associated with long-standing sinus from periapical lesion of a mandibular incisor.

colour and translucency; a tooth with a necrotic pulp is commonly less translucent than the adjoining teeth, and is sometimes discoloured also (*Fig*. 5). The presence of fractures, caries and fillings is noted. The incisal or occlusal surfaces of adjacent crowns are compared to determine if a tooth has been extruded; similarly, the alinements of the incisal edges and labial surfaces are examined for evidence of displacement.

When the source of pain has been localized to a particular tooth, the amount of access to the crown and the possibility of restoring this are considered, and the periodontal condition of the tooth is assessed to ensure that its retention is justified.

b. Diagnostic tests

The following diagnostic tests may be used to supplement visual examination: Percussion, Palpation, Mobility Test, Radiographic Examination, Vitality Tests, Anaesthetic Test, Transillumination and Investigation of Restorations and Carious Lesions. Usually when diagnostic tests are indicated, only a few are needed, but occasionally many of them have to be used.

i. PERCUSSION

In percussion the crown of a tooth is tapped with the tip of a finger or with an instrument. A painful response to percussion denotes inflammation of the peri-odontal membrane, but the converse is not necessarily true. Sometimes, especially with a root-filled tooth, although percussion does not cause pain, the sensation it evokes is different from that experienced with other teeth.

In performing the test, several teeth are percussed in a random order, so elimina-ting the possibility of bias on the patient's part. Initially, a suspect tooth must be tapped very gently, since the periodontal membrane may be extremely tender; if

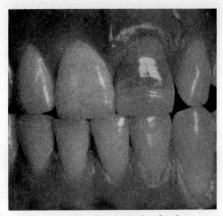

Fig. 5. |1. Discoloration of crown following necrosis of pulp.

there is no response, a sharper tap is given. Percussion at right-angles to the long axis of the crown will occasionally evoke pain where none was felt from tapping along the long axis. Multi-rooted teeth are percussed over each root.

It must be borne in mind that tenderness to percussion does not necessarily denote pulpal disease. A tooth with a healthy pulp may develop an acute apical periodontitis from a blow on the face or premature occlusal contact; alternatively, an acute periodontitis may occur as a sequel to food packing between two teeth (*Fig*. 6) or to established periodontal disease. It is only when all other causes have been excluded that pain from percussion may be regarded as indicative of pulpal disease.

If a metallic instrument is used, the sound produced by percussing a tooth with periapical disease is sometimes obviously duller than that given by a tooth with an intact periapex.

ii. PALPATION

In palpation, light pressure is applied with the fingertips to the soft tissues. The region which most commonly yields positive information in response to this test, and which is therefore tested most often, is the buccal sulcus.

The object of the test is to determine the shape and consistency of the tissues and, from the patient's reaction, their sensitivity. If a swelling is present, the operator will be able to tell if it is hard or soft, and, if soft, whether or not it is fluctuant.

Tenderness over the root apex of a tooth indicates inflammation of the periodontal membrane. As already pointed out, however, this may result from other causes besides pulpal disease. Also, absence of tenderness does not preclude the presence of inflammation of the periodontal membrane.

Excluding abscess formation associated with periodontal disease, swelling of the mucosa over the root apex of a tooth denotes partial or complete necrosis of its pulp.

Palpation is also used to detect submandibular or submental lymphadenitis following on periapical or periodontal disease.

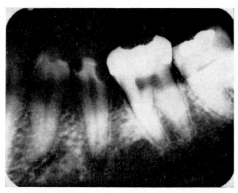

Fig. 6. ⌐6. Mesial root—acute periodontitis due to food packing between ⌐5 and ⌐6, accentuated by mesial tilt of ⌐6.

iii. MOBILITY TEST

The mobility test consists of gripping the crown of a tooth and moving it in a buccolingual direction; either the fingers or an instrument, or both, may be used. The object is to assess from the amount of movement of the crown how firmly the root is attached to the alveolar bone. Incidental information is also gained on the sensitivity of the periodontal membrane.

The mobility test *per se* gives no direct information about the state of the pulp. Whilst pronounced mobility is commonly associated with an acute periapical abscess, it may also result from advanced periodontal disease.

iv. RADIOGRAPHIC EXAMINATION

Probably no single factor has contributed more to improving the standard of endodontic treatment than the introduction of the X-ray machine. Intraoral radiographs of the periapical regions are often indispensable in the diagnosis of pulpal and periapical disease, and should always be taken prior to pulpotomy or root canal treatment.

Although such a valuable aid in diagnosis and treatment, much information which a radiograph would otherwise yield can be lost through incorrect angulation of the tube, or incorrect exposure of the film or through faulty processing. It is a mistake to use fewer films than are really necessary. Thus, the common practice of relying on one film for a view of four incisor teeth often results in relatively little information being gained about any of them. On occasions it is useful to take additional films using different vertical or horizontal angulations of the tube. For example, a change in horizontal angulation is usually necessary to separate completely the images of the different roots of a posterior tooth (*Fig.* 7) and two or three radiographs often have to be taken. Again, although a root fracture may not be visible on a film when the normal vertical angulation for the tooth is used, it can sometimes be detected when the angulation is changed. Similarly, deliberately

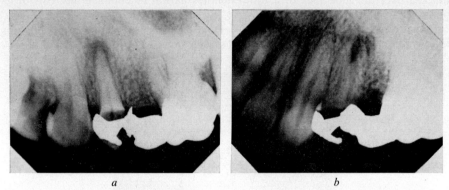

a	*b*

Fig. 7. |4. *a*, View with normal horizontal angulation to tube; *b*, View with tube angled distally. Two roots are now apparent.

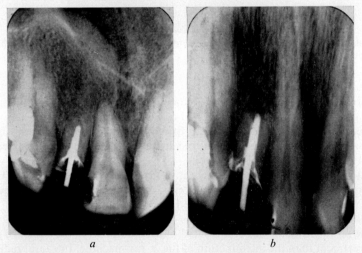

a	*b*

Fig. 8. 2|. *a*, View with normal vertical angulation to tube. No periapical lesion visible; *b*, View with tube angled more horizontally. Periapical lesion visible.

angulating the tube so as to elongate the image may reveal a small zone of periapical radiolucency which would otherwise have remained undetected (*Fig.* 8).

Where the origin of a sinus is not immediately apparent, a radiograph taken with a gutta percha point inserted into the sinus tract may show it leading to a periapical lesion some distance away (*see Fig.* 25).

EXAMINATION OF RADIOGRAPHS

In viewing a radiograph, different structures are examined in turn, and not all at once.

The crown of each tooth is inspected for caries, fillings and evidence of lining material beneath fillings. The size and shape of the pulp chamber are determined; whilst with posterior teeth a bite-wing film will generally provide more information, with anterior teeth a periapical view combined with visual examination in the mouth will give a good idea of the proximity of fillings to the pulp chamber.

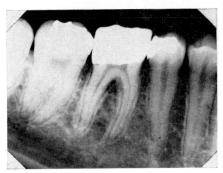

Fig. 9. 6̅|. Mesial root—widening of apical periodontal membrane.

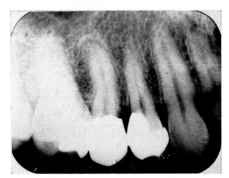

Fig. 10. 5̲|. Loss of demarcation between apical periodontal membrane and adjoining bone.

Next, the entire length of each root is examined for the presence of resorption, fracture and perforation. The course of each root canal is followed from the pulp chamber to its apical end; the width of the canal and its anatomy apically are noted. More than one main root canal may be present within the root, and occasionally a lateral branch from the main canal may be seen. The presence of pulp calcifications should not be overlooked. Other radio-opaque bodies in the canal, including root-filling materials, are usually obvious. Often the radiographic appearance provides a good guide to the composition of a root filling.

The periodontal membrane of each root is now traced from the gingival region to the root apex both mesially and distally. In this way a widening of the periodontal membrane apically (*Fig.* 9), or a loss of demarcation between the membrane and the adjoining bone (*Fig.* 10), is easier to detect. Also, a separate bone lesion alongside the lateral surface of the root—arising from a lateral canal, a perforation, or a root fracture, or from periodontal disease—is less likely to be overlooked (*Fig.* 11). The periodontal membrane rather than the lamina dura is traced, since the latter is often not visible in the apical region.

Finally, the supporting bone of each tooth is examined, both periapically and interdentally.

DIAGNOSIS OF PERIAPICAL DISEASE

In viewing bone, it must be remembered that although bone destruction, and therefore radiolucency, is the typical sequel of periapical irritation, bone sclerosis with resultant increased radiopacity occasionally occurs in response to very chronic irritation (*Fig.* 12). Also, radiolucent zones around the apices of teeth are not necessarily indicative of periapical disease. Thus, normal anatomical structures, including the mental foramen, the incisive fossa and extensions of the maxillary antrum, show as zones of radiolucency. The positions of these structures should

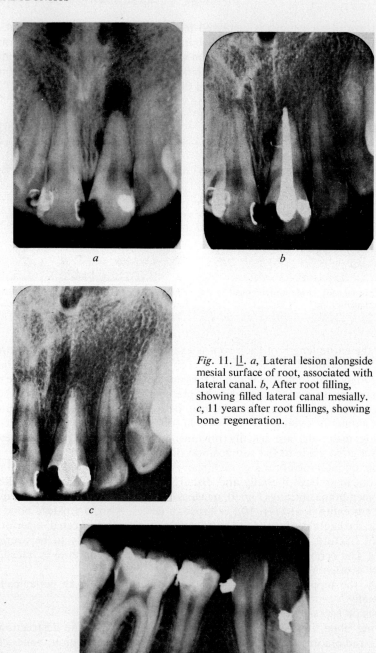

Fig. 11. |1. *a*, Lateral lesion alongside mesial surface of root, associated with lateral canal. *b*, After root filling, showing filled lateral canal mesially. *c*, 11 years after root fillings, showing bone regeneration.

Fig. 12. 3|. Periapical sclerosis resulting from pulpal disease.

be determined when examining films, and if necessary their precise relations to the apices of the roots assessed by tracing their outlines.

Where a radiolucent zone represents one of these anatomical structures and not a periapical lesion, it is possible to trace a well-defined periodontal membrane around the root apex. Also, a positive response from the tooth to vitality tests helps in ruling out the possibility of periapical disease. When doubt still exists, further radiographs are taken using different horizontal angles. A zone which represents a normal structure changes in position according to the angulation used (*Fig.* 13); where it results from periapical disease, it is in all views associated with

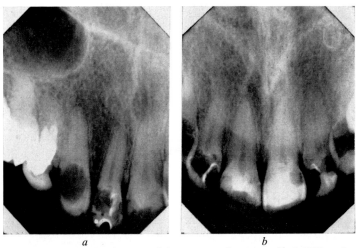

a   *b*

Fig. 13. *a*, Incisive fossa showing as radiolucent area above apex 1⌋; *b*, With a change in horizontal angulation to tube, incisive fossa shows between apices of 1⌋ and ⌊1.

the root of the tooth. The same criteria are used to differentiate lesions following on pulpal disease from other lesions of the jaws, such as developmental cysts.

Very occasionally, zones of radiolucency unassociated with normal anatomical structures, periapical disease or cystic conditions develop around the apices of teeth with healthy pulps. One such condition is periapical cemental dysplasia. This is seen most commonly in the mandibular incisor region, usually involving several teeth (*Fig.* 14). Eventually, following the radiolucent stage, masses of cementum may be deposited on the roots involved or within the lesion itself, or new bone may be laid down. Periapical zones of radiolucency may also develop in patients suffering from hyperparathyroidism, hyperthyroidism, fibrous dysplasia, Paget's disease, multiple myeloma, Gaucher's disease and Hand–Schüller–Christian disease (Seltzer, 1971). None of these conditions results in pulpal disease, and therefore root canal treatment is not called for.

Although a large periapical lesion may, from radiographic examination, appear to involve more than one tooth, only one of the teeth may in fact have a necrotic pulp (*Fig.* 15). Where this is so, the tooth corresponding to the mesiodistal centre of the lesion is often, but not invariably, the offender (*Fig.* 16); with careful inspection an intact periodontal membrane can usually be traced around each of the other roots.

From the foregoing comments, it is obvious that a periapical zone of radio-lucency is not always associated with disease of the pulp of the adjacent tooth. Unless there are clinical manifestations which leave no doubt as to the offender,

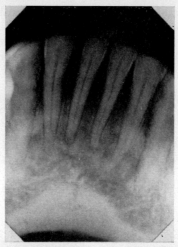

Fig. 14. Periapical cemental dysplasia of $\overline{21|12}$ region. The pulps of all the teeth were vital.

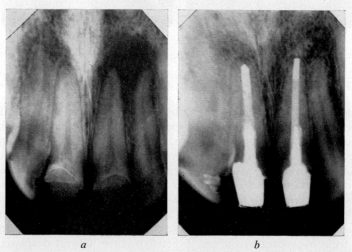

a   *b*

Fig. 15. *a*, Periapical lesion apparently associated with both $\underline{1}$ and $\underline{2}$; *b*, Complete repair of lesion 5 years later. $\underline{2}$ had a vital pulp and did not need treatment.

therefore, a suspect tooth should always be tested for vitality and the results compared with those from other teeth before either endodontic treatment or extraction is performed.

v. VITALITY TESTS

The following vitality tests may be used to assess the state of a pulp: Heat Test, Cold Test, Electric Pulp Test and the Test Cavity. The equipment necessary for these tests is illustrated in *Fig.* 17. If the patient's pain is brought on by hot or cold foods, the offending tooth may often be located by using the heat or cold test to stimulate the type of pain experienced.

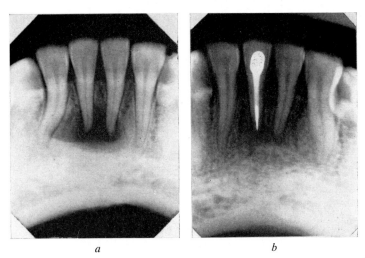

a   *b*

Fig. 16. *a*, Periapical lesion of T̄|T̄ region, with T̄| apex opposite centre of lesion; *b*, Almost complete repair of lesion 4 years later. |T̄ had a vital pulp and did not need treatment.

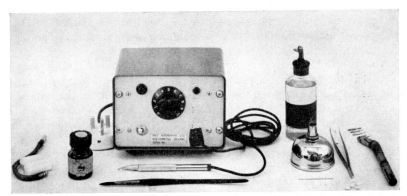

Fig. 17. From left to right, equipment and materials needed for isolation: Electric Pulp Test, Heat and Cold Tests and Test Cavity.

In the first three of these tests, it is important that the tooth is dried and isolated with wool rolls from the lip or cheek. With each, the object of the test and the manner in which it will be performed are explained to the patient. To provide controls, and to have the patient experience the sensation which may be felt, teeth in which there is no reason to suspect pulpal disease are tested first. If possible, the corresponding teeth on the opposite side of the same arch are used as controls.

With each of the three tests—heat, cold and electric—the stimulus is applied to a similar region on each tooth, so as to obtain comparative results. With anterior teeth, the stimulus is normally applied to the labial enamel of the incisal third of the crown. With multi-rooted teeth the stimulus is applied in line with each particular root. Since there is no means of confining the stimulus to the pulp of the root under test, however, differences in pulpal status between the various roots of a multi-rooted tooth make interpretation difficult (*Fig.* 18).

In vitality testing, exposed dentine should be avoided, otherwise an accelerated and probably exaggerated response is likely. Also, the stimulus should not be applied against restorations unless unavoidable. Non-metallic restorations are relatively poor conductors and a test made through such a material will therefore

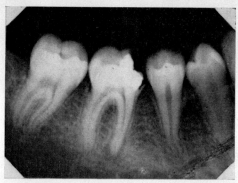

Fig. 18. ⅋|. Although the mesial root had a necrotic pulp and was associated with a periapical lesion, the distal root had a vital pulp.

lead to a delayed response, or to no response at all. Conversely, metallic restorations, being good conductors, may result in responses at low levels of stimulation; they may also cause misleading results by conducting the stimulus to an adjoining metallic restoration in another tooth, although this effect may be reduced by the insertion of a celluloid strip between the teeth. From these considerations it is evident that if the tooth has a porcelain or acrylic crown, it cannot be properly tested unless an area of exposed tooth substance is available for the test, or unless it is made available by cutting a hole through the crown into dentine; in interpreting the results of such a test, due allowance has to be made for the fact that the stimulus is applied to dentine. Applying the test through a hole cut into dentine is also occasionally of value where the crown is of metal, although misleading results can occur.

Heat Test: In this test the end of a stick of gutta percha is heated until it is soft and just begins to burn. It is then allowed to cool for a few seconds before being placed on the tooth. Immediately the patient indicates sensation, the gutta percha is removed. The response, which according to the patient may range from slight to moderate pain, should occur in a few seconds and last no more than a few seconds. Where there is no reaction, the test is repeated on the middle one-third of the crown.

Instead of gutta percha, a heated plastic instrument may be used.

Where a gold crown is present, heat may be applied by 'polishing' the crown with an abrasive rubber disc.

Cold Test: The cold test is conducted in a similar manner to the heat test. Either ethyl chloride on a wool roll or a wool pledget, or a piece of ice, is applied to the teeth. A convenient method of using ice, described by Grossman (1960) is to fill a used local anaesthetic cartridge with water and to freeze this in a refrigerator. Ehrmann (1973) describes the use of a dry ice pencil. Again, a response should occur within a few seconds and last only a few seconds.

Electric Pulp Test: The advantage claimed for the electric pulp test over the heat and cold tests is that the degree of stimulation necessary to evoke a response may be measured and so a quantitative result obtained. A special apparatus, the electric pulp tester, is used to conduct the test.

Two types of electric pulp tester are available, one in which the current is varied and one in which the voltage is varied. The former is considered preferable, since a given voltage may lead to different amounts of current due to variation in the electrical resistance of the tissues, especially enamel. By the incorporation of a scale and the use of a control knob to vary the current or the voltage, the amount of stimulation needed to evoke a response may be measured. Either a high-frequency or a low-frequency signal may be used. Both battery- and mains-operated testers are available.

With some pulp testers, one electrode is placed against the tooth and the other is held in the patient's hand. With other testers, only one electrode is used; this is applied to the tooth, and the circuit is completed by the operator holding his hand against the patient's cheek or under the chin, or retracting the lip or cheek with the fingers.

When explaining the electric pulp test, the patient is asked to raise the hand immediately a tingling or painful sensation is felt in the tooth. The teeth are now isolated with wool rolls. The crowns are thoroughly dried to prevent a response from a flow of current along the periodontal membrane, although, in terms of current, this structure has a higher threshold to stimulation than the pulp. A good conductor of electricity, such as colloidal graphite, is applied to part of the incisal or occlusal one-third of the tooth buccally to provide an effective pathway for the flow of current between the electrode and the curved enamel surface (*Fig.* 19).

After ensuring that the control knob is set at zero, the apparatus is switched on and the electrode placed firmly against the graphite and held steadily in position. The electrical stimulus is now gradually increased until the patient responds, when the reading is noted. Before the electrode is removed from the tooth, either the current is switched off or the control knob is reset at zero. For each tooth the test is repeated at least once to verify the first reading.

In general, the greater the bulk of enamel and dentine through which current has to pass to reach the pulp, the greater the amount of current needed for stimulation. Thus, anterior teeth respond at a lower level of stimulation than posterior teeth. On a scale of 10 units, a variation of up to 2·0 units between the readings for different anterior teeth, or between readings for the same anterior tooth at different times, is usually regarded as within the range of normal. Similarly, with both premolars and molars variations of up to 3·0 units may be normal.

After pulpotomy has been performed, an increase in stimulation of two or more units may be necessary to evoke a response. Factors tending to influence the degree of nervous excitability, such as fatigue or the administration of analgesics, may alter the threshold to stimulation. Cooke and Rowbotham (1952) have pointed out that a tooth with an incompletely formed root and a wide apical foramen sometimes gives no response to the electric pulp test, even though its pulp is vital.

Electrical limitations associated with the design of electric pulp testers have been demonstrated by the studies of Civjan et al. (1973) and Matthews and Searle (1974).

Electric pulp testers should not be used on patients with cardiac pacemakers, since interference with the action of the pacemaker is possible.

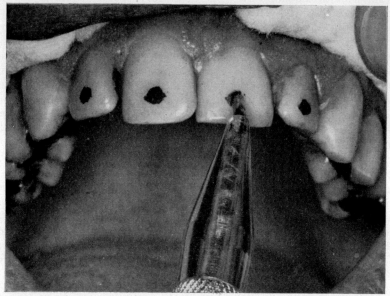

Fig. 19. Labial surfaces of 21|12 painted with colloidal graphite. |1 is being pulp tested.

Test Cavity: Occasionally the results obtained from thermal and electrical tests are not sufficiently conclusive to assess a pulp as vital or necrotic. This occurs especially when a great deal of dentine has been deposited in the pulp chamber. In these cases a test cavity may be prepared in the crown of the tooth with the object of stimulating the pulp, at least in the first instance, merely by the act of cutting dentine. The cavity is normally made on the lingual or occlusal surface of the tooth; if a small filling is already present, it may be removed and later replaced. Where there is tenderness to percussion of the tooth, care has to be taken not to confuse pain from pressure on the periodontal membrane during cavity preparation with that arising from the pulp.

Where cavity preparation fails to evoke pain, thermal and electrical tests may be applied through the base of the cavity. Obviously, they must be performed with great care. If these also are without effect, it is almost certain that the pulp is necrotic.

Other Vitality Tests: Howell et al. (1970) and Stoops and Scott (1976) have reported favourably on the diagnosis of pulpal vitality by measuring the surface temperature of teeth with the aid of liquid crystals and thermistors respectively, whilst Barber et al. (1969) have suggested the measurement of ultrasonic transmission and reflection from the dentine-pulp interface. At the present time these methods must be regarded as experimental.

vi. ANAESTHETIC TEST (Diagnostic injection)

The anaesthetic test is used in an attempt to determine the source of pain where the results of other tests have failed to localize the offending tooth. In this test, to which the term 'diagnostic injection' is sometimes applied, a local anaesthetic is injected to anaesthetize the pulp and periapex of a particular tooth, or the pulps and periapices of a group of teeth. Elimination or appreciable reduction of the pain indicates that the source is in the anaesthetized region, whilst persistence of the pain indicates that the source lies in some other region. It follows that the test is of no use unless pain is present at the time of examination.

Because of the possibility of misinterpretation due to the diffusion of local anaesthetic solution, the anaesthetic test is of most value when the suspect teeth are not immediately adjacent. Where an infiltration injection is used, the solution is deposited subperiosteally so as to limit its spread. The test is particularly useful where it is uncertain whether the pain arises from the mandible or the maxilla; depending on the position of the possible source of pain, either a mental or an inferior dental injection is given.

vii. TRANSILLUMINATION

A tooth with a necrotic pulp is commonly less translucent than the adjoining teeth, due to the presence of breakdown products of the pulp. Whilst this difference can often be detected during normal visual examination under good lighting conditions, it can if wished be made more obvious if the teeth are examined in a darkened room with the aid of a mouth lamp.

Transillumination may be used in a similar manner to examine the periapical region also, but is not usually employed for this purpose.

viii. INVESTIGATION OF RESTORATIONS AND CARIOUS LESIONS

The removal of one or more restorations or the excavation of carious cavities is sometimes necessary in locating or confirming the source of a pain suspected of arising from pulpal disease, particularly where the pain is of a chronic and long-standing nature. The main object of the procedure is to determine if the pulp of a tooth has been exposed. However, it must be pointed out that although the finding of an exposure may suggest strongly that a particular tooth is the offender, the absence of a clinically visible exposure is not necessarily indicative of a healthy pulp. Some exposures are doubtless too small to be detected clinically. Also, it has already been pointed out that pulpitis may precede carious exposure of the pulp. Despite these limitations, the procedure often constitutes an indispensable aid to diagnosis.

When it is necessary to test a number of teeth in this way, the order in which the teeth are investigated is determined from the results of other tests, including the radiographic appearances of restorations and carious lesions. In investigating a restored tooth, the restorative material, including any lining which may be present, must be removed in its entirety. Fragments of material, even if minute, must not be allowed to remain. Particular care is needed when removing silicate, composite or acrylic fillings, since it is easy to overlook a layer of one of these materials in the base of a cavity. Similarly, carious lesions in the tooth, including those under restorations, are eliminated. Overhanging enamel must not be left—albeit only temporarily until the tooth is permanently restored—if it prevents inspection of part of the cavity. Although not imperative, there is some advantage in avoiding wherever possible the injection of a local anaesthetic, since by preventing or reducing pain or haemorrhage this makes detection of an exposure more difficult.

When caries and restorative material have been eliminated, each cavity is dried and then examined under a good light. Each cavity wall in turn is inspected and then explored with a probe, particular attention being paid to axial and side walls, and the junction of the latter with the cavity floor. Suspect areas are best explored with an instrument finer than a probe, such as the tip of a very small reamer. Such an instrument is applied with gentle pressure and at different angles to the area. For relatively inaccessible areas, the reamer may be bent a few millimetres from its tip.

In searching for an exposure, it must be borne in mind that, even though the bulk of the pulp is vital, necrosis may have taken place in the region of the exposure. In consequence, haemorrhage and pain may not occur when an exposure is uncovered.

Other Diagnostic Tests: Certain specialized tests have been suggested for the differentiation of radicular cysts from other periapical lesions. Howell et al. (1968) have described a method of aspirating fluid from a periapical lesion by way of the root canal or through the overlying cortical plate. The aspirated material is stained by the Papanicolaou technique for the presence of epithelial cells, so providing a guide to cyst formation.

The test described by Morse et al. (1973) also uses fluid aspirated from a periapical lesion. The aspirated fluid is examined by polyacrylamide-gel electrophoresis. Compared with other periapical lesions, cysts give more intense albumin patterns, together with patterns in the globulin region.

Although the results of these methods are promising, neither seems readily applicable as yet to routine dental practice.

EVALUATION OF DIAGNOSTIC METHODS IN ASSESSING PULPAL STATES

The possibility of differentiating the various pathological states of the pulp on the basis of clinical criteria has been much overrated in the past, as various studies have shown (Stephan, 1937; Mitchell and Tarplee, 1960; Seltzer et al., 1963; Baume, 1970).

Before considering the classification of pulpal states, therefore, it is necessary to evaluate further some of the diagnostic methods employed. Much of the following account is based on the reports of Seltzer et al. (1963, 1965) and Seltzer (1972).

1. Clinical features of pulpal pain

An exposure of the pulp may be anticipated in the majority of teeth with a history of pulpal pain. Conversely, most teeth with exposed pulps are painful. The more advanced the degree of pulpal inflammation, the greater is the likelihood of pain, but when the entire pulp has become necrotic, pain is less likely.

Advanced pulpal damage is more likely where there is a history of previous pain from the tooth, and possibly where the patient is aware of the nature of the pain, or where the pain is associated with an existing restoration. However, there seems no correlation between the precise nature of the pain and the histological state of the pulp.

A history of increased pain with external stimuli—such as heat or cold, or sweet or sour foods, or when lying down—is more common where the pulp has undergone pathological change, but occurs no more commonly in any one pathological state.

The more frequent or intense the pain, and the longer an episode of pain lasts, the more advanced is the degree of pulpal inflammation likely to be.

2. Percussion

A painful response to percussion, denoting inflammation of the periodontal membrane, is much more likely where the pulp is partly or completely necrotic.

3. Vitality test

a. Heat and cold tests
Partially or completely necrotic pulps are far less likely to respond to heat and cold tests than pulps without necrotic change. A normal response—that is, the cessation of pain a few seconds after withdrawing the stimulus—is much more likely with pulps without necrosis, whether healthy or inflamed, than where there is partial or complete necrosis. Most uninflamed pulps give a normal response to thermal tests.

b. Electric pulp test
Although a tooth with an inflamed pulp is more likely to respond to the electric pulp test at a different level, higher or lower, than the control tooth, the tendency is not marked. Thus, although the electric pulp test is of some value in suggesting inflammation, it is far from reliable in this respect.

Most teeth react to the electric pulp test so long as partial or complete necrosis of the pulp has not occurred. Thus, absence of response, or response only at a very high level of stimulation, almost certainly indicates that the pulp is partly or completely necrotic, probably the latter; however, the converse is not true, since some teeth with completely necrotic pulps react to the test (Johnson et al., 1970).

4. Radiographic examination

Inflammation of the pulp does not end abruptly at the apical foramen, but progresses to involve the periapical tissues before complete pulpal necrosis has occurred. Thus, extensive pulpal inflammation is invariably associated with periapical inflammation, so that a zone of periapical radiolucency may sometimes be seen where the pulp is chronically inflamed and the apical pulp still vital (*see Figs.* 1, 9 and 10).

CLASSIFICATION OF PULPAL STATES

It is apparent from the previous comments that in assessing the pulpal status the diagnostic methods available are of limited value. In particular, tests of pulpal vitality are considerably less reliable than is sometimes realized. The vitality of a pulp is ultimately dependent on its blood supply. However, each of the commonly used vitality tests relies on stimulating the nervous tissue of the pulp which, as Cahn (1930) and Mullaney et al. (1970) have pointed out, can persist long after the adjacent structures are hopelessly diseased. Furthermore, Langeland (1976) has shown that even when the tooth is associated with a periapical granuloma or cyst, some vital pulp tissue, including nerves, may still be present in the root canal.

Also, in interpreting the results of thermal and electric tests, the assumption is made that the pulps of the control teeth are normal, but this may not in fact be so. Thus, the results of vitality tests should not be the only criteria for assessing the state of a pulp. Instead, the information yielded by these tests should be considered in conjunction with that gained from other diagnostic measures.

In the past, inflammatory conditions of the pulp have generally been classified into four states—acute serous pulpitis, acute suppurative pulpitis, chronic ulcerative pulpitis and chronic hyperplastic pulpitis. Each of these states has been regarded as clinically recognizable. Before pulpitis became definitely established, a condition of hyperaemia was thought to be clinically recognizable; in favourable cases, and with suitable treatment, this condition, unlike pulpitis, could resolve.

However, Seltzer et al. (1963) and Baume (1970) concluded that hyperaemia is merely part of an inflammatory process, and does not constitute a histological entity, let alone a clinical one. Nor do acute serous and acute suppurative pulpitides constitute histological entities, unless occurring as direct sequels to operative procedures, in which case they are often painless and therefore remain clinically undiagnosed. Instead, they develop to affect part of a pulp already chronically inflamed. Thus, different histological conditions may exist in different parts of the pulp. From a clinical viewpoint, therefore, it is doubtful if the terms 'hyperaemia', 'acute pulpitis', 'acute serous pulpitis' and 'acute suppurative pulpitis' can be accurately used. Where there are acute symptoms present, the use of the term 'pulpitis with acute symptoms', or some similar term, is preferable. The term 'chronic pulpitis' is also better avoided in clinical descriptions, since an absence of acute symptoms does not preclude acute inflammation of part of the pulp.

In view of these considerations, and bearing in mind the limited value of the diagnostic methods available, it is clear that only two pathological states of the pulp may be reliably diagnosed clinically, namely pulpitis and necrosis of the pulp. A clinical diagnosis of an uninflamed pulp cannot be made with complete certainty. Even if this were possible, the fact that a pulp is without inflammation does not preclude the possibility of atrophic changes.

CLASSIFICATION OF PERIAPICAL STATES

Both acute and chronic inflammatory processes of the periapex are recognizable clinically.

1. Acute periapical disease

There are two acute inflammatory conditions of the periapical tissues, namely acute apical periodontitis and acute periapical abscess, the latter following upon the former. The difference between them is one of degree, and in consequence it is not always possible to differentiate between the two with certainty.

The treatment of both conditions is dealt with in Chapter 10.

a. Acute apical periodontitis

Acute inflammation of the apical periodontal membrane may be caused by irritation from the root canal, or by trauma to the crown of the tooth or the periodontal membrane. In the former event, the pulp will be inflamed or necrotic. In the latter event, the condition occurs independently of the state of the pulp, so that, initially, this is usually not inflamed.

When acute apical periodontitis is caused by irritation from the root canal, it may develop as an exacerbation of a chronic periapical lesion, or it may represent the initial periapical response to inflammation and necrosis of the pulp or to operative procedures in the pulp cavity. In the former event, periapical radiolucency is apparent. In the latter, however, although there may eventually be radiographic evidence of widening of the periodontal membrane space if the condition progresses to abscess formation, no such radiolucent zone is visible. The work of Bender and Seltzer (1961) and Wengraf (1964) suggests that this is because erosion of cortical bone is necessary for the production of a radiolucent area, with the result that an early lesion confined to cancellous bone may not be visible radiographically when the patient is first seen (*Fig. 20*).

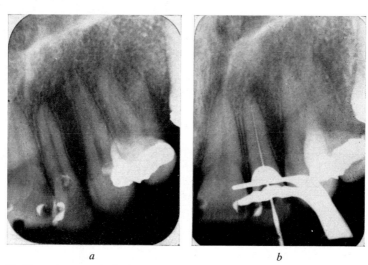

a   *b*

Fig. 20. |2. *a*, Acute periapical abscess, but virtually no bone destruction evident; *b*, Obvious bone rarefaction apparent 10 days later, following destruction of cortical bone.

In acute apical periodontitis there is pain on percussion. The tooth may or may not show increased mobility, and the patient may or may not find it tender to eat on. Although there may be some inflammation and tenderness to palpation of the soft tissues overlying the root apex, there is no obvious swelling.

b. Acute periapical abscess

An acute periapical abscess is a localized collection of pus under pressure in the vicinity of the root apex of a tooth. It is associated with disease and necrosis of the pulp and is the sequel to acute apical periodontitis.

The condition is associated with severe pain. The tooth shows a considerable increase in mobility and is extremely sensitive to percussion. As the condition progresses, the pain increases and the inflamed soft tissues overlying the root apex swell and eventually become fluctuant. Usually the adjoining lip or cheek, or both, also swell, sometimes considerably. The tooth tends to be extruded from its socket, so that the patient may be aware of a premature contact on closure; on occasions the degree of extrusion may be marked (*Fig.* 21). The adjoining teeth may become more mobile. At this stage the patient may feel and look exhausted

2

and ill. The pulse and temperature may be elevated. A regional lymphadenitis is usually detectable.

In the absence of treatment, drainage of the abscess may occur by a number of routes. The most common of these is into the mouth following progressive thinning

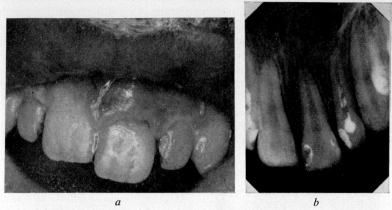

a   b

Fig. 21. *a*, Acute periapical abscess showing marked extrusion of |1; *b*, Radiographic appearance.

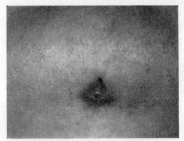

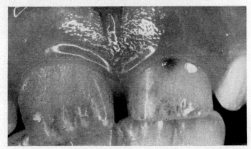

Fig. 22. Sinus opening onto surface of chin a few days after drainage of an acute periapical abscess of a mandibular incisor.

Fig. 23. |1. Blood-stained pus at gingival margin following drainage of an acute periapical abscess along periodontal membrane into gingival crevice.

and eventual rupture of the mucoperiosteum overlying the lesion. Sometimes the swelling is mainly extra-oral and a sinus opening onto the surface of the skin is formed (*Fig.* 22). Occasionally a sinus develops along the periodontal membrane and the lesion drains into the gingival crevice (*Fig.* 23). Very rarely drainage into the antrum or nasal cavity occurs.

The formation of a sinus and the drainage of pus lead to abatement of the acute symptoms which, with the establishment of a chronic periapical lesion, may disappear completely. However, if the sinus closes, acute abscess formation may recur at any time.

2. Chronic periapical disease

Chronic periapical disease may develop following drainage of an acute periapical abscess, or may result directly from extension of a pulpitis into the periapical region.

Apart from radiographic change, which will be dealt with presently, it is not uncommon for chronic periapical disease to exist with no clinical manifestations whatsoever (*Fig.* 24). On other occasions, manifestations are present, although some may not be immediately apparent.

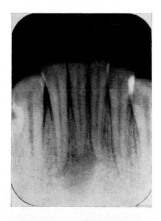

Fig. 24. Chronic periapical lesion ⊤⌐ with no clinical manifestations, discovered only from full-mouth radiographs.

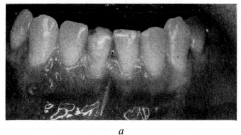

a

Fig. 25. *a*, Sinus from chronic periapical lesion of ⊤⌐ opens between ⌐2⌐ and ⌐3⌐; *b*, Radiographic appearance, with gutta percha point inserted into sinus.

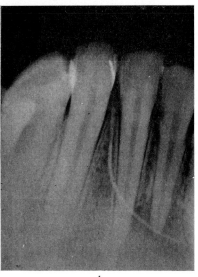

b

One of the commonest manifestations, unless there is drainage by way of the root canal into a cavity in the crown of the tooth, is a sinus. This usually opens intraorally close to the labial or buccal sulcus over the root of the tooth, but sometimes some distance from it (*Fig.* 25). Although the sinus may open flush with the surrounding mucous membrane, the latter is often elevated in the immediate vicinity of the opening, forming a so-called 'gumboil', which may be quite large (*Fig.* 26). There may be evidence, in the form of raised nodules of tissue, of previous sinuses which have closed and healed.

Occasionally the sinus opens onto the palate; this occurs especially when the involved root is closer to the palatal than the buccal cortex, as with lateral incisors and the palatal roots of molars. Similarly, sinuses from mandibular incisors sometimes open lingually; these same teeth also seem to be associated with extraoral drainage more commonly than most other teeth. Sinus formation into the gingival crevice sometimes occurs (*Fig.* 27), but drainage into the nasal cavity or antrum is a rarity. Where there is no drainage by way of the root canal and no evidence of

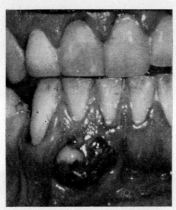

Fig. 26. An unusually large 'gumboil' in mandibular incisor region.

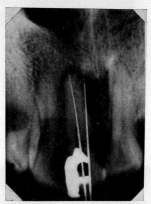

Fig. 27. 1|. Two silver points, one inserted into the root canal and the other into a sinus leading to the gingival crevice from the periapical region.

a sinus, the lesion is sometimes called a 'blind abscess'. On rare occasions, two sinuses from the same lesion may exist simultaneously (*Fig.* 28).

Usually there is no pain, or only slight pain. Sometimes pain occurs only as tenderness on eating. There may be some swelling in the region of the apex of the involved root, in which case slight tenderness can usually be elicited on palpation. The tooth itself may be a little loose and may show discoloration or loss of translucency. A duller sound than normal is sometimes audible when the tooth is percussed, and slight or moderate discomfort may be elicited by this procedure. Where the crowns of the immediately adjoining teeth appear to have been deflected from their positions in the arch, cystic change may be suspected; in these cases, the radiographs should be carefully examined for evidence of root movement, and the appearance compared with that on the opposite side of the arch.

Sometimes the manifestations of periapical disease are more acute than has just been described, but not so severe as to form an acute periapical abscess. Such a condition is sometimes called a 'subacute periapical abscess', and commonly occurs as a minor exacerbation of a chronic periapical lesion.

Limitations of radiographic examination in chronic periapical disease

Radiographic examination plays a very important role in diagnosing the presence of chronic periapical disease. It is therefore relevant to consider at this stage certain limitations of radiographs of the periapical region, besides those referred to previously in this chapter.

First, the radiograph presents only a two-dimensional picture. The buccolingual positions and depths of structures, and of changes within them, are not depicted. For example, it is not possible to assess the buccolingual extent of a periapical lesion, except indirectly and very roughly from its degree of radiolucency relative to other structures.

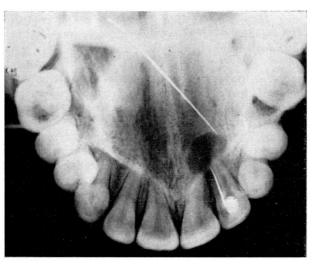

Fig. 28. |2. Silver points inserted into two sinuses from the same lesion. One opens into the gingival crevice and the other onto the palate.

Secondly, as has already been pointed out, destruction of periapical bone may not be apparent radiographically until cortical bone has been eroded. Thus, although there is evidence that bone destruction associated with established chronic periapical disease can usually be detected radiographically (Nicholls, 1963; Brynolf, 1967; Rowe and Binnie, 1974), this may not apply to the early stages of periapical involvement. Furthermore, the image of a lesion alongside the buccal or lingual aspect of the root will be partly or completely obscured.

Thirdly, the radiographic appearance of the periapical region gives no indication whether bone destruction has been caused by infection or by chemical or physical sources of irritation. Also, where periapical breakdown has resulted from the presence of micro-organisms in the pulp cavity, it does not follow that the bone lesion itself contains organisms. Indeed, it will be pointed out in Chapter 3 that usually it does not. It is therefore incorrect, from the radiographic appearance alone, to call a periapical zone of radiolucency an 'infected area'. Furthermore, the available evidence indicates no correlation between the species of organisms isolated from pulp cavities and the radiographic appearances of associated periapical lesions (Berwick, 1921; Burket, 1937).

Fourthly, there is a similar lack of correlation between the radiographic and histological appearances of periapical lesions. In the past, periapical lesions have usually been classified into three main groups—chronic periapical abscesses, granu-lomas and radicular cysts. However, the radiographic differentiation between these groups is not satisfactory. Radiographic differentiation between a chronic abscess and a granuloma is not possible, and even the histological differentiation is dubious; indeed, the former term has largely fallen into disuse. Any distinction between them is in any case of doubtful clinical significance. As recent studies have shown, the identification of a radicular cyst from its radiographic appearance is also un-satisfactory and, within the size range of lesions for which root canal treatment is normally contemplated, cannot, by normal methods, reliably be made (Priebe et al., 1954; Wais, 1958; Sommer et al., 1961; Linenberg et al., 1964; Bhaskar, 1966). From the clinical standpoint, therefore, specific descriptions should be avoided and instead the terms 'chronic periapical lesion' or 'chronic periapical disease' used.

Sometimes a zone of periapical bone destruction associated with a root-filled tooth is discovered only by chance, as a result of routine radiographic examination. In the absence of clinical manifestations of chronic periapical disease, it is difficult to decide whether such a zone represents an active lesion or one which has resolved and is healing, unless of course a series of preceding radiographs is available for comparison. Where the radiolucent zone is large and it is known that the tooth was root filled some years previously, it is reasonable to assume that resolution has not occurred. Similarly, where it is important for medical reasons to eliminate all possible foci of sepsis, then treatment is indicated. With these exceptions, how-ever, in the absence of preceding radiographs it is necessary to defer a firm decision for a few months, when further radiographs may be taken for comparison.

REFERENCES

Barber F. E., Lees S. and Lobene R. R. (1969) Ultrasonic pulse-echo measurements in teeth. *Arch. Oral Biol.* **14**, 745.
Baume L. J. (1970) Diagnosis of diseases of the pulp. *Oral Surg.* **29**, 102.
Bender I. B. and Seltzer S. (1961) Roentgenographic and direct observation of experimental lesions in bone, 1. *J. Am. Dent. Assoc.* **62**, 152.
Bender I. B., Seltzer S. and Kaufman I. J. (1959) Infectibility of the dental pulp by way of the dental tubules. *J. Am. Dent. Assoc.* **59**, 466.
Berwick C. C. (1921) The bacteriology of peridental tissues radiographically suggesting infection. *J. Infect. Dis.* **29**, 537.
Bhaskar S. N. (1966) Oral Surgery–Oral Pathology Conference No. 17, Walter Reed Army Medical Centre. Periapical lesions: types, incidence and clinical features. *Oral Surg.* **21**, 657.
Brannstrom M. and Nyborg H. (1972) Pulp reaction to composite resin restorations. *J. Prosthet. Dent.* **27**, 181.
Brown A. C. (1968) Pulp tissue pressure and blood flow. In: Finn S. B. (ed.), *Biology of the Dental Pulp Organ : A Symposium.* Alabama, University of Alabama Press, pp. 381–95.
Brynolf I. (1967) A histological and roentgenological study of the periapical region of human upper incisors. *Odontol. Revy* **18**, Suppl. 11.
Burket L. W. (1937) Studies of the apices of teeth. A correlation of the bacteriological, roentgeno-logical and gross anatomical findings in human necropsies. *Yale J. Biol. Med.* **9**, 271, 347.
Cahn L. R. (1930) Neuritis of the dental pulp. *Dent. Items* **52**, 699
Civyan S., Barone J. J. and Vaccaro G. J. (1973) Electric pulp vitality testers. *J. Dent. Res.* **52**, 120.
Cooke C. and Rowbotham T. C. (1952) An Electric Pulp Tester. *Br. Dent. J.* **92**, 147.
Dickey D. M., El-Kafrawy A. H. and Mitchell D. F. (1974) Clinical and microscopic pulp response to a composite restorative material. *J. Am. Dent. Assoc.* **88**, 108.
Ehrmann E. H. (1973) Four-handed sit-down endodontics. In: Grossman L. I. (ed.), *Transactions of the 5th International Conference on Endodontics.* Philadelphia, University of Pennsylvania, pp. 158–75.

Eriksen H. M. (1974) Pulpal response of monkeys to a composite resin cement. *J. Dent. Res.* **53,** 565.

Friend L. A. and Glenwright H. D. (1968) An experimental investigation into the localization of pain from the dental pulp. *Oral Surg.* **25,** 765.

Gier R. E. and Mitchell D. F. (1968) Anachoretic effect of pulpitis. *J. Dent. Res.* **47,** 564.

Grossman L. I. (1960) *Endodontic Practice,* 5th ed. London, Kimpton, p. 26.

Hansen H. P. and Bruun C. (1971) Long-term pulp reaction to silicate cement with an intradental control. *Scand. J. Dent. Res.* **79,** 422.

Harris W. E. (1973) Endodontic pain referred across the midline: report of a case. *J. Am. Dent. Assoc.* **87,** 1240.

Howell F. V., de la Rosa V. M. and Abrams A. M. (1968) Cytologic evaluation of cystic lesions of the jaws: a new diagnostic technique. *J. S. Calif. Dent. Assoc.* **36,** 161.

Howell R. M., Duell R. C. and Mullaney T. P. (1970) The determination of pulp vitality by thermographic means using cholesteric liquid crystals: a preliminary study: *Oral Surg.* **29,** 763.

Johnson R. H., Dachi S. F. and Haley J. V. (1970) Pulpal hyperemia—a correlation of clinical and histologic data from 706 teeth. *J. Am. Dent. Assoc.* **81,** 108.

Langeland K. (1967) The histopathologic basis in endodontic treatment. *Dent. Clin. North Am.* **11,** pp. 491–520.

Langeland K. and Langeland L. K. (1968) Indirect capping and the treatment of deep carious lesions. *Int. Dent. J. Lond.* **18,** 326.

Linenberg W. B., Westfield N. J., Waldron C. A. and DeLaune G. F. (1964) A clinical, roentgenographic and histopathologic evaluation of periapical lesions. *Oral Surg.* **17,** 467.

Logan T. H. (1964) Pain apparently referred across the midline from a perforated lower second molar. *Oral Surg.* **18,** 593.

Matthews B. and Searle B. N. (1974) Some observations on pulp testers. *Br. Dent. J.* **137,** 307.

Mitchell D. F. and Tarplee R. E. (1960) Painful pulpitis. A clinical and microscopic study. *Oral Surg.* **13,** 1360.

Morse D. R., Patnik J. W. and Schacterle G. R. (1973) Electrophoretic differentiation of radicular cysts and granulomas. *Oral Surg.* **35,** 249.

Mullaney T. P., Howell R. M. and Petrich J. D. (1970) Resistance of nerve fibers to pulpal necrosis. *Oral Surg.* **30,** 690.

Nicholls E. (1963) Assessment of the periapical status of pulpless teeth. *Br. Dent. J.* **114,** 453.

Plant C. G. (1970) The effect of polycarboxylate cement on the dental pulp. *Br. Dent. J.* **129,** 424.

Plant C. G. (1973) The effect of polycarboxylate containing stannous fluoride on the pulp. *Br. Dent. J.* **135,** 317.

Priebe W. A., Lazansky J. P. and Wuehrmann A. H. (1954) The value of the roentgenographic film in the differential diagnosis of periapical lesions. *Oral Surg.* **7,** 979.

Qvist V. (1975) Pulp reactions in human teeth to tooth-colored filling materials. *Scand. J. Dent. Res.* **83,** 54.

Reeves R. and Stanley H. R. (1966) The relationship of bacterial penetration and pulpal pathosis in carious teeth. *Oral Surg.* **22,** 59.

Rowe A. H. R. and Binnie W. H. (1974) Correlation between radiological and histological inflammatory changes following root canal treatment. *J. Br. Endodont. Soc.* **7,** 57.

Seltzer S. (1971) *Endodontology: Biologic Considerations in Endodontic Procedures.* New York, McGraw-Hill, pp. 125–40.

Seltzer S. (1972) Classification of pulpal pathosis. *Oral Surg.* **34,** 269.

Seltzer S., Bender I. B. and Nazimov H. (1965) Differential diagnosis of pulp conditions. *Oral Surg.* **19,** 383.

Seltzer S., Bender I. B. and Ziontz M. (1963) The dynamics of pulp inflammation: correlations between diagnostic data and actual histologic findings in the pulp. *Oral Surg.* **16,** 846, 969.

Shovelton D. S. (1968) A study of deep carious dentine. *Int. Dent. J., Lond.* **18,** 392.

Sommer R. F., Ostrander F. D. and Crowley M. C. (1961) *Clinical Endodontics,* 2nd ed. London, Saunders, p. 444.

Stanley H. R., Going R. E. and Chauncey H. H. (1975) Human pulp response to acid pretreatment of dentine and to composite restoration. *J. Am. Dent. Assoc.* **91,** 817.

Stephan R. M. (1937) Correlation of clinical tests with microscopic pathology of the dental pulp. *J. Dent. Res.* **16,** 267.

Stoops L. C. and Scott D. (1976) Measurement of tooth temperatures as a means of determining pulp vitality. *J. Endodontol.* **2**, 141.

Suzuki M., Goton G. and Jordan R. E. (1973) Pulpal response to pin placement. *J. Am. Dent. Assoc.* **87**, 636.

van Hassel H. J. (1971) Physiology of the human dental pulp. *Oral Surg.* **32**, 126.

Wais F. T. (1958) Significance of findings following biopsy and histologic study of 100 periapical lesions. *Oral Surg.* **11**, 650.

Wengraf A. (1964) Radiologically occult bone cavities: an experimental study and review. *Br. Dent. J.* **117**, 532.

FURTHER READING

Langeland K., Dowden W. E., Tronstad L. and Langeland L. K. (1971) Human pulp changes of iatrogenic origin. *Oral Surg.* **32**, 943.

Shovelton D. S. (1972) The maintenance of pulp vitality. *Br. Dent. J.* **133**, 95.

Shovelton D. S. (1976) Pulp protection. *J. Br. Endodont. Soc.* **9**, 57.

Chapter 2

Endodontic treatment and the maintenance of pulpal vitality

Where the pulp of a tooth is vital but is exposed, or is in imminent danger of becoming exposed, it is sometimes possible by suitable treatment to maintain it in a vital, healthy state; in some cases the entire pulp is retained, whilst in others the coronal part is removed. In pulp capping, or direct pulp capping, a protective material is applied to the exposure and the entire pulp is retained. Where there is no visible exposure and the dentine immediately over the pulp is left undisturbed and covered with a protective material, the procedure is sometimes called 'indirect' pulp capping; this method of treatment is connected closely with the conservative treatment of deep carious lesions. In pulpotomy, or vital amputation, part of the pulp is removed; the cut surface of the remainder, constituting most or all of the radicular pulp, is covered with a suitable material and is left undisturbed and in a vital state.

Many aspects of both direct and indirect pulp capping are empirical. This is due to some considerable degree to our present inability to determine with reasonable accuracy from clinical criteria the state of a pulp. Thus, it is difficult not only to assess the pulpal state following capping, and therefore the result of such treatment, but also the pulpal state beforehand. It is hardly surprising, therefore, that there are differences of opinion on such fundamental issues as, for example, the indications for, and contraindications to, pulp capping. In this connection, the apparently favourable clinical results obtained with capping materials containing cortico-steroid drugs have, in the opinion of some, radically expanded the scope of pulp capping, and in consequence restricted the indications for partial or complete removal of the pulp. A separate account of the use of these materials will be given.

CONSERVATIVE TREATMENT OF DEEP CARIOUS LESIONS: INDIRECT PULP CAPPING

It was pointed out in Chapter 1 that chronic pulpitis, although not apparent clinically, develops before the pulp is exposed by caries. However, provided there is no exposure and the process of restoring the tooth removes the source of pulpal irritation and does not cause undue additional damage to the pulp, this inflammation may be expected to resolve.

Normally, to ensure the complete elimination of the original source of pulpal irritation, all softened dentine associated with the carious process is removed.

Sometimes, however, it may be felt that even though the lesion has not reached the pulp, removal of the last traces of softened dentine at the base of the lesion could not be accomplished without a serious risk of also removing the remaining sound dentine covering the pulp. The operator is thus faced with the problem either of leaving a little softened dentine which may contain micro-organisms, or of removing this dentine and perhaps exposing the pulp.

1. Microbiological state of cavity floor

For the most part, the evidence that is available indicates that as a carious lesion enlarges demineralization of dentine precedes its invasion by micro-organisms, so that the softened dentine at the base of a lesion is usually sterile or only lightly contaminated (Stephan et al., 1943; MacGregor et al., 1956; Sarnat and Massler, 1965; Fusayama et al., 1966).

However, in those teeth where residual softened dentine is contaminated, if the cavity is merely filled with a 'non-antiseptic' material such as amalgam, some micro-organisms, especially lactobacilli, may remain viable under the filling for many months or even years (Schouboe and MacDonald, 1962; Fisher, 1966, 1969). Although it is uncertain whether these organisms could cause further carious invasion, the possibility cannot be ruled out.

2. Treatment of cavity floor

Various preparations may be applied to the cavity floor in an attempt to sterilize softened, and supposedly contaminated, dentine. These preparations are divisible into chemical antiseptics, and calcium hydroxide and zinc oxide–eugenol compounds used as lining or base materials.

a. Treatment with chemical antiseptics

In the past it was sometimes advocated that a chemical antiseptic—for example, silver nitrate, beechwood creosote or monochlorphenol—be applied to residual softened dentine, either by placing the drug in the cavity for a short time immediately prior to filling, or by actually sealing it in the cavity. In discussing the advisability of using such drugs, three main factors merit consideration: first, the power of diffusion of the drug through decalcified and normal dentine; secondly, the antiseptic efficiency of the drug within dentine, especially in relation to the duration of its application; and thirdly, the effect of the drug should it reach the pulp.

So far as the first two factors are concerned, the studies of Seltzer (1942a, b) and that of Muntz et al. (1943) emphasized the inadequacy of most of the drugs advocated at that time. The fact that a drug diffuses to a certain depth in dentine does not denote sterilization to the same depth, or indeed to any depth at all.

The third factor, the effect of the drug should it reach the pulp, is significant in that chemical antiseptics kill not only micro-organisms but also tissue cells, and are therefore capable of causing further irritation to a pulp which, because of the cavity depth, is probably already inflamed. Thus, a mixture of camphorated mono-chlorphenol and penicillin, which had previously been advocated for cavity sterilization, was shown by Langeland et al. (1968) to cause acute pulpitis when applied to the dentine of experimental cavities.

For these reasons the use of chemical antiseptics in the treatment of deep cavities is now largely obsolete.

b. Treatment with calcium hydroxide compounds
There is considerable evidence that the application of calcium hydroxide, at least in the form of a paste with water or methyl cellulose, leads to sterilization, or near-sterilization, of residual softened dentine (King et al., 1965; Aponte et al., 1966; Fisher, 1972). It has also been shown that proprietary calcium hydroxide cements and pastes have no deleterious effect on the pulp when applied to deep cavities (Berk, 1950; Tronstad and Mjor, 1972).

There is also reason to believe that an increase in mineralization may occur in the dentine remaining under calcium hydroxide pastes and cements. Some evidence to this effect is provided by the radiographic studies of Sowden (1956), Law and Lewis (1961) and Jordan and Suzuki (1971), and by a television densitometric evaluation carried out by Kerkhove et al. (1967). Rather more conclusive evidence was provided by Mjor (1967) using microradiographic techniques, whilst the study by Eidelman et al. (1965), in which the dentine base of the cavity was analysed for phosphorus content, apparently leaves no doubt that an increase in mineralization does occur under calcium hydroxide.

c. Treatment with zinc oxide–eugenol
Sterilization of residual softened dentine may occur not only under calcium hydroxide but also under zinc oxide–eugenol cement (King et al., 1965).

Similarly, the application of zinc oxide–eugenol may also be followed by an increase in mineralization of the underlying dentine. Stewart and Richardson (1968), Kerkhove et al. (1967) and Jordan and Suzuki (1971) conclude that there is little if any difference between the effects of calcium hydroxide and zinc oxide–eugenol in this respect. The study of Ehrenreich (1968) is apparently the only one to report a definite superiority for zinc oxide–eugenol over calcium hydroxide for the purpose of rehardening carious dentine.

3. Selection of teeth for indirect capping: pulp state

Where there is positive evidence that the pulp is vital, and there are no clinical signs or symptoms indicative of pulpitis, such as spontaneous pain, it is usually assumed that caries has not reached the pulp. Although all softened dentine should be removed from the side walls of such a cavity, that at the base of the lesion is normally left undisturbed if its removal would entail a significant risk of pulp exposure (*Figs. 29* and *30*). As the preceding discussion has shown, application of a calcium hydroxide or zinc oxide–eugenol preparation prior to filling should be followed by arrest of the carious process and an increase in mineralization of the cavity floor.

It should be noted that in most of the reports of increased mineralization following the application of calcium hydroxide or zinc oxide–eugenol, it is specifically stated that the treated teeth either had no history of pain suggesting a pulpitis or were non-carious with experimentally prepared cavities. Where there is clinical evidence of pulpitis, it is probable that decalcification has reached or is very close to the pulp. Thus, Shovelton (1968) found marked pulpal inflammation when the remaining sound dentine was less than 0·3 mm thick, whilst micro-organisms were found in the pulp when the dentine was 0·2 mm or less in depth. Under these circumstances, continued pulpal health with sterilization and remineralization of the carious dentine seems improbable, and the removal of all softened dentine is indicated. Precautions should be taken to avoid unnecessary contamination of the pulp in the event of exposure. The tooth is isolated from saliva and the cavity cleaned of debris and washed with a mild antiseptic solution such as sodium hypochlorite. The last layers of softened dentine are removed with care in case exposure has not yet occurred. In view of the risk of forcing micro-organisms and their toxins into the pulp, as little pressure as possible is exerted on the base of the cavity.

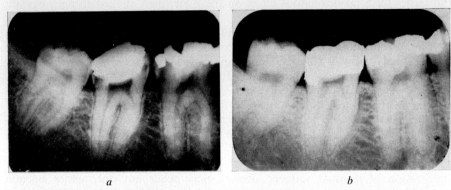

a   *b*

Fig. 29. ⑺. *a*, Softened dentine left in base of cavity; *b*, Two years later the pulp still responds to vitality tests and the tooth is symptomless and without evidence of periapical change.

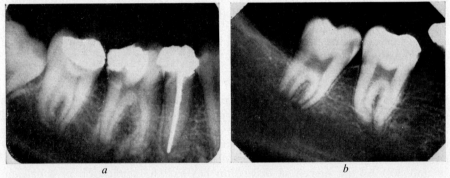

a   *b*

Fig. 30. ⑺. *a*, Softened dentine left in base of cavity; *b*, Three years later the pulp still responds to vitality tests and the tooth is symptomless and without evidence of periapical change. ⑹ was extracted.

4. Subsequent removal of softened dentine

Following the application of a calcium hydroxide or zinc oxide–eugenol preparation to the base of a cavity, the need later to remove the formerly softened dentine is questionable.

Those operators who attempt to remove softened dentine at a later date base their approach on two beliefs: first, that following on previous treatment of the cavity the pulp will have laid down sufficient reparative dentine to make its exposure by further excavation improbable; and, secondly, that the decalcified dentine at the base of the cavity contains micro-organisms which are continuing to invade the dentine over the pulp, or are likely to at some future date. There are two objections to this approach. The first is that until more tissue is excavated it is not possible to tell if sufficient reparative dentine has been formed. The second, which has already been discussed, is that sterilization or near-sterilization of the cavity floor should have occurred.

It therefore seems that there is little to be gained by deliberately opening the cavity at a later date in order to complete the removal of the original base of the carious lesion, unless of course the tooth is to support an expensive restoration such as a crown or bridge, which could be mutilated should pulpal disease and the need for root canal treatment become apparent later. If the tooth is to serve such a function, it is advisable to wait at least 3 months, and preferably 6 months, for reparative dentine formation before excavating the original base of the cavity.

5. Selection of base material; restoration of deep cavities

Calcium hydroxide, but not zinc oxide–eugenol, has other potentially beneficial effects besides those already described. For example, it may encourage calcific repair of a small exposure which has been overlooked, or is so small as to be undetectable by clinical examination. It is also feasible that, by virtue of its highly alkaline pH, it may help to allay pulpal irritation by neutralizing the acidic products of the micro-organisms responsible for decalcification of the dentine. For these reasons, and because of the greater weight of evidence regarding its sterilizing action on residual contaminated dentine, calcium hydroxide is considered preferable to zinc oxide–eugenol as the base material in the treatment of deep cavities.

To ensure that caries does not recur in the base of the cavity, it is important that the overlying restoration provide as effective a seal as possible. Particular care is taken to ensure that the enamel is soundly supported, and that there is no suspicion of decalcification or caries of the side walls. From this viewpoint, the use of zinc oxide–eugenol cement over the calcium hydroxide base is preferable to zinc phosphate cement, since it provides a better seal. Also, it avoids neutralization of the calcium hydroxide, which could occur if phosphate cement were applied directly to a thin layer of calcium hydroxide paste.

The lining of the cavity should provide a firm base so that the pulp cannot be injured during insertion of the overlying restoration by the transmission of pressure through a thin layer of dentine. If necessary, a layer of zinc phosphate cement is applied to give additional strength to the zinc oxide–eugenol lining already present. To prevent possible transmission of pressure to the base of the cavity during mastication, some workers consider there should be a shelf of sound dentine around and occlusal to the deepest part of the cavity. If the cavity has been correctly prepared so that the minimal amount of sound tissue has been removed, this shelf is usually present.

6. Postoperative observation: prognosis

It is desirable that the tooth be examined radiographically and by vitality tests some time following restoration—say 1 year afterwards—to check the state of the pulp.

Because of the limitations of vitality tests, and also because the original state and proximity of the cavity floor to the pulp obviously cannot be determined, incontrovertible conclusions on the prognosis of indirect pulp capping are not possible. Within these limitations, however, and with appropriate case selection, the available reports indicate a favourable prognosis. Using a calcium hydroxide paste, Law and

Lewis (1961) reported that 44 (77 per cent) out of 57 teeth treated were successful after 2 years. Jordan and Suzuki (1971) obtained 236 successes (97 per cent) out of 243 teeth treated with various calcium hydroxide preparations or zinc oxide–eugenol cement; there was no evidence that the result varied according to the agent used. Kerkhove et al. (1967) reported 70 successes (92 per cent) out of 76 teeth treated with calcium hydroxide paste or zinc oxide cement and observed for 12 months; again, the agent used seemed to have little effect on the prognosis.

There is some evidence from comparative studies that the prognosis for indirect capping is better than that for direct pulp capping or pulpotomy. Of a total of 1048 teeth followed for up to 4 years, Hawes et al. (1964) report failure rates of 3, 7 and 19 per cent respectively; calcium hydroxide paste was used in all instances. Similarly, Delaney and Seyler (1966), using a calcium hydroxide cement, obtained a success rate of 88 per cent with indirect capping and 77 per cent with direct capping; the teeth were observed for 6–18 months. In this last study, complete excavation of caries with resultant near, but not actual, exposure gave a success rate of 95 per cent.

DIRECT PULP CAPPING

1. Diagnosis of pulpal exposure

The diagnosis of pulpal exposure was dealt with in Chapter 1. It is made preferably on the basis of visual observation of a defect in the wall of the pulp cavity, from which there is often haemorrhage. Probing suspect areas to determine their sensitivity may also have to be relied upon, but directly the diagnosis is made the exposure should not be probed again.

2. Selection of teeth for pulp capping

Capping of pulp exposures should be restricted to those cases where there is no reason to suppose that the reparative ability of the pulp has been seriously reduced. This implies that inflammation of the pulp is non-existent or minimal. Thus, exposures resulting from the injudicious use of instruments during cavity preparation, rather than directly from caries of the dentine, may be favourable for capping.

The contraindications to pulp capping are illustrated in *Fig.* 31. If the pulp has obviously been penetrated by an instrument, rather than merely nicked, it should not be capped, since the amount of tissue damage, and therefore the inflammatory response, is likely to be considerable. Also, it is probable that dentine chips have been driven into the pulp, and there is some evidence that this makes for a worse prognosis (Kalnins and Frisbie, 1960). Moreover, in such a case contamination by micro-organisms is less likely to be restricted to the exposed surface of the pulp. On the same basis, capping should not be performed when exposure results from an instrument plunging first through a mass of carious dentine and then through a layer of sound dentine covering the pulp. Contamination of an exposure by a film of saliva is of less consequence, provided immediate steps are taken to isolate the tooth and eliminate the saliva.

Capping is rarely a warrantable form of treatment for an exposure resulting from fracture of the crown. It is contraindicated if the tooth is that of a child and has an open apex, since the main objective in such a case is to ensure continued development of the root apex. It is generally agreed that whereas pulpotomy provides a reasonably certain means of eliminating the contaminated region of the pulp, capping does not. However, it should be pointed out that there seems to have been no large-scale study into the prognosis of capping such teeth.

With tooth fracture in an older patient, the root apex will already be sufficiently developed to constitute no problem should root canal treatment later become necessary as a consequence of pulpal disease. Provided that a post crown or some

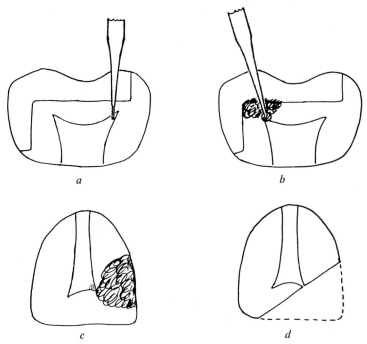

Fig. 31. Contraindications to pulp capping—*a*, Penetration of pulp; *b*, Exposure from instruments plunging through caries; *c*, Exposure and breakdown of pulp from caries; *d*, Exposure due to fracture of crown.

other complex restoration is not indicated, that there is no apical periodontitis to cause further embarrassment to the pulp, and that the patient is treated within a few hours of the accident whilst contamination of the pulp by micro-organisms is still superficial, capping may be tried. However, few cases are seen in which all of these conditions are fulfilled, and even when they are pulp capping must be regarded as a far less certain method of treatment than pulpectomy and root canal therapy.

Where exposure is a direct result of caries and there is clinical evidence of pulpitis, it is generally agreed that the prognosis of pulp capping is unfavourable, and the study of Nyborg (1958) lends both clinical and histological support to this view. However, this should not be taken to mean that a successful outcome is completely out of the question. Sometimes the operation may be successful, especially if there is reason to believe the pulpitis is limited in extent. Copious haemorrhage or a serous or purulent exudate from the exposure implies the very reverse, of course, and therefore makes for a distinctly unfavourable prognosis.

As in the treatment of an exposure resulting from fracture of the crown, capping should not be performed where the pulp of a tooth with an incompletely formed apex has been exposed by caries; instead, pulpotomy is indicated.

The validity of certain factors commonly held in the past to be contraindications to pulp capping is questionable. For example, it has often been stated that larger exposures have a worse prognosis than smaller ones. In consequence it was advised that capping should not be attempted where the exposed part of the pulp was more than, say, 0·5 mm in diameter, although different operators' estimates of 0·5 mm when viewing an exposure probably vary considerably. Also, older patients were reputed to constitute poorer risks, as were exposures which did not bleed. Studies by Shankle and Brauer (1962) and Berk (1963) suggest that the size of the exposure and the age of the patient are not by themselves major factors in determining the outcome of treatment. The absence of haemorrhage from the exposure, assuming it has not resulted from the previous injection of a local anaesthetic, is more difficult to evaluate, but would seem to be of significance only when it denotes degeneration or necrosis of the pulp.

A final point to bear in mind when deciding whether to cap an exposure concerns the nature of the restoration. When this is likely to be complex, then pulp capping, like the retention of decalcified dentine in the base of a cavity, is unwise.

Even though it may be decided that pulp capping is contraindicated, it is often used as a temporary measure, so that at a subsequent visit pulpotomy or root canal treatment may be performed as an elective rather than an emergency procedure.

3. Pulp-capping materials

Many substances, often in combination or with other additives, have been tested or advocated at one time or another for pulp capping. They include anorganic bone, antibiotics, calcium hydroxide, cyanoacrylates, corticosteroids, crystalline substances based on thymol, dentine chips, polycarboxylate cements, tricalcium phosphate ceramic, zinc oxide–eugenol and various cements based on this, and the sulphonamides. With the exception of the corticosteroids, which will be discussed later under a separate heading, the most popular of these and the one for which there is most support histologically is undoubtedly calcium hydroxide.

a. Calcium hydroxide preparations

Calcium hydroxide may be used as a powder alone, or it may be made into a paste by the addition of sterile water, physiological saline solution, local anaesthetic solution, or an aqueous solution of methyl or hydroxyethyl cellulose, or it may be used in the form of various cements. Of these, the most commonly used are probably the cements and calcium hydroxide and methyl or hydroxyethyl cellulose paste, since they are the easiest to apply. It is irrational to incorporate antibiotics within the preparation, since the high degree of alkalinity of calcium hydroxide destroys, or at least severely reduces, their activity. Barium sulphate may be added to make calcium hydroxide preparations radiopaque.

There seems no firm evidence that any one form of calcium hydroxide preparation gives significantly better results (Weiss and Bjorvatn, 1970; Rowe and Binnie, 1975). However, one particular cement, namely Hydrex, has been shown to cause pulpal inflammation and necrosis when used as a dressing for pulpotomy wounds (Phaneuf et al., 1968; Hirschfeld et al., 1972). It has also been shown to give inferior results compared with other calcium hydroxide preparations when used for pulp capping

(Sekine et al., 1971). There is evidence that the irritant effects of Hydrex result from the catalyst paste and not the base paste (Sela et al., 1973).

In successful cases of capping with calcium hydroxide, a calcified barrier is formed in the region of the exposure. This barrier, within which may be many spaces, is apparent 4–6 weeks following treatment and walls off the underlying pulp, which should show little or no evidence of infiltration in the vicinity of the original lesion. Between the barrier and the original exposure is a superficial layer of pulpal tissue which has undergone necrosis from the action of the calcium hydroxide. However, with at least one calcium hydroxide cement, namely Dycal, it has been shown that a calcific barrier forms in direct contact with the cement (Stanley and Lundy, 1972; McWalter et al., 1973; Tronstad, 1974). In the study of Stanley and Lundy (1972), it is pointed out that the width of the pulp opposite the exposure in relation to the potential depth of tissue devitalization immediately following capping may be a relevant factor in case selection. Thus, where the pulp is exceptionally narrow, as at the base of a deep approximal box, pulp capping with calcium hydroxide may be contraindicated.

b. Zinc oxide–eugenol cements

With zinc oxide–eugenol there is little tendency for calcific bridging of the exposure, and the pulp, although probably symptomless, remains chronically inflamed (Weiss and Bjorvatn, 1970; Nixon and Hannah, 1972). However, it is feasible that the failure of the pulp to wall itself off with a calcific barrier is associated with impurities in the zinc oxide, since both radiological proof (Cooke and Rowbotham, 1956) and histological proof (Sekine et al., 1960) have been presented that show that the use of analytical zinc oxide–eugenol as the capping material in pulpotomy is commonly followed by the formation of a calcific bridge.

c. Cyanoacrylates

The efficacy of cyanoacrylates for pulp capping is uncertain. Some studies have reported favourable results using isobutyl cyanoacrylate, with the formation of a calcific bridge in direct contact with the capping material, the absence of a necrotic zone under the material and less pulpal inflammation than occurs with calcium hydroxide preparations (Bhaskar et al., 1969; Berkman et al., 1971; Bhaskar et al., 1972). Other studies, however, have reported relatively poor results with both isobutyl cyanoacrylate (Rowe and Binnie, 1975) and n-butyl cyanoacrylate (Nixon and Hannah, 1972).

d. Other materials

Although polycarboxylate cement produces only a mild pulpal reaction when applied to an exposure, a calcific bridge is seldom formed (McWalter et al., 1973).

Recently, promising results with a mixture of tricalcium phosphate ceramic and physiological saline solution have been reported (Heller et al., 1975).

4. Significance of calcific bridging of exposure

It must be pointed out that the formation of a calcific barrier at the site of exposure does not necessarily mean that the underlying pulp is uninflamed, and is therefore not necessarily indicative of success. An advantage which a calcific barrier may confer, assuming it to be complete, is to make contamination of the pulp less likely in the event of subsequent leakage of the overlying restoration. This may well be important to the ultimate success of the procedure.

5. Technique

Where a carious tooth is under treatment, certain measures should be taken as soon as it is realized that exposure of the pulp is likely. Before proceeding further with the cavity wall which is suspect, all carious tissue is eliminated from the remainder of the cavity. Before any more caries is removed from the suspect wall, the tooth is isolated and the cavity is cleaned of debris and washed with a mild antiseptic solution, such as sodium hypochlorite, the solution then being absorbed with wool pledgets. Where possible, the instruments used to remove the remaining carious dentine are first treated in a hot salt sterilizer to eliminate gross contamination. If burs are employed for this purpose, they are used with the lightest of pressures in a brushing manner, so that an instrument cannot penetrate the surface of the pulp. Although there is conflicting evidence on the effect of dentine fragments on pulpal healing, most operators try to avoid forcing them into the pulp or leaving them on the exposed pulpal surface. Thus, if exposure does occur, any debris in the vicinity of the pulpal wound or on its surface is gently lifted away with excavators or wiped away with a wool pledget moistened with sterile saline or water. The exposure should be kept moist pending capping.

Sometimes exposure occurs when it is not anticipated, usually as a result of over-zealous instrumentation. Here, the same precautions are instituted as when an exposure is foreseen. The tooth is isolated immediately, the cavity is washed free of debris and any carious dentine remaining in the vicinity of the exposure is removed. Pending capping the exposed part of the pulp should if possible be kept covered with a wool pledget moistened with sterile saline to prevent unnecessary contamination or desiccation.

The pulp is now capped. At no time prior to capping should caustic drugs be applied to the cavity. In order that the capping material contacts the pulpal wound and is not lifted away from it, haemorrhage should have ceased by the time it is applied. Usually, this will have occurred without any special treatment; if it has not, it may easily be brought about by applying a moist wool pledget with light pressure to the exposure for a minute or so. Although Kalnins (1957) and Kalnins et al. (1964) have produced evidence that, with calcium hydroxide at any rate, firm pressure may, by controlling haemorrhage, promote a favourable response, it is usually agreed that as little pressure as possible should be used in applying the capping material.

Calcium hydroxide powder may be applied by means of an insufflator or after compacting it into an amalgam carrier, or sometimes with a plastic instrument. The excess material to the sides of the exposure, but not immediately around it, is removed with excavators. When a paste of calcium hydroxide is used it is applied with the aid of college forceps or a plastic instrument, or from a pre-loaded syringe (see Chapter 13). The paste may be dried by directing a gentle stream of warm air over it, the excess then being removed. Calcium hydroxide cements take the form of a two-paste system; the base and catalyst are mixed to a creamy consistency and the resultant cement 'painted' over the exposure and adjoining dentine with a fine plastic instrument.

6. Restoration of the tooth

Since there is a definite breach in the dentine covering the pulp, there must be no leakage of saliva into the cavity after the patient is dismissed. This is of obvious importance immediately following capping, but may also be important even in the event of a calcific barrier forming, since this barrier may not be complete. As with indirect capping, due precautions are taken to ensure that restoration of the tooth does not result in pressure on the pulp. The restoration, be it temporary or permanent, must not make premature contact during mastication.

It is advisable wherever possible to complete the preparation and restore the tooth directly after capping. If a temporary restoration is necessary, it should be placed carefully to ensure that it is not broken or lost before the patient is next seen. If the tooth is badly broken down, a temporary crown is fitted. On no account is unsupported enamel left at the margins of the preparation.

As with indirect capping, it is better to line the floor of the cavity with a fast-setting zinc oxide–eugenol cement than with a phosphate cement, especially when the pulp has been capped with calcium hydroxide and only a thin layer has been used. If there is doubt that this will provide sufficient strength, a layer of phosphate cement may be placed above the zinc oxide–eugenol (*Fig.* 32). Placing a disc of

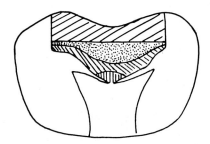

Fig. 32. Above the pulp-capping material, layers of restoration are fast-setting zinc oxide–eugenol cement, phosphate cement and overlying restoration.

metal or celluloid immediately above the pulp-capping material, although popular at one time as a means of protecting the pulp from pressure during restoration of the cavity, is now seldom done, but there is no objection to the practice.

7. Postoperative observation: prognosis

Most teeth are quite comfortable following pulp capping. If there is hypersensitivity to temperature change, it should last for no more than a couple of days. There should be no actual pain. If hypersensitivity persists or if the tooth is actually painful, failure may be assumed.

It is not uncommon, however, for failure to occur without pain, and for symptoms to arise only after necrosis of the pulp has led to obvious involvement of the periapical tissues (*Figs.* 33 and 34). The tooth should therefore be observed postoperatively and the pulp tested for vitality periodically. If local anaesthesia has been used and it has not been possible to perform an electric pulp test before or immediately after exposing the pulp, such a test is made soon after any hypersensitivity has ceased, say 2 weeks after capping; the reading from this test then provides a basis for comparison with the results of subsequent tests. If a subsequent test suggests failure, a radiograph of the tooth is taken; loss of periapical bone will confirm a diagnosis of failure. The studies of Simon (1942) and Feitelson (1956) suggest that most failures which can be diagnosed by clinical tests become apparent within 12 months; however, Shovelton et al. (1971) found that a considerable number of failures became apparent 1–2 years after pulp capping.

Based on clinical assessment, including vitality tests and radiographic examination, and with careful selection of cases, the prognosis of pulp capping is good (*Figs.* 35 and 36). Indeed, some workers estimate the success rate to be about 90 per cent (Nyborg, 1958; Hawes et al., 1964). However, the success rate when

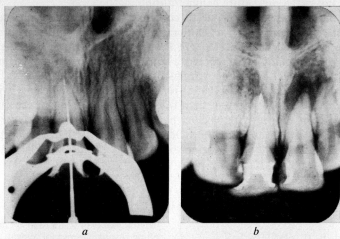

a   *b*

Fig. 33. |1. *a*, Shortly after pulp capping; *b*, Seven months later, showing periapical lesion.

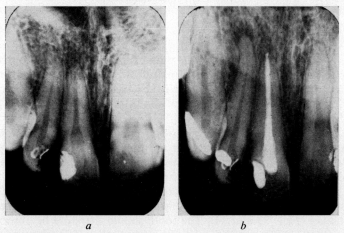

a   *b*

Fig. 34. 2|. *a*, Shortly after pulp capping; *b*, Fourteen months later, showing periapical lesion.

assessed histologically is considerably less, as would be expected. This is shown by the study of Nyborg (1958). The same study also indicates that although histological examination may show that a clinically successful result is really a failure, it almost always agrees with a clinical diagnosis of failure.

Although the presence of a calcific barrier is sometimes included in the criteria of success in studies on the prognosis of pulp capping, it must be pointed out that this test, like tests of pulpal vitality, has definite limitations. The fact that a barrier may be demonstrated radiographically is no indication that it is complete. Also, even where there are no overlying metallic restorations to hamper the radiologic assessment, radiographic examination may not always reveal a barrier which is present; thus, a higher percentage of calcific barriers may be demonstrated by

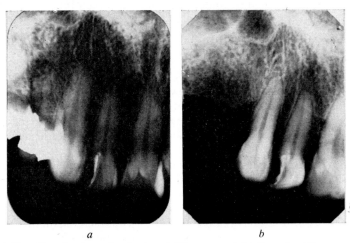

| a | b |

Fig. 35. 2|. *a*, Shortly after pulp capping; *b*, Three years later the pulp still responds to vitality tests and the tooth is symptomless and without evidence of periapical change.

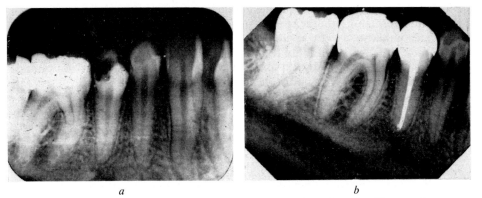

| a | b |

Fig. 36. 6|. *a*, Shortly after pulp capping; *b*, Three years later the pulp still responds to vitality tests and the tooth is symptomless and without evidence of periapical change.

removing the restorations and examining visually the sites of the original exposures than by radiographic examination. It has already been pointed out, moreover, that the formation of a calcific barrier does not necessarily indicate that the underlying pulp is without inflammatory change.

TREATMENT WITH CORTICOSTEROID DRUGS

In recent years corticosteroid drugs have been used for pulp capping. The effect of these drugs is to prevent an inflammatory reaction to irritation, or to suppress an inflammatory process which already exists. As a consequence of their anti-inflammatory effect, the tissue defences in the region of their application are also suppressed, so that if micro-organisms are already present in the tissues there is little resistance to their spread. When corticosteroid drugs are applied to exposed pulps, therefore, they should be combined with either a suitable chemical antiseptic or an antibiotic.

1. Efficacy of corticosteroids

Many of the studies of the efficacy of corticosteroids for indirect or direct pulp capping have been based on clinical assessment. These studies, apparently without exception, have reported favourable results. For example, Cowan (1966) reports a clinical success rate of 90 per cent. There have also been favourable reports on the use of these preparations in the treatment of pain arising from extensive cavity preparations.

Histological studies have conflicted somewhat in their conclusions, however. In the study of Fiore-Donno and Baume (1962), which is probably the most extensive to be reported, various preparations containing different corticosteroids were used as capping materials following partial pulpotomy. It was found that the favourable clinical results obtained with corticosteroid-containing preparations were not confirmed when the teeth were extracted and examined histologically. With the exception of one preparation, which included calcium hydroxide, no solid barrier was formed. Instead, there was fibrosis and chronic pulpitis. It was concluded that corticosteroids either inhibited formation of the elements necessary for dentine formation or accelerated their maturation into connective tissue.

A later publication (Baume and Fiore-Donno, 1968) confirmed and enlarged upon these findings. Application of various corticosteroid–antibiotic compounds to cap previously intact pulps led to metaplastic changes in the pulp, with stunting of dentine formation and congestion of blood vessels in the apical region; when calcium hydroxide was included in the compound, some osteoid formation eventually occurred, but never sealed the exposure completely. Application of the same compounds to exposed and previously painful pulps also led to metaplastic changes, together with a slowly progressive but symptomless chronic pulpitis. These workers conclude that permanent contact of corticosteroids with an exposed pulp whose vitality is to be maintained is contraindicated.

Lawson and Mitchell (1964) used a preparation which did not include calcium hydroxide, and also failed to demonstrate the formation of a hard-tissue barrier after capping. Barker and Ehrmann (1969) reported on the use of Ledermix cement, which does contain calcium hydroxide; application to exposed normal pulps for up to 727 days failed to induce complete bridging, whilst application to previously painful pulps tended to be followed by chronic pulpitis. Both Mjor and Nygaard-Ostby (1966) and Barker and Ehrmann (1969) noted a localized deposition of dentine leading to narrowing of the root canal apical to the exposure. Similarly, Cowan (1966), who also used Ledermix, reported chronic pulpitis with absence of calcific bridging. Both Rowe (1967) and Paterson (1976a, b) found that necrosis was common following the use of corticosteroid–antibiotic preparations in rats, whilst Uitto et al. (1975) have demonstrated that Ledermix paste suppresses collagen synthesis in the pulp.

On the other hand, Turell et al. (1958), using a preparation containing calcium chloride, reported that a transformation into dentinoid of the fibrous connective tissue formed postoperatively could be seen 5 or 6 weeks after capping. Also, Vigg (1962) was able to demonstrate, by visual examination of the original exposure sites, calcific barriers in 14 out of 18 cases; in the same way, Fry et al. (1960) demonstrated barriers in 3 teeth. In neither of these last two studies did the capping material contain calcium hydroxide.

Hansen (1969) tested various preparations for capping experimentally exposed teeth; 7 out of 48 teeth treated with a corticosteroid or a corticosteroid–antibiotic combination showed calcific bridging, and in 6 of these calcium hydroxide was included in the capping material. Schroeder (1968) in a small-scale study showed that pre-treatment of an exposed pulp with Ledermix paste for 3–4 days, followed by removal of the paste and application of calcium hydroxide, may enhance the likelihood of bridging of the exposure.

2. Corticosteroid preparations used

Various preparations containing corticosteroids have been described. Not only have cortisone and hydrocortisone been used, but also much more powerful members of this group, such as prednisolone, dexamethasone, and triamcinolone

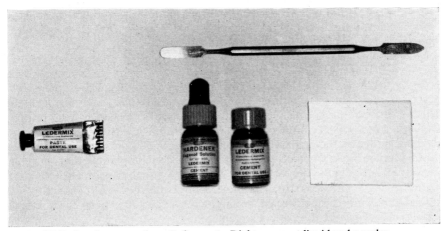

Fig. 37. Ledermix preparations. Left—paste. Right—cement liquid and powder.

acetonide. The anti-inflammatory effect of the last-named drug is stated to be between twenty and thirty-five times that of hydrocortisone (Kutscher et al., 1961). In general, because of the possibility of contamination or actual infection of the exposed region of the pulp, an antiseptic, usually an antibiotic, has been included in the preparation.

In Great Britain, probably the best known corticosteroid–antibiotic combination is Ledermix (triamcinolone acetonide) (Cyanamid of Great Britain Ltd.). The preparation is presented in two forms, a paste and a cement (*Fig.* 37). The paste consists of a mixture of triamcinolone acetonide and demethylchlortetracycline calcium in a water-soluble cream; the latter consists of calcium chloride, zinc oxide, sodium sulphate, carbowax and water (Paterson, 1976a). The cement is available in slow- and fast-setting forms; the powder contains triamcinolone acetonide, demethylchlortetracycline hydrochloride, zinc oxide, canada balsam, rosin and calcium hydroxide, whilst the liquid consists of eugenol and rectified turpentine oil, and, in the slow-setting form, polyethylene glycol. The instructions for use indicate that in treating an exposed, inflamed pulp, the paste is sealed against the exposure for 2–3 days, during which time the triamcinolone is continuously released (Schroeder, 1963). At the end of this period the paste is removed and replaced by the cement, the hardening mechanism of which regulates the release of triamcinolone (Schroeder, 1963). In cases of pulpal irritation where no exposure is present, treatment with the paste is omitted, and the cement is applied directly to the floor of the cavity.

3. Present status of corticosteroids

In the capping of cariously exposed pulps, there is no doubt that corticosteroid preparations are effective in eliminating pulpal pain, but the elimination of pain is not necessarily synonymous with elimination of its cause. In a carefully controlled clinical study, Shovelton et al. (1971) found no significant difference in the rates of success 2 years after pulp capping with Ledermix cement and calcium hydroxide paste, although there was some indication that the application of Ledermix paste to the exposure for 3 days was beneficial. However, the limitations of clinical tests in assessing pulpal status have already been referred to. The available histological evidence indicates that the final outcome of capping these teeth with corticosteroid preparations is probably chronic pulpitis and necrosis.

In the capping of traumatic exposures occurring during caries removal, there seems no definite evidence that corticosteroids are any superior to calcium hydroxide. In the study of Shovelton et al. (1971) there was no significant difference in the success rates obtained with Ledermix cement and other materials, including calcium hydroxide paste. On the existing histological evidence, calcific bridging would seem more likely following the use of calcium hydroxide, and the latter must be regarded as the preparation of choice.

It was pointed out in Chapter 1 that where the inflammatory process has extended to involve the apical periodontal membrane, as manifested by pain when the tooth is percussed, it is probable that part of the pulp is necrotic. In such a case pulp capping should not be performed, even though application of a corticosteroid preparation may relieve the patient's pain.

Although Leonard and Cotton (1971) were unable to demonstrate the penetration of prednisolone or cortisone through dentine, Langeland and Langeland (1968) in an extensive investigation found that prednisolone did penetrate dentinal tubules when applied to the floor of a cavity, but report that it was engulfed by macrophages in the pulp and accordingly did not exert an anti-inflammatory effect; pulpal inflammation resulting from operative procedures or caries persisted despite the application of corticosteroids to the cavity. These findings cast some doubt on the anti-inflammatory value of corticosteroids in indirect capping and following extensive cavity preparations.

PULPOTOMY

The main objective of pulpotomy is to enable formation of the root apex to be completed. The part of the pulp in which the tissue defences have localized the infecting micro-organisms—and which is therefore inflamed—is removed with the object of maintaining the vitality and health of the remainder of the pulp which is not infected or obviously inflamed.

Partial pulpotomy, or pulp curettage, denotes the removal of only a part of the pulp within the pulp chamber (*see Fig.* 46, p. 59). Total pulpotomy denotes the removal of all of the coronal pulp, and often a minor portion of that within the root canal also (*see Figs.* 44 and 45, pp. 57, 58). Since removal of the inflamed part of the pulp is more likely with total pulpotomy, this procedure is usually considered preferable to partial pulpotomy.

As in pulp capping, the formation of a calcific barrier to wall off the remaining pulp is not necessarily synonymous with a successful result. However, the studies of James et al. (1957) and Schroder (1973) indicate that the likelihood of such a barrier forming is related to the severity of postoperative inflammation of the pulp. Apart from this consideration, the presence of a calcific barrier is considered important in that it makes contamination of the pulp less likely should there be leakage of the overlying restoration later.

1. Selection of teeth for pulpotomy (*Figs.* 38 *and* 39)

The advisability of pulpotomy in preference to pulp capping where the pulp of a tooth with an open apex has been exposed by fracture of the crown or by caries

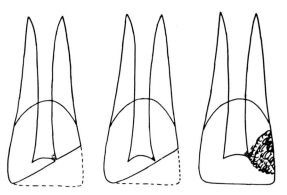

Fig. 38. Indications for pulpotomy—teeth with open apices and vital pulps, exposed or nearly exposed as a result of fracture of the crown, or exposed by caries.

was discussed in an earlier part of this chapter. Where exposure has resulted from fracture of the crown, it is usually held that the chance of a successful pulpotomy diminishes the longer the tooth has been left untreated, particularly where more than 2–3 days have elapsed. However, provided there is evidence of pulpal vitality and no strong suspicion of involvement of the radicular part of the pulp, pulpotomy should be performed, even though several days have elapsed since the accident. In addition, pulpotomy is generally advocated where an extensive fracture has left only a thin covering of dentine over the pulp, even though it has not actually exposed it; merely applying a protective covering to the exposed dentine in such cases is not uncommonly followed by necrosis of the pulp.

It has already been pointed out in Chapter 1 that the narrower the apical foramen the more susceptible is an inflamed pulp to necrosis from the accumulation of inflammatory exudate. For this reason, most workers consider the prognosis following pulpotomy appreciably worse when the apex is fully formed than when it is open, since the operation itself results in some degree of pulpal inflammation. However, there is some evidence (Masterton, 1966) that pulpotomy may be successful in the former type of case, and under certain circumstances, therefore, it may be

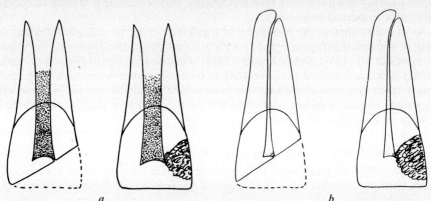

Fig. 39. Contraindications to pulpotomy; *a*, Teeth with open apices and largely necrotic pulps; *b*, Teeth with closed apices and exposed pulps.

indicated. Thus, where exposure occurs during cavity preparation and capping is contraindicated by obvious inflammation or contamination of the coronal part of the pulp, and pulpectomy is precluded by root canal anatomy, then pulpotomy may be tried. Again, when the crown of a tooth has been fractured and capping is thought unwise because the patient is not seen until the pulp has been exposed to the saliva for some hours, pulpotomy may be performed, provided of course that a post crown will not be needed to restore the tooth and that there is no apical periodontitis to interfere with the pulpal circulation. Few cases fulfil these conditions, however, and in consequence the pulp is generally removed and root canal treatment performed.

Since the immediate aim of pulpotomy is to eliminate the infected and inflamed part of the pulp, the operation is contraindicated where there is evidence that the radicular part of the pulp to be left is infected. Pain on percussion or evidence of periapical rarefaction attributable to extension of pulpal disease to the periodontal membrane are therefore contraindications. Where these changes result from displacement of a tooth by a blow, however, they do not contraindicate pulpotomy provided the apex is open and the degree of displacement is not severe. The treatment of traumatized anterior teeth is considered in greater detail in Chapter 16.

2. Materials used to cover the pulpal wound

Many of the materials advocated for pulp capping have also been used to cover the pulp wound in pulpotomy.

As with pulp capping, probably the most popular material, and the one for which there is the greatest support, is calcium hydroxide. However, the unfavourable results obtained by Phaneuf et al. (1968) in applying Hydrex to pulpotomy wounds indicate that this material should not be used. Also, it must be emphasized that the use of calcium hydroxide, or indeed of any calcium compound, is not essential to successful pulpotomy with the formation of a calcific bridge, as has been proved by a number of histological investigations. The studies of James et al. (1957) and of Sekine et al. (1960) have demonstrated bridging in human teeth after the use of antibiotics. Sekine and his colleagues also reported a high incidence of bridging following the use of chemically pure zinc oxide–eugenol, a finding confirmed radiologically by Cooke and Rowbotham (1956). Via (1955) showed bridges after pulpotomies of monkey teeth when barium sulphate was used, whilst Massler and his co-workers have proved in a number of studies that bridging is part of the normal pattern of healing in the rat and occurs with various materials (Massler and Miyamoto, 1963). Similarly, in pulp capping dogs' teeth, Hunter (1955) found that the application of magnesium hydroxide was followed by bridging.

The results of studies such as these leave no doubt that the use of calcium hydroxide is not essential to walling off of the pulpal wound by hard tissue and the maintenance of a healthy pulp. Furthermore, there is evidence that various other materials, including zinc oxide–eugenol, are just as effective as calcium hydroxide in maintaining the vitality, if not the normality, of the pulp. However, so far as the production of a calcified bridge is concerned, the material for which there is the greatest support is undoubtedly calcium hydroxide. Thus, in the comparative histological study of Sekine et al. (1960), the percentages of teeth showing bridging after pulpotomy using calcium hydroxide, zinc oxide–eugenol, tetracycline and penicillin were 86, 51, 22 and 11 respectively. James et al. (1957) also found the incidence of bridging to be less under antibiotics, or combinations of an antibiotic and a calcium compound, than under calcium hydroxide. Mills (1953) tested human teeth for their pulpal response to a number of preparations and found that appreciable pulpal metaplasia occurred only under calcium salts. On the basis of comparative studies on rats, Massler and Miyamoto (1963) concluded that although calcium hydroxide or some other calcium compound is not essential for the formation of a calcific bridge, the use of calcium hydroxide results in a wider calcific reaction which occurs earlier.

More recently, Hannah (1972) has reported favourable results using a paste of calcium hydroxide powder and 5 per cent glutaraldehyde. The antiseptic action of glutaraldehyde and its fixative effect on the superficial layer of pulp may be advantageous.

3. Pattern of pulpal healing

The calcific barrier formed after pulpotomy varies in its nature and is not necessarily complete. In successful cases, it consists of an irregularly calcified outer layer, pulpal to which is a layer of tubular dentine which completely walls off the pulp and is lined by odontoblasts. This appearance, together with an underlying pulp which is normal, constitutes an ideal result. It may be visible radiographically 6 weeks after pulpotomy, although with some teeth it cannot be seen for a few months (Hallett and Porteous, 1963). The work of Masterton (1966) led him to conclude that, although tubular dentine is formed in the majority of posterior teeth, callus is usually formed in incisors.

In other cases, the pulp is only partly walled off from the cavity beyond because the calcific barrier is incomplete and contains many spaces. Such a result is less favourable. Ulmansky et al. (1971) investigated the effect of applying Ledermix paste to pulpotomy wounds for various periods before replacing it with a calcium hydroxide paste. The formation of dentine bridges traversed by vascular channels was demonstrated, but the underlying pulp was chronically inflamed or necrotic when Ledermix paste had been applied for longer than 24 hours. The effect of treating cariously exposed posterior teeth by pulpotomy and the application of Ledermix cement has been studied by Barker (1975). In general, the remaining pulp tissue was normal, but there was only partial calcific bridging of the pulpal wound, even though the teeth were observed for up to 868 days. The nature of the calcific material varied from aberrant dentine to cementum or bone-like substance.

The mechanism of healing following the capping of exposed pulps with calcium hydroxide was investigated by Glass and Zander (1949). The superficial part of the pulp was found to become necrotic, and under this a layer of calcium proteinate was formed, as a result, it was thought, of a reaction between the calcium hydroxide and the pulp. Underneath this there occurred a fibrous proliferation with subsequent calcification, with the resultant formation of an irregularly calcified layer. Later, new odontoblasts proliferated, and reparative dentine was formed on the pulpal aspect of the calcified layer. The results of the studies of Berman and Massler (1958) and Kozlov and Massler (1960) on rats are in broad agreement with this, but suggest that the calcium ions both for the superficial layer of dystrophic calcification and for the dentine underneath come from the pulp itself. This view, which accords with the previously quoted findings that calcium compounds are not necessary for the formation of a calcific bridge, has been confirmed by the experimental work of Sciaky and Pisanti (1960) and Pisanti and Sciaky (1964). However, Stark et al. (1964) concluded that in using calcium hydroxide for pulpotomy, most of the calcium in the dentine bridge originated from the capping material.

The origin of the newly formed odontoblasts under a dentine bridge is not entirely clear, but the results of Mills (1953) suggest they arise by the differentiation of fibroblasts in the pulp.

4. Technique

a. Preliminary treatment
It is preferable that pulpotomy be performed as a deliberately planned procedure rather than as an emergency form of treatment, since this permits an adequate amount of time to be set aside for the operation, and enables all necessary measures to be taken to ensure that treatment is performed in an aseptic manner, a factor which is most important to success.

Where the exposure is due to caries, the pulp is allowed to bleed for a few minutes, since this helps to clean the area of debris and micro-organisms and to relieve any congestion of the pulpal blood vessels. The exposure is cleaned of any remaining debris and protected from further contamination whilst all remaining caries is removed from the cavity. The pulp is now capped with calcium hydroxide, prior to the insertion of a temporary filling of fast-setting zinc oxide–eugenol cement. Should a metal band be necessary to support the temporary filling or to allow later isolation of the tooth by a rubber dam, it is applied immediately after capping the pulp. An appointment for pulpotomy is made for within 1 week's time, during which period the treatment given will have relieved the patient's pain, besides reducing contamination of the exposure site by organisms.

With an exposure resulting from fracture of the crown, most operators, provided there are not more serious injuries to be seen to, perform pulpotomy when the patient is first seen. So long as the necessary time is available, and provided the patient is not so upset as to make the procedure damaging psychologically, there is no objection to this. Often, however, this is not so and it is better to defer the operation for a day or so. Under these circumstances, only the emergency treatment described in Chapter 16, such as attention to minor injuries of the soft tissues, together with certain preliminary work to be described presently, is done at this first visit. Where indicated, a metal band may be fitted and cemented to the tooth after first capping the pulp.

Whatever the cause of the exposure, certain other preliminary procedures, which can also be done at a first visit, are necessary. It is essential that a periapical radiograph be taken of the tooth. This is necessary to preclude the possibility of root fracture, and also shows the state of root formation, the state of the periapex and the anatomy of the pulp chamber.

An electric pulp test of the tooth should also be done; the reading is recorded so as to provide a basis for comparison with the results of subsequent tests. With an exposure due to fracture, the current used during the test must not greatly exceed that normally needed to evoke a response from such a tooth, since the pulp, although still vital, may be in a state of shock in which it ceases temporarily to respond to stimuli. Also, as Cooke and Rowbotham (1952) point out, a tooth with an incompletely formed apex sometimes does not respond to an electric pulp test, even though the pulp is vital. Unless these facts are borne in mind, damage to the pulp, and perhaps a mistaken diagnosis, may result. It is also better not to use heat to test the pulp, since the transfer of heat to the latter does not cease immediately the source is removed from the tooth.

b. Operation proper

The actual operation of pulpotomy is performed in its entirety at one visit. The following account assumes that the entire coronal pulp is to be removed, that is, that total pulpotomy is to be performed. A brief account of partial pulpotomy will be given separately.

Detailed accounts of certain aspects of the operation—such as the technique of isolation, the maintenance of asepsis and the gaining of access to the pulp chamber —are given in later chapters dealing with root canal treatment.

Following the application of a dressing to the exposed pulp, the tooth should be comfortable when the patient attends. The pulp of the tooth is anaesthetized by a subperiosteal injection of local anaesthetic solution, or, where appropriate, by a nerve-block injection. The tooth is then isolated, using a rubber dam whenever possible, and its surface is scrubbed with a wool pledget moistened with a suitable antiseptic solution and dried.

The roof of the pulp chamber is now removed in its entirety, as if for root canal treatment. The burs used for this are largely a matter of personal preference, but normally they will comprise inverted cone and round patterns. They should not be run at such a speed that overheating of the pulp is likely, otherwise with the reduced circulation resulting from the local anaesthetic damage may result to the radicular part of the pulp. With posterior teeth, the approach is through the occlusal aspect of the tooth and the initial penetration is towards the centre of the pulp chamber. With fractured anterior teeth, the approach is through the dentine exposed by the fracture. The initial penetration is over the centre of the pulp chamber. Alternatively, the exposure itself may be used as the starting point, provided it has not been covered by a temporary restoration (*Fig.* 40). Where the pulp of an anterior tooth has been exposed not by a fracture but by caries, the approach is through the palatal or lingual surface.

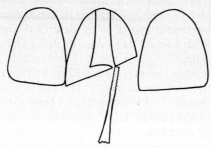

Fig. 40. Using exposure of fractured anterior tooth as starting point for removing pulp-chamber roof.

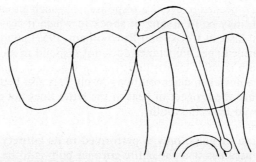

Fig. 41. In pulpotomy on a molar tooth, an excavator may be rested against the floor of the pulp chamber and guided by it as it cuts the pulp.

Debris is now removed from the vicinity of the bleeding pulp surface, after which the coronal part of the pulp is removed. This may be done either with a sharp, long-shank excavator, or with a round or fissure bur. Since it is thought that a bur does not give such a clean cut and is more likely to disturb the radicular pulp, it is usually recommended that an excavator be used. This is generally possible with molar teeth, since the excavator may be rested against and guided by the floor of the pulp chamber as it cuts the pulp (*Fig.* 41). With these teeth, the pulp is severed just within each root canal.

With a single-rooted tooth, however, the absence of a floor to the pulp chamber makes the use of an excavator difficult, and in consequence a bur is generally employed. If, as with single-rooted posterior teeth, it is necessary to use right-angle rather than straight instruments, a long-shank bur is preferable. The bur should be slightly wider than the coronal part of the root canal, and is applied with light pressure against the pulp and the root dentine. It is run slowly in reverse until a level about 2·0 mm apical of the cemento-enamel junction buccally is reached, due allowance being made for the degree of eruption of the tooth. If the appearance of the pulp suggests that necrotic tissue is still present, the root canal must be penetrated further. Unless tissue of normal appearance has been encountered by the time the middle one-third of the root has been reached, pulpotomy is abandoned and root canal treatment instituted.

Removal of the pulp of a single-rooted tooth to this level corresponds roughly, in relation to the alveolar border, to the levels worked to in a multi-rooted tooth. It usually ensures that all infected tissue has been eliminated. Another object in removing the pulp to this level rather than to a more coronal one is that it provides enough room for the application of a thick layer of capping material over the pulp stump; thus, by using a material which does not set, such as calcium hydroxide paste, some room may be provided for oedema of the pulp stump following the operation. Also, the remaining pulp is less susceptible to irritation from subsequent mesial or distal caries of the crown.

To ensure that pressure is not exerted on the pulp during closure of the pulp cavity later, some workers cut a shelf in the dentine at the level of the cemento-enamel junction, using a fissure bur (*Fig.* 42). This may be done before the pulp within the coronal part of the canal is removed.

After the pulp has been amputated to the desired level, it is allowed to bleed for 2 or 3 minutes so as to eliminate debris and micro-organisms and to reduce any congestion present. The cavity is then irrigated with sterile saline or local anaesthetic solution to remove remaining debris, dried, and inspected to ensure that all debris has been removed and that no shreds of pulpal tissue have been left.

Attention is now directed to the arrest of bleeding from the pulp stump, if this has not already occurred. A variety of methods may be used to bring about clotting on the cut surface of the pulp, but usually the application of a wool pledget moistened with sterile normal saline is sufficient. Following the formation of a clot, any residual blood on the walls of the cavity is removed.

It must be pointed out that although the importance of the presence of a clot seems generally agreed upon, the actual influence that postoperative bleeding has on the ultimate outcome is uncertain. Nyborg and Slack (1960) point out that if bleeding occurs into the pulp itself, the extravasated blood constitutes a foreign body and may perhaps lead to areas of necrosis. Also, it may lift the capping material out of contact with the pulpal surface.

It is also to ensure close contact between the capping material and the pulp that some workers advise that only a thin blood clot be allowed to form. The techniques of applying the various calcium hydroxide materials which may be used to cover pulpal wounds have already been described in the section on pulp capping; pastes are generally used in preference to cements, which are difficult to apply to pulpotomy wounds. Just as in pulp capping, there is some disagreement on the degree of pressure which should be employed, but most operators use only enough to bring the material into close contact with the pulp. The thickness of material used is at least 1·0 mm, and usually nearer to 2·0 mm. Excess capping material on the sides of the cavity is eliminated; where a shelf in the dentine has been cut, material is removed to this level (*Fig.* 42).

The importance to pulpal healing of an effective seal to the cavity has been stressed by Berman and Massler (1958), and to this end it is advisable to seal the base of the cavity with a layer of zinc oxide–eugenol cement. If it is wished, zinc phosphate cement may be placed over this to provide a strong base for a subsequent restoration (*Fig.* 42).

After removing the rubber dam and checking that the filling material does not interfere with the occlusion, a radiograph of the tooth is taken to serve as a basis for comparison with later films.

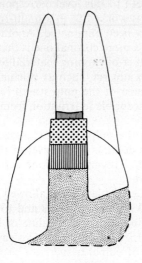

Fig. 42. Coronal to the material covering the pulpotomy wound are fast-setting zinc oxide–eugenol cement, which rests against any shelf present, phosphate cement and overlying restoration.

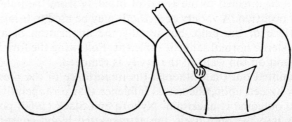

Fig. 43. With exposure of a pulp horn, partial pulpotomy may be performed to remove the entire horn.

c. Partial pulpotomy

Sometimes, partial pulpotomy (*see Fig.* 46) is advocated in preference to total pulpotomy. Its major advantages compared with the latter operation are that it conserves tooth tissue and is a much simpler form of treatment. The disadvantage of partial pulpotomy, namely, that elimination of the infected part of the pulp is less certain, has already been pointed out. For this reason, the operation is best reserved for cases in which contamination of the pulp by micro-organisms is minimal but for which pulp capping is contraindicated, as, for example, where the pulp has been penetrated rather than nicked by careless cavity preparation.

The operation is performed with the same attention to asepsis as total pulpotomy. After any necessary preliminary treatment has been performed, a round bur obviously larger than the exposure, often about a size 6 or 8, is revolved slowly against the exposed pulp until it has penetrated as far as its own radius. Where exposure has occurred in the vicinity of a pulp horn, the entire horn is cut away (*Fig.* 43). Haemorrhage is allowed to continue for a minute or so, and the cavity then irrigated. The wound is inspected to check that no necrotic material remains, after which clotting is allowed to occur and the capping material is applied. The cavity is then sealed.

If when the pulp wound is inspected there is still evidence of necrosis, some operators merely extend the area of operation and remove more tissue until the pulp appears intact. As already indicated, however, total pulpotomy is a more certain method of treatment for such cases.

5. Postoperative observation: prognosis

There should be no more than transient discomfort following pulpotomy, and the tooth should be quite comfortable after the first postoperative day. It is checked

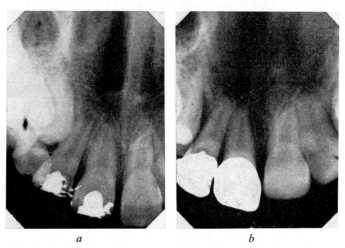

a   *b*

Fig. 44. 2̲1̲|. *a*, Directly after pulpotomy; *b*, Some months later, showing continued development of the root apices and the formation of calcific bridges, with no evidence of pathology.

clinically and radiographically and tested for vitality of its pulp 6–8 weeks following treatment, and every few months thereafter, if possible for a period of not less than 2 years.

The criteria of success, besides the absence of symptoms, are that the pulp remains vital and that the radiographs show the formation of a calcific bridge and the continued development of the apical part of the root, with no evidence of internal resorption of the root or of periapical disease (*Figs.* 44, 45 and 46). When interpreting vitality tests, their limitations must be borne in mind. It has been pointed out elsewhere that a tooth with an incompletely formed root may not respond to an electric pulp test, even though the pulp is vital. Where there is a response, an increase in the degree of stimulation will be needed to evoke a reaction after pulpotomy; an increase in the region of about 3 or 4 units may be regarded as normal.

3

The limitation of the radiograph for detecting the presence of a calcific bridge, and the fact that the formation of a bridge is not necessarily indicative of a healthy pulp, has also been noted. When viewing radiographs and assessing whether a calcific bridge has formed, due allowance must be made for the radiographic

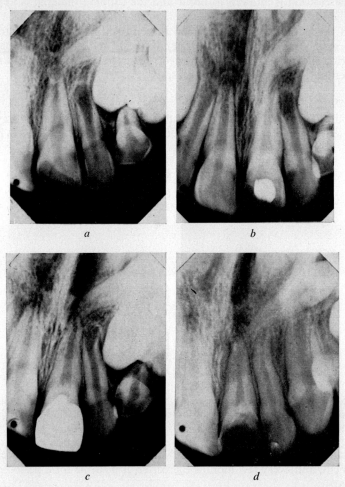

Fig. 45. |1. *a*, Immediately before pulpotomy; *b*, Four months later. A calcific bridge is just visible; *c*, Ten months later. The calcific bridge is thicker and root apex formation is more advanced. There is no evidence of pathology; *d*, Three years later. Root apex formation has continued. The pulp should be removed and root canal treatment performed.

density of the material used to cover the pulp stump. A series of radiographs of a tooth treated by pulpotomy will show a progressive increase in thickness of the calcific bridge (*Fig.* 45).

Studies on the prognosis of pulpotomy indicate that, on the basis of clinical and radiologic assessment, a success rate of 70 per cent or more may be anticipated

(Slack, 1953; Hallett and Porteous, 1963; Hawes et al., 1964; Masterton, 1966). Studies reporting an appreciably lower rate of success have usually been concerned with the treatment of primary teeth, and for these there is evidence of a high incidence of internal resorption following treatment.

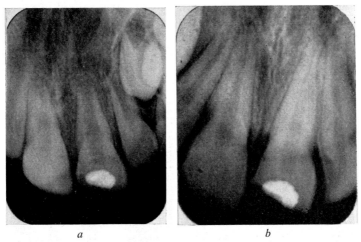

a   *b*

Fig. 46. |1. *a*, Shortly after partial pulpotomy; *b*, Almost 3 years later, with the formation of a calcific bridge and completion of root apex formation. There is no evidence of pathology.

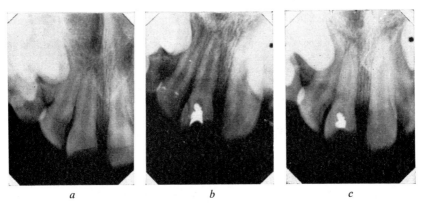

a   *b*   *c*

Fig. 47. 1|. *a*, Immediately before pulpotomy; *b*, A few weeks later; *c*, Seven months later. The root canal is largely obliterated by calcification.

It has been pointed out by a number of workers, for example Luks (1954) and Moodnik (1963), that after development of the root apex is completed there is a distinct tendency for calcification to proceed and gradually to obliterate the canal (*Fig.* 47). When this occurs ultimate necrosis of the pulp, with the development of a periapical lesion, is common. In such a tooth, the extent of the calcification may prevent location of the canal, so that root canal treatment by way of the crown is impossible. Thus, unless it is possible to expose the root apex surgically and to treat and fill the root canal from its apical end, extraction is unavoidable. In other cases, evidence of pulpal necrosis and periapical disease occurs in the absence of widespread pulpal calcification (*Fig.* 48). Not only should these teeth be observed postoperatively, therefore, but there is also a strong case for regarding pulpotomy as an interim procedure and instituting root canal treatment directly root apex formation has been completed. Root canal treatment is indeed often mandatory, since many of these teeth will eventually need post crown restorations.

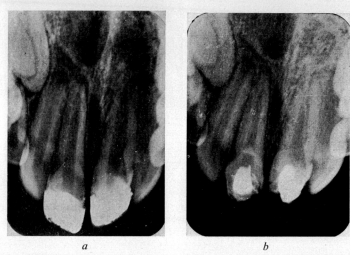

a   *b*

Fig. 48. 1|. *a*, Immediately before pulpotomy; *b*, Nine months later. A calcific bridge is visible. Although there is no evidence of widespread pulpal calcification and root apex formation has continued, a periapical lesion is apparent. Root canal treatment should be performed.

Another complication, but fortunately an uncommon one with permanent teeth, is for the root to be perforated, and even ultimately destroyed, by resorption proceeding from within the root canal. If obvious radiographical evidence of internal resorption becomes apparent, the remaining pulp must be removed as soon as possible.

REFERENCES

Aponte A. J., Hartsook J. T. and Crowley M. C. (1966) Indirect pulp capping success verified. *J. Dent. Child.* **33**, 164.

Barker B. C. W. (1975) Conservative treatment of cariously exposed vital pulps in posterior teeth with a glucocorticosteroid–antibiotic compound. *J. Br. Endodont. Soc.* **8**, 5.

Barker B. C. W. and Ehrmann E. H. (1969) Human pulp reactions to a glucocorticosteroid–antibiotic compound. *Aust. Dent. J.* **14**, 104.

Baume L. J. and Fiore-Donno G. (1968) The use of corticosteroid–antibiotic preparations in endodontic therapy. In: Grossman L. I. (ed.), *Transactions of the 4th International Conference on Endodontics.* Philadelphia, University of Pennsylvania, pp. 62–82.

Berk H. (1950) The effect of calcium hydroxide-methyl cellulose paste on the dental pulp. *J. Dent. Child.* **17**, 65.

Berk H. (1963) Pulp capping: re-evaluation of criteria based on clinical and histological findings. *Int. Dent. J., Lond.* **13**, 577.

Berkman M. D., Cucolo F. A., Levin M. P. and Brunelle L. J. (1971) Pulpal response to isobutyl cyanoacrylate in human teeth. *J. Am. Dent. Assoc.* **83**, 140.

Berman D. S. and Massler M. (1958) Experimental pulpotomies in rat molars. *J. Dent. Res.* **37**, 229.

Bhaskar S. N., Beasley J. D., Ward J. P. and Cutright D. E. (1972) Human pulp capping with isobutyl cyanoacrylate. *J. Dent. Res.* **51**, 58.

Bhaskar S. N., Cutright D. E., Boyers R. C. and Margetis P. N. (1969) Pulp capping with isobutyl cyanoacrylate. *J. Am. Dent. Assoc.* **79**, 640.

Cooke C. and Rowbotham T. C. (1952) An electric pulp tester. *Br. Dent. J.* **92**, 147.

Cooke C. and Rowbotham T. C. (1956) A review of a technique for pulpotomy and report on 175 cases. *Br. Dent. J.* **100**, 174.

Cowan A. (1966) Treatment of exposed vital pulps with a corticosteroid–antibiotic agent. *Br. Dent. J.* **120**, 521.

Delaney J. M. and Seyler A. E. (1966) Hard set calcium hydroxide as a sole base in pulp protection. *J. Dent. Child.* **33**, 13.

Eidelman E., Finn S. B. and Koulourides T. (1965) Remineralisation of carious dentin treated with calcium hydroxide. *J. Dent. Child.* **32**, 218.

Ehrenreich D. W. (1968) A comparison of the effects of zinc-oxide eugenol and calcium hydroxide on carious dentin in human primary molars. *J. Dent. Child.* **35**, 451.

Feitelson N. (1956) Pulp capping with calcium hydroxide and penicillin. *J. Dent. Child.* **23**, 214.

Fiore-Donno G. and Baume L. J. (1962) Effect of capping compounds containing corticosteroids on the human dental pulp. A long-term histologic study. *Helv. Odontol. Acta* **6**, 23.

Fisher F. J. (1966) The viability of micro-organisms in carious dentine beneath amalgam restorations. *Br. Dent. J.* **121**, 413.

Fisher F. J. (1969) The viability of micro-organisms in carious dentine beneath amalgam restorations: an appendix. *Br. Dent. J.* **126**, 355.

Fisher F. J. (1972) The effect of a calcium hydroxide/water paste on microorganisms in carious dentine. *Br. Dent. J.* **133**, 19.

Fry A. E., Watkins R. F. and Phatak N. M. (1960) Topical use of corticosteroids for the relief of pain sensitivity of dentine and pulp. *Oral Surg.* **13**, 594.

Fusayama T., Okuse K. and Hosoda H. (1966) Relationship between hardness, discoloration and microbial invasion in carious dentin. *J. Dent. Res.* **45**, 1033.

Glass R. L. and Zander H. A. (1949) Pulp healing. *J. Dent. Res.* **28**, 97.

Hallett G. E. M. and Porteous J. R. (1963) Fractured incisors treated by vital pulpotomy. A report on 100 consecutive cases. *Br. Dent. J.* **115**, 279.

Hannah D. R. (1972) Glutaraldehyde and calcium hydroxide: a pulp dressing material. *Br. Dent. J.* **132**, 227.

Hansen H. (1969) Pulp capping with corticoid-containing materials. *Odont. Tidskr.* **77**, 223.

Hawes R. R., Dimaggio J. and Sayegh F. (1964) Evaluation of direct and indirect pulp capping. (Abstract.) *J. Dent. Res.* **43**, 808.

Heller A. L., Koenigs J. F., Brilliant J. D., Melfi R. C. and Driskell T. D. (1975) Direct pulp capping of permanent teeth in primates using a resorbable form of tricalcium phosphate ceramic. *J. Endodontol.* **1**, 95.

Hirschfeld Z., Sela J. and Ulmansky M. (1972) Hydrex and its effect on the pulp: preliminary findings on the rat molar. *Oral Surg.* **34**, 364.

Hunter H. A. (1955) A study of the mechanism concerned in the deposition of lime salts in bridging over a pulp exposure (Abstract.). *J. Dent. Res.* **34**, 697.

James V. E., Englander H. R. and Massler M. (1957) Histologic response of amputated pulps to calcium compounds and antibiotics. *Oral Surg.* **10**, 975.

Jordan R. E. and Suzuki M. (1971) Conservative treatment of deep carious lesions. *J. Canad. Dent. Assoc.* **37**, 337.

Kalnins V. (1957) The effect of pressure on the healing of the exposed human dental pulp. *J. Dent. Res.* **36**, 437.

Kalnins V. and Frisbie H. E. (1960) The effect of dentine fragments on the healing of the exposed pulp. *Archs Oral Biol.* **2**, 96.

Kalnins V., Masin L. F. and Kisis A. (1964) Healing of exposed dental pulps under various pressure dressings. *Oral Surg.* **18**, 381.

Kerkhove B. C., Herman S. C., Klein A. I. and McDonald R. E. (1967) A clinical and television densitometric evaluation of the indirect pulp capping technique. *J. Dent. Child.* **34**, 192.

King J. B., Crawford J. J. and Lindahl R. L. (1965) Indirect pulp capping: a bacteriologic study of deep carious dentine in human teeth. *Oral Surg.* **20**, 663.

Kozlov M. and Massler M. (1960) Histologic effects of various drugs on amputated pulps of rat molars. *Oral Surg.* **13**, 455.

Kutscher A. H., Zegarelli E. V., Silvers H. F. and Piro J. D. (1961) Clinical laboratory studies on a new topical corticosteroid—triamcinolone acetonide. *Oral. Surg.* **14**, 938.

Langeland K. and Langeland L. K. (1968) Indirect capping and the treatment of deep carious lesions. *Int. Dent. J., Lond.* **18**, 326.

Langeland K., Tobon G. and Langeland L. K. (1968) The effect of corticosteroids on the dental pulp. In: Grossman L. I. (ed.), *Transactions of the 4th International Conference on Endodontics.* Philadelphia, University of Pennsylvania, pp. 15–44.

Law D. B. and Lewis T. M. (1961) The effect of calcium hydroxide on deep carious lesions. *Oral Surg.* **14**, 1130.

Lawson B. F. and Mitchell D. F. (1964) Pharmacologic treatment of painful pulpitis. A preliminary, controlled, double-blind study. *Oral Surg.* **17**, 47.

Leonard E. P. and Cotton W. R. (1971) Dentine in vivo impermeability to radioactively labeled prednisolone. *Oral Surg.* **31**, 104.

Luks S. (1954) Pulpotomy—a critical evaluation. *J. Dent. Child.* **21**, 249.

MacGregor A., Marsland E. A. and Batty I. (1956) Experimental studies of dental caries. 1, The relation of bacterial invasion to softening of the dentine. *Br. Dent. J.* **101**, 230.

McWalter G. M., El-Kafrawy A. H. and Mitchell D. F. (1973) Pulp capping in monkeys with a calcium-hydroxide compound, an antibiotic, and a polycarboxylate cement. *Oral Surg.* **36**, 90.

Massler M. and Miyamoto O. (1963) Pulpotomy: a reappraisal. In: Grossman L. I. (ed.), *Transactions of the 3rd International Conference on Endodontics.* Philadelphia, University of Pennsylvania, pp. 1–28.

Masterton J. B. (1966) The healing of wounds of the dental pulp of man: a clinical and histological study. *Br. Dent. J.* **120**, 213.

Mills J. S. (1953) The evocation and production of protective secondary dentine. *Aust. J. Dent.* **57**, 241.

Mjor I. A. (1967) Histologic studies of human coronal dentine following the insertion of various materials in experimentally prepared cavities. *Arch. Oral Biol.* **12**, 441.

Mjor I. A. and Nygaard-Ostby B. (1966) Experimental investigations on the effect of Ledermix on normal pulps. *J. Oral Therap. Pharmacol.* **2**, 367.

Moodnik R. M. (1963) Clinical correlations of the development of the root apex and surrounding structures. *Oral Surg.* **16**, 600.

Muntz J. A., Dorfman A. and Stephan R. M. (1943) *In vitro* studies on sterilization of carious dentin. I. Evaluation of germicides. *J. Am. Dent. Assoc.* **30**, 1893.

Nixon G. S. and Hannah C. McD. (1972) N-butyl cyanoacrylate as a pulp capping agent. *Br. Dent. J.* **133**, 14.

Nyborg H. (1958) Capping of the pulp. The processes involved and their outcome. *Odont. Tidskr.* **66**, 293.

Nyborg H and Slack G. L. (1960) Clinical evaluation of pulpotomy. *Int. Dent. J., Lond.* **10**, 452.

Paterson R. C. (1976a) Corticosteroids and the exposed pulp. *Br. Dent. J.* **140**, 174.

Paterson R. C. (1976b) Bacterial contamination and the exposed pulp. *Br. Dent. J.* **140**, 231.

Phaneuf R. A., Frankl S. N. and Ruben M. P. (1968) A comparative histological evaluation of three calcium hydroxide preparations on the human primary dental pulp. *J. Dent. Child.* **35**, 61.

Pisanti S. and Sciaky I. (1964) Origin of calcium in the repair wall after pulp exposure in the dog. *J. Dent. Res.* **43**, 641.

Rowe A. H. R. (1967) Reaction of the rat molar pulp to various materials. *Br. Dent. J.* **122**, 291.

Rowe A. H. R. and Binnie W. H. (1975) Cyanoacrylate, calcium hydroxide, antibiotic/steroid preparations as pulp capping agents. (Abstract.) *Q. Dent. Rev.* **9**, 23.

Sarnat H. and Massler M. (1965) Microstructure of active and arrested dentinal caries. *J. Dent. Res.* **44**, 1389.

Schouboe T. and MacDonald J. B. (1962) Prolonged viability of organisms sealed in dentinal caries. *Arch. Oral Biol.* **7**, 525.

Schroder U. (1973) Reaction of human dental pulp to experimental pulpotomy and capping with calcium hydroxide. *Odont. Revy* **24**, Suppl. 25.

Schroeder A. (1963) The application of corticosteroids in endodontia. *Dent. Practnr Dent. Rec.* **13**, 420.

Schroeder A. (1968) Indirect capping and the treatment of deep carious lesions. *Int. Dent. J., Lond.* **18**, 381.

Sciaky I. and Pisanti S. (1960) Localization of calcium placed over amputated pulps in dog's teeth. *J. Dent. Res.* **39**, 1128.

Sekine N., Asai Y., Nakamura Y., Tagami T. and Nagakubo T. (1971) Clinico-pathological study of the effect of pulp capping with various calcium hydroxide pastes. *Bull. Tokyo Dent. Coll.* **12**, 149.

Sekine N., Hasegawa M. and Saijo Y. (1960) Clinico-pathological study of vital pulpotomy. *Bull. Tokyo Dent. Coll.* **1**, 29.

Sela J., Hirschfeld Z. and Ulmansky M. (1973) Reaction of the rat molar pulp to direct capping with the separate components of Hydrex. *Oral Surg.* **35**, 118.

Seltzer S. (1942a) Effective duration of some agents used for dentin sterilization. *J. Dent. Res.* **21**, 115.

Seltzer S. (1942b) Effectiveness of antibacterial agents used in cavity sterilization. *J. Dent. Res.* **21**, 269.

Shankle R. J. and Brauer J. S. (1962) Pulp capping. *Oral Surg.* **15**, 1121.

Shovelton D. S. (1968) A study of deep carious dentine. *Int. Dent. J., Lond.* **18**, 392.

Shovelton D. S., Friend L. A., Kirk E. E. J. and Rowe A. H. R. (1971) The efficacy of pulp capping materials: a comparative trial. *Br. Dent. J.* **130**, 385.

Simon W. J. (1942) Pulp capping. *NW. Dent.* **21**, 134.

Slack G. L. (1953) Vital pulpotomy in the treatment of fractured incisors. *Br. Dent. J.* **94**, 32.

Sowden J. R. (1956) A preliminary report on the recalcification of carious dentine. *J. Dent. Child.* **23**, 187.

Stanley H. R. and Lundy T. (1972) Dycal therapy for pulp exposures. *Oral Surg.* **34**, 818.

Stark M. M., Myers H. M., Morris M. and Gardner R. (1964) The localisation of radioactive calcium hydroxide Ca45 over exposed pulps in rhesus monkey teeth: a preliminary report. *J. Oral Therap. Pharmacol.* **1**, 290.

Stephan R. M., Muntz J. A. and Dorfman A. (1943) *In vitro* studies on sterilization of carious dentin. III. Effective penetration of germicides into carious lesions. *J. Am. Dent. Assoc.* **30**, 1905.

Stewart D. J. and Richardson A. (1968) Effect of calcium hydroxide and zinc oxide–eugenol on young, noncarious dentine. (Abstract.) *J. Dent. Res.* **47**, 978.

Tronstad L. (1974) Reaction of the exposed pulp to Dycal treatment. *Oral Surg.* **38**, 945.

Tronstad L. and Mjor I. A. (1972) Pulp reactions to calcium hydroxide-containing materials. *Oral Surg.* **33**, 961.

Turell J. C., Areco N. and Morales E. C. (1958) Reacciones iniciales de la pulpa dentaria frente al acetato de cortisona. *Odont. Urg.* **12**, 404. Abstracted in *Dent. Abst., Chicago* **4**, 31 (1959).

Ulmansky M., Sela J., Langer M. and Yaari A. (1971) Response of pulpotomy wounds in normal human teeth to successively applied Ledermix and Calxyl. *Arch. Oral Biol.* **16**, 1393.

Uitto V.-J., Antila R. and Ranta R. (1975) Effects of topical glucocorticoid medication on collagen biosynthesis in the dental pulp. *Acta Odont. Scand.* **33**, 287.

Via W. F. (1955) Barium sulfate and antibiotic mixture in pulpotomy. *J. Dent. Child.* **22**, 195.

Vigg J. (1962) Hydrocortisone in pulp therapy. *Dent. Prog.* **2**, 285.

Weiss M. B. and Bjorvatn K. (1970) Pulp capping in deciduous and newly erupted permanent teeth of monkeys. *Oral Surg.* **29**, 769.

FURTHER READING

Shovelton D. S. (1968) Maintenance of pulp vitality. *J. Br. Endodont. Soc.* **2**, 38, 60.

Chapter 3

Rationale of root canal treatment: selection of teeth for treatment

Root canal treatment denotes the removal of a vital or necrotic pulp from a root canal and its replacement by a filling. Its object is to prevent the extension of disease from the pulp to the periapical tissues, or, where this has already occurred and periapical disease exists, to encourage resolution and the return of the periapical tissues to normal. Thus, successful root canal treatment enables the tooth to be conserved and retained as a useful member of the arch without constituting a danger either to the health of the supporting structures or to the general health of the patient.

RATIONALE OF ROOT CANAL TREATMENT

1. Pathogenesis of periapical irritation

The immediate aim of root canal treatment is to eliminate the causes of periapical irritation. These causes comprise micro-organisms and their toxins, and physical and chemical agents; they may operate singly or in combination.

a. Microbial agents

The experimental work of Fish (1939) showed that in bone infection there are four zones of reaction. The central of these is termed the 'zone of infection', since it is the only one in which the infecting micro-organisms are found. Besides organisms, it is made up of dead bone and large numbers of polymorphonuclear leucocytes. These ingest organisms everywhere except where they are out of reach, namely in the spaces of the Haversian system left empty by the death of the osteocytes. Around the zone of infection is the 'zone of contamination', in which, as a result of irritation from toxins diffusing from the zone of infection, the osteocytes have also died; although this zone contains no organisms, it is heavily infiltrated by round cells. Around this is the 'zone of irritation', in which the toxins diffusing from the centre of the lesion are sufficiently dilute to allow the survival of histiocytes and osteoclasts; these cells remove the collagenous matrix and the bone itself, resulting in resorption. Finally, forming the outer part of the lesion, is the 'zone of stimulation', in which the concentration of toxins, although very low, is sufficient to stimulate fibroblasts and osteoblasts to lay down new bone, albeit imperfectly formed.

In pulpal infection the invading organisms are non-motile, and, as the work of Figg et al. (1944) suggests, are found only in regions of necrotic pulpal tissue. In consequence, by the time the entire pulp has become necrotic and micro-organisms have grown along the root canal, the toxins produced by these organisms have diffused ahead and evoked a cellular response in the periapical tissues. Thus, the tissue immediately adjoining the apical foramen, although heavily infiltrated by inflammatory cells, is normally devoid of micro-organisms.

The state which exists when a chronic periapical lesion has developed following pulp disease is illustrated by *Fig.* 49, the root canal forming the zone of infection (A), with the zone of contamination (B) immediately beyond the apical part of the

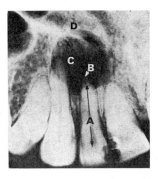

Fig. 49. Showing zones which exist with a chronic periapical lesion: A, The root canal constitutes the zone of infection; B, The zone of contamination immediately around the apical foramen; C, The zone of irritation, corresponding to the bulk of the periapical lesion; D, The zone of stimulation around the periphery of the lesion.

root. The polymorphonuclear leucocytes around and just within the apical end of the canal cannot get far inside, however, since as they do so they get farther from their source of nutrition and become surrounded by an increasingly high concentration of bacterial toxins. Similarly, organisms within the canal have little chance of survival when they grow beyond its confines, since they are immediately engulfed by the waiting cells. Thus, a stalemate ensues.

Some accident resulting in pressure on the contents of the root canal may lead to the sudden passage of a large number of organisms beyond the apical foramen, with the result that the zone of infection extends into the periapical region and an acute periapical abscess forms. Commonly, however, the stalemate persists and toxins continue to pass from the root canal and through the surrounding zone of contamination into the tissue beyond, so leading to the formation of a zone of irritation (C). Here, bone is resorbed, so that a radiolucent area is formed. Beyond this, where the toxins are more dilute, fibroblasts and osteoblasts may sometimes be stimulated to form a fibrous capsule with a layer of sclerotic bone to wall off the lesion, the two constituting a zone of stimulation (D).

It is hardly surprising, therefore, that various studies, including those of Grossman (1959), Shindell (1961) and Andreasen and Rud (1972), have shown that most chronic periapical lesions are sterile. Furthermore, as will be discussed presently, the fact that bone is resorbed does not necessarily mean that the irritant is microbial in nature. Thus, it is wrong to regard periapical lesions as regions of infection. Such a lesion represents a defensive reaction of the tissues to irritation from the pulp cavity.

To rid the pulp cavity of micro-organisms, it is necessary both to clean it and to apply some form of bactericidal agent to its walls. In the process of cleaning, not only is pulpal tissue removed, but also the superficial dentine forming the walls of the pulp cavity is eliminated. Besides resulting in a smooth-sided cavity suitable for filling, this has the added advantage of removing the majority of the organisms which have succeeded in penetrating the dentinal tubules. As different investigations, including those of Chirnside (1958) and Shovelton (1964), have shown, invasion of the dentinal tubules from a necrotic pulp is often surprisingly limited in extent. Where organisms are present, they are found mostly in the root canal and in the dentine immediately surrounding the canal. There seems no evidence that they penetrate cementum; indeed, the study of Furseth (1974) indicates that peripheral root dentine contains very few dentinal tubules. Any organisms which are situated deeply within the dentinal tubules and which are not removed by cleaning will, it is hoped, be reached and eliminated by the antiseptic agent applied to the pulp cavity.

Following the elimination of organisms, the pulp cavity is filled. If it is merely sealed from the mouth, but otherwise allowed to remain empty, organisms within necrotic material inadvertently left in the root canal may recommence growth. Also, in the absence of a root filling, reinfection of the canal and renewed periapical irritation may result from leakage of the coronal restoration, or exposure of lateral branches of the root canal as a consequence of gingival recession or periodontal disease. Furthermore, at some later date it may be necessary to utilize part of the root canal to restore the crown of the tooth, with the result that unless its apical part has been obliterated by a filling, periapical disease will recur.

Before leaving this aspect of root canal treatment, it must be emphasized that pulpal infection need not necessarily imply root canal infection. With an exposed vital pulp, micro-organisms are confined, initially at any rate, to the superficial part of the pulp which undergoes necrosis in the region of the exposure (*Fig.* 50).

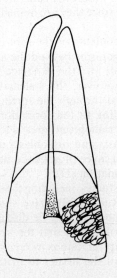

Fig. 50. With an exposed vital pulp, organisms are confined initially to the pulp which becomes necrotic in the region of the exposure.

The pulp within the root canal may remain free of micro-organisms for some time. Therefore, if the superficial part of the pulp containing the micro-organisms is destroyed by heat, or sterilized in some other way before the radicular pulp is removed, infection of the root canal may be prevented.

b. Physical and chemical agents

The control of infection is not the only factor to be considered in root canal treatment. Physical and chemical sources of periapical irritation are also of considerable importance, and it is mainly during root canal treatment that the danger of irritation from these sources exists. The more common ways in which it arises will now be considered.

i. INSTRUMENTATION BEYOND THE APICAL FORAMEN

The passage of instruments beyond the apical foramen, unless essential for the drainage of an acute periapical abscess, is inadvisable. There are four reasons for this. First, it injures and therefore irritates the periapical tissues. Secondly, by widening the apical foramen it makes the extrusion of material into the periapical tissues more likely during root filling. Alternatively, in ensuring that material is not extruded periapically, inadequate condensation of the filling, and therefore incomplete obliteration of the root canal, tends to occur. In either event, the result is a poorer prognosis. Thirdly, it increases the risk of driving debris and micro-organisms from the pulp cavity into the periapical tissues, so extending the zone of infection into the latter and sometimes leading to the formation of an acute periapical abscess. Fourthly, in vital pulp removal, instrumentation beyond, rather than short of, the apical foramen has been shown not only to cause much more severe periapical inflammation (Seltzer et al., 1968), but also to be followed more often by epithelial proliferation, with possible cyst formation (Seltzer et al., 1969).

ii. INSERTION AND DIFFUSION OF DRUGS INTO THE PERIAPICAL TISSUES

Many antiseptic drugs formerly used in root canal treatment, such as phenol and combinations of cresol and formalin, are very irritant to living tissues. Since there is no practicable way of preventing the diffusion of drugs from the root canal into the adjoining periapical tissues, highly irritant ones, such as those just mentioned, should not be used as root canal antiseptics.

Even those antiseptics previously thought to be relatively bland in their action, such as beechwood creosote and camphorated paramonochlorphenol, may under certain circumstances cause considerable irritation (Schilder and Amsterdam, 1959; Harrison and Madonia, 1971). In consequence, root canal antiseptics should not be inserted beyond the apical end of the canal. This applies especially to preparations in the form of a paste or cream, since the pressure of these on the adjacent tissues will lead to physical irritation also. The insertion of antiseptics into a periapical lesion is in any event unnecessary, since the causative micro-organisms—with the exception of those occasionally passing beyond the apical foramen and being phagocytosed—are confined to the pulp cavity. Proof that it is unnecessary is provided by the study of Hedman (1951).

iii. INCOMPLETE OBLITERATION OF THE APICAL PART OF THE ROOT CANAL

At one time it was believed that if a treated root canal were left unfilled or incompletely filled, tissue fluid entering the canal by way of the apical foramen would stagnate and form breakdown products and these in turn would diffuse back into the periapical region and lead to renewed periapical irritation. This stagnation or 'hollow tube' concept held sway for many years and was based on the experimental work of Rickert and Dixon (1931). However, it has now been shown to be untenable (Selye, 1959; Goldman and Pearson, 1965; Torneck, 1966; Phillips, 1967).

Nonetheless, at least one study (Goldman and Pearson, 1965) supports the belief that tissue fluid, whilst not stagnating and forming breakdown products, may circulate by way of the apical foramen between the periapical tissues and the prepared root canal. Thus, in an unfilled or incompletely filled root canal, the presence of tissue fluid could enable residual organisms within the dentinal tubules

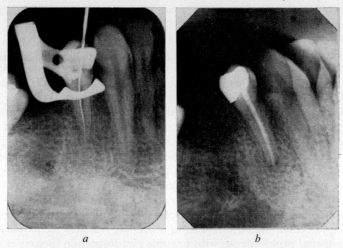

Fig. 51. ⊼|. *a*, During root canal treatment; *b*, Three years later, failure is evident. There is a periapical lesion with resorption of the root apex. A gap is visible along the entire length of the root filling distally.

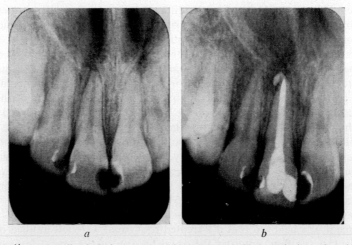

Fig. 52. 1|. *a*, Immediately before root canal treatment; *b*, Six months later there is an obvious periapical lesion, with an excess of cement in the periapical tissues.

or actually in the canal to recommence growth and cause a recurrence of periapical irritation. It is hardly surprising, therefore, that it has been shown (Strindberg, 1956; Harty et al., 1970; Adenubi and Rule, 1976) that the prognosis of root canal treatment is poorer where there are voids apically between the filling and the walls of the canal than where the canal is completely filled (*Fig.* 51).

iv. EXTRUSION OF FILLING MATERIAL INTO THE PERIAPICAL REGION

Extrusion of filling material beyond the apical foramen results in pressure on the periapical tissues, and therefore leads to irritation. Unless the material is rapidly resorbed, the irritation is likely to be of a long-standing nature. Depending on the nature of the material, there may be some degree of chemical irritation also. Furthermore, where the filling beyond the apical foramen remains in rigid continuity with that within the root canal, the degree of irritation may be more severe, since the excess material moves with the tooth during mastication. It is not surprising, therefore, that overfilling the root canal with a material which is not rapidly resorbed, as in *Fig.* 52, is associated with a poorer prognosis (Strindberg, 1956; Grahnen and Hansson, 1961; Nicholls, 1961; Seltzer et al., 1963). It has also been shown that the presence of excess filling material periapically enhances the tendency to epithelial proliferation and cyst formation (Seltzer et al., 1973; Binnie and Rowe, 1974).

To summarize, the essential stages of root canal treatment are cleaning, antiseptic medication and filling. To these must be added the need for asepsis throughout treatment to avoid needless contamination of the root canal. Provided treatment eliminates all existing sources of irritation and does not lead to severe or permanent new sources of irritation, the outcome should be successful. Where the periapical tissues were originally normal, they should remain so afterwards, although occasionally a slight temporary deterioration is clinically detectable during and for a short time after treatment, as described in Chapter 9. Where there was periapical disease prior to treatment, resolution of the lesion with the deposition of new bone should occur, but again there may be a temporary deterioration.

It must be pointed out, however, that with acute periapical conditions, cleaning should be deferred until the zones defined previously have become more definitely established and the defences of the periapical region fully mobilized against the spread of organisms. The preliminary treatment which is given in these cases is therefore directed to this end, with conversion of the acute condition into a chronic one. If this is not first achieved, the instrumentation entailed by cleaning may result in the spread of organisms into tissues whose defences are not yet mobilized fully.

2. Influence of root canal anatomy on treatment

To ensure complete elimination of the root canal as a source of irritation to the periapical tissues, cleaning, antiseptic medication and filling ideally should extend as far as its apical end, namely the apical foramen.

Numerous studies on root canal anatomy have shown that in fully developed roots the apical foramen is generally to one side of the root, and is therefore a little short of the root apex (Kuttler, 1955; Green, 1955, 1956, 1973; Pineda and Kuttler, 1972; Burch and Hulen, 1972; von der Lehr and Marsh, 1973). As *Figs.* 53 and 54 show, Kuttler found that the distance between the centre of the foramen and the root apex varies from 0·5 mm in a young to 0·7 mm in an older person. The narrowest part of the root canal, the position of which also varies with age, is about 0·5–0·7 mm short of the centre of the apical foramen, usually just coronal to the dentinocemental junction within the canal. The narrowest part of the canal is therefore about 1·0–1·5 mm from the root apex. Between this level and the apical foramen the canal is funnel-shaped and is at an angle to the long axis of the remainder of the root canal.

Thus, there are obvious difficulties in using the apical foramen as a level to which to work. Neither radiographic examination nor the tactile sensation transmitted by instruments within the root canal can enable accurate localization of the apical foramen. Because of the deflection of the extreme apical end of the root canal, if successively larger instruments are used beyond its narrowest part there is the possibility of instrument breakage or penetration of the side of the canal, and even

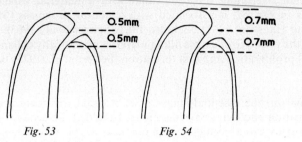

Fig. 53   Fig. 54

Fig. 53. The anatomy of the root apex and the apical region of the canal in a young person.

Fig. 54. The anatomy of the root apex and the apical region of the canal in an older person.

of perforation of the root. Even though the apical bend may be negotiated, the farther the canal is instrumentated beyond its narrowest part the more difficult it becomes to fill completely the prepared part of the canal without forcing material beyond the apical foramen. It would in any case be virtually impossible to seal the apical foramen without forcing filling material into the periapical tissues, not only because the apical part of the canal is funnel-shaped, but also because the rim of the apical foramen varies in level from point to point according to the form of the root.

On balance, therefore, it seems doubtful that there is any advantage in attempting to clean or fill the canal beyond its narrowest level, about 1·0–1·5 mm from the root apex, even though a more apical level is sometimes advocated. The results of investigations by Strindberg (1956), Grahnen and Hansson (1961), Nicholls (1961), Seltzer et al. (1963), and Adenubi and Rule (1976) lend support to this attitude. They indicate that with both vital and necrotic pulps the prognosis of treatment is just as good when the root canal is cleaned and filled to a millimetre or so short of the root-end as when the end of the root filling is flush with the latter. Root filling to either of these levels gives a better prognosis than filling beyond the root-end.

3. Significance of certain technical limitations in root canal treatment

In view of the fact that neither the extreme apical part of the root canal nor the branches of the canal can be adequately cleaned or filled, it is pertinent to ask how any non-surgical form of treatment can be successful.

First, it must be pointed out that these parts of the pulp cavity, although they may contain necrotic tissue, do not necessarily contain micro-organisms. They may not even contain necrotic tissue, even though the pulp has undergone necrosis. Thus, various workers, amongst them Thoma (1918) and more recently Shovelton (1964), have demonstrated that the apical part of the root canal may be filled with granulation tissue extending from an associated periapical lesion; indeed, Barrett (1925) found this to be the rule with pulpless teeth. Also, as a sequel to pulpal disease, calcification of branches of the root canal may occur, so that they become reduced in size and even obliterated.

Other factors to be considered are the diffusibility of the antiseptic drug, or drugs, applied to the pulp cavity, and the effects of capillary action. For example, the study of Wach et al. (1955) demonstrates that penicillin sealed within a rootc anal travels into the adjoining dentinal tubules, whilst both Martin et al. (1968) and Avny et al. (1973) have shown parachlorphenol preparations to penetrate root dentine. It would seem reasonable to assume that a similar diffusion occurs into the extreme apical end of the root canal as well as into its branches. The fine calibres of these branches, and to a lesser extent the narrowness of the apical end of the canal, assuming the root of the tooth to be fully formed, will encourage penetration of the drug by capillary action.

Probably the most obvious factor, however, is the state of the remaining pulp. Where this is necrotic it will offer no resistance to invasion, and is therefore likely to contain micro-organisms. Provided that cleaning has extended to within a short distance of the apical foramen, the volume of necrotic material which remains is relatively small, so that there is a good chance that any organisms present are eliminated by the antiseptic drug employed. However, there is obviously a limit to which an antiseptic drug may diffuse before becoming so diluted that it no longer destroys micro-organisms. Besides being related to the length and calibre of the uncleaned part of the root canal, this depends also on the number of organisms present and their resistance, as well as on the drug which is used. Although it is therefore difficult to lay down hard-and-fast rules, it is probably fair to say that the prognosis is distinctly unfavourable if it is not possible to approach the root apex closer than 2·5–3·0 mm in cleaning and filling.

On the other hand, where vital pulp is present in the apical part of the root canal, invasion by micro-organisms will be limited by the tissue defences present. Also, if the precaution described previously is taken, namely, to destroy by heat the coronal part of the pulp before entering the radicular part, the root canal will probably contain few or no organisms. In this type of case, therefore, the proximity of cleaning and filling to the apical foramen is probably not so critical as with a necrotic pulp, especially as the residual pulpal tissue may undergo calcification (Barker, 1976). Indeed, indirectly it is no doubt a testimony to the powers of recovery and healing of this residual pulp that various levels in the apical one-third of the root have been advocated for the removal of a vital pulp. However, in the light of our present knowledge, a level about 1·0–1·5 mm from the root apex should be reached wherever possible.

4. Apical limit

It will have become apparent from the foregoing description that a root filling should not stop short of the level to which the canal has been cleaned, otherwise a space is left in which tissue fluid can accumulate, so detracting from the prognosis (Muruzabal and Erausquin, 1973).

Conversely, if the root filling passes beyond the level to which the canal has been cleaned, it is likely to cause undue pressure, either directly on the periapical tissues or on whatever occupies the apical part of the canal. Should the apical part of the canal contain vital pulpal or granulation tissue, this tissue will be irritated. Should it be occupied by necrotic pulpal tissue, this will be compressed against, and probably driven into, the periapical tissues, and periapical irritation will occur. Whatever the condition of the uncleaned apical part of the canal, even if it is devoid of tissue, it is most unlikely that it can be adequately filled unless a large excess of material is used.

It is obvious, therefore, that the level to which the canal is filled should correspond to that to which it has been cleaned, that is, the apical limit to filling should correspond to the apical limit to cleaning. For convenience of description, the term *apical limit* will be used in all subsequent accounts. Wherever possible, this will be about 1·0–1·5 mm from the root apex.

SELECTION OF TEETH FOR TREATMENT

In discussing the suitability of a tooth for root canal treatment, it is assumed that the patient's attitude and oral hygiene warrant treatment, that the crown is freely accessible and can be restored, and that the tooth is not better extracted for orthodontic or prosthetic purposes. It is also assumed that the proximity of the root apex to adjacent major anatomical structures, such as the maxillary antrum, has been determined. Where there is rampant caries or widespread periodontal disease, the response to treatment of these diseases should be assessed before beginning root canal treatment, except of an emergency nature.

1. Indications: pulpectomy

The term *pulpectomy* indicates the removal of a pulp. Generally a vital pulp is referred to, although some workers employ the term whether the pulp is vital or necrotic.

Pulpectomy is indicated wherever there is clinical evidence of pulpitis and where it is thought that the health of the pulp cannot be restored or maintained by pulp capping or pulpotomy. It is usually indicated where the pulp of a tooth with a fully developed root has been exposed by caries or by fracture of the crown, or where the pulp has not only been exposed but also penetrated by careless cavity preparation. In a tooth with an incompletely formed root and a wide apical foramen, pulpectomy is indicated where necrosis of the radicular part of the pulp precludes pulpotomy.

Since the object of root canal treatment is to ensure the health of the periapical tissues, it will of course be indicated wherever it has been decided to retain a tooth with a necrotic pulp. However, there are occasional cases of an exceptional nature where treatment may not be attempted and yet such a tooth is retained. A patient with a terminal illness who is not inconvenienced by the tooth provides an obvious example. Another is the case in which adequate root canal treatment, with or without surgical intervention, is not possible, such as a molar tooth with root canals almost completely obliterated by calcification. Provided that there is no discomfort and no evidence of periapical disease, and that the patient has no systemic disease which might be adversely affected by its presence, such a tooth may be retained.

However, it should be checked clinically and radiographically from time to time to ensure that the position does not change.

Occasionally, even though there is no exposure and no reason to suspect pulpal disease, it is necessary to perform root canal treatment on a tooth with a healthy pulp to enable its restoration, as, for example, after fracture of the crown. In this connection, the considerable buccal reduction of tooth substance needed in the preparation for a porcelain-bonded to gold crown should be considered. With mandibular central incisors, for example, Stanley et al. (1975) found that the average distance from the pulp to the cemento-enamel junction labially was 1·96 mm. Where the tooth is smaller than normal, and therefore the labial dentine thinner, an obvious problem arises. Either less than the required labial reduction is made, and in consequence the labial porcelain reduced in thickness, or the pulp is endangered. Unless the patient is prepared to accept the aesthetic limitation imposed by the former approach, pulpectomy and root canal treatment are indicated if a porcelain-bonded to gold crown is to be used.

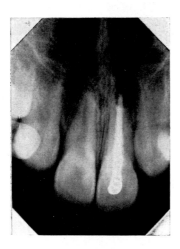

Fig. 55. The root filling in ⌊1 contains voids apically and should be replaced by a new filling before a post crown is made.

Where a post crown has to be constructed, root canal treatment should be repeated wherever an existing root filling contains voids which could result in periapical contamination during preparation of the crown (*Fig.* 55), even though there is no evidence of periapical disease at the time.

2. Contraindications

Before deciding to perform root canal treatment, various factors relating to the patient and to the tooth and its periodontium should be considered. A well-taken periapical radiograph is essential for this purpose. If this fails to show each root of the tooth, together with the associated periapical region, clearly and completely, additional radiographs are taken.

Throughout the following account, root canal treatment denotes treatment without surgical intervention. It must be emphasized that hardly any of the contraindications to be discussed are absolute. Although they may seriously detract from the prognosis of non-surgical treatment, they do not necessarily make it hopeless.

a. Factors relating to the patient

Any systemic disease which might reasonably be expected to reduce the powers of tissue defence and repair, and which has not yet been successfully controlled,

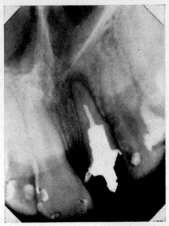

Fig. 56. |2. Has periapical disease, but a post crown obstructs access to the apical region of the canal.

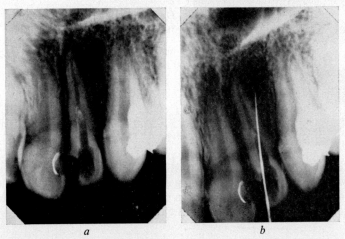

         a   *b*

Fig. 57. |2. *a,* Access to apical region of canal is obstructed by cement; *b,* In trying to cut through the cement the root was perforated.

constitutes a contraindication to treatment. Fortunately, patients suffering from such conditions are rarely seen in a dental surgery, at least as far as the dentist is aware. Where the disease has been adequately controlled and there is no reason to suspect an unfavourable tissue response, there is no contraindication to treatment. Bender et al. (1963) go so far as to state that they know of no systemic disorder which negates treatment.

    The possibility of a systemic disease, or its sequelae, being adversely affected by root canal instrumentation must also be considered. Thus, a patient with endocardial damage could develop bacterial endocarditis from a bacteraemia caused by instrumentation within an infected root canal, and will therefore need appropriate antibiotic therapy if treatment is undertaken (Chapter 14).

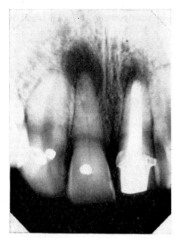

Fig. 58. Access to apical region of 1| root canal obstructed by diffuse calcification. Although a root canal is just apparent radiographically, it could not be found.

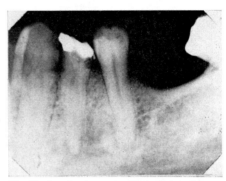

Fig. 59. A pulp stone one-third of way along |4 root canal obstructs passage of instruments apically.

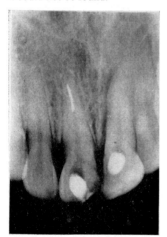

Fig. 60. Obstruction by a broken instrument in apical region of 1| root canal.

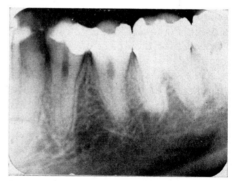

Fig. 61. Obstruction due to a bifid root canal |4.

b. Factors relating to the tooth and its periodontium

Almost all the conditions which detract from the prognosis of treatment fall under this heading. Most of these conditions prevent adequate cleaning, antiseptic medication or filling of the pulp cavity. Although some of them may be diagnosed from clinical examination alone, many can only be detected from radiographs of the periapical region. In some cases the factor detracting from the prognosis may be eliminated by combining treatment of the root canal with periapical surgery or with some other surgical procedure; the conditions where this may apply are marked with an asterisk (*). With other teeth this solution may not be possible, either because surgical treatment is not practicable or because it would not leave

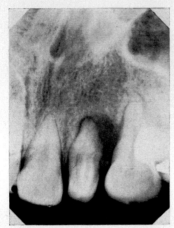

Fig. 62. Dens in dente |2, with periapical disease.

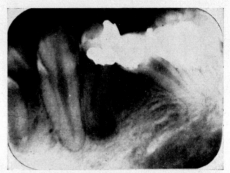

Fig. 63. Curvature of /4 root obstructs access to apical region canal.

enough periodontal attachment to support the tooth; such teeth obviously have to be extracted.

i. INACCESSIBILITY OF APICAL REGION OF CANAL*

Inaccessibility of the apical region of the root canal to cleaning and filling by way of the pulp chamber is the commonest contraindication to non-surgical root canal treatment. Periapical surgery is indicated in the treatment of such cases, and is performed with the object of removing, or facilitating effective treatment of, the inaccessible part of the canal.

Access to the apical region of the root canal may be prevented by an obstruction which cannot be bypassed or removed, or by division, curvature or perforation of the canal. As already noted, the proximity of the apical limit to the apical foramen is less critical where the pulp is vital than where it is necrotic. Thus, if the extreme apical part of the pulp is vital and uninfected, treatment is sometimes successful even though 4·0 mm or 5·0 mm of the pulp have to be left. Where the pulp is necrotic, however, the prognosis of treatment must be considered unfavourable if a level within at least 2·5 mm or 3·0 mm of the apex cannot be reached.

An obstruction may consist of a calcification of the pulp cavity, a restoration such as a post crown (Fig. 56) or a layer of impenetrable root filling or some other foreign body in the root canal (Fig. 57). Calcification may be distributed throughout the pulp cavity (Fig. 58), or it may be localized in the form of a pulp stone (Fig. 59). The commonest foreign body to cause obstruction, other than a root filling or a post crown, is probably a broken instrument (Fig. 60).

Division of a root canal some distance short of the root apex to form two or more branches of roughly equal calibre is occasionally seen (Fig. 61). When it occurs, both branches are often impenetrable. Adequate root canal treatment of the type of *dens in dente* depicted in *Fig.* 62 is not possible.

Excessive curvature of a root canal occurs most commonly with posterior teeth (*Fig.* 63). In cleaning a curved root canal, the root is sometimes perforated. When this happens, instruments, instead of following the course of the apical part of the

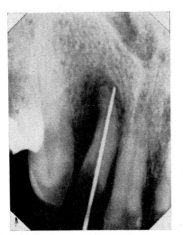

Fig. 64. Perforation of curved root canal 2| acts as an obstruction to instrumentation of root canal beyond.

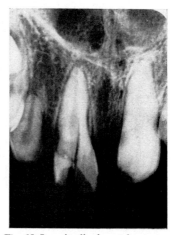

Fig. 65. Longitudinal root fracture involving the root canal of 1| provides pathway for continual contamination from gingival sulcus.

root canal, tend to catch against and enter the perforation, since this is in line with the coronal part of the canal (*Fig.* 64).

ii. LONGITUDINAL ROOT FRACTURE

Irrespective of pulpal status, extraction is indicated where a traumatized tooth has a longitudinal fracture involving the gingival sulcus and extending through the root canal in an apical direction (*Fig.* 65). The prognosis for repair of such a fracture is distinctly unfavourable (Michanowicz et al., 1971). Moreover, the fracture in effect splits the tooth and provides a route for continual contamination of the pulp cavity and the periapical region from the gingival sulcus.

iii. PERFORATION OF THE ROOT*

Where the root has been perforated, whether as a result of resorption or of trauma from dental instruments, cleaning, medication and filling of the perforation, as well as of the root canal itself, are necessary. Whilst some perforations can be satisfactorily treated by way of the pulp chamber, others can be treated adequately only by way of a surgical approach. In some cases satisfactory treatment is not possible by either approach, and extraction is indicated.

The classification and treatment of perforations are dealt with in Chapter 14.

iv. PERIAPICAL DISEASE ASSOCIATED WITH A FOREIGN BODY PERIAPICALLY*

Periapical surgery or extraction is indicated where there is evidence of periapical disease associated with a foreign body which cannot be removed from the periapical region by way of the pulp chamber.

The commonest foreign body is undoubtedly an excess of root-filling material. The removal of such an excess by way of the pulp chamber may not be possible, particularly where the material within the canal is not continuous with that beyond (*Fig.* 66).

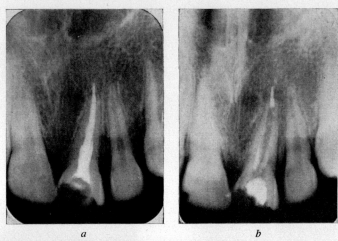

a   *b*

Fig. 66. *a*, There is a break in the gutta percha root filling just short of the root apex of |1, which was giving pain; *b*, The apical fragment of filling material could not be removed through the pulp chamber.

Where the foreign body consists of a broken instrument (*Fig.* 67), its removal is especially important.

v. FAILURE OF PREVIOUS ROOT CANAL TREATMENT*

Where previous treatment of the root canal was performed adequately but has failed, there is little point in repeating it. Under such circumstances the treatment of choice is periapical surgery, the object being to eradicate some unfavourable factor—such as a root fracture—which has previously remained undetected.

vi. PERSISTENCE OF PERIAPICAL IRRITATION DURING TREATMENT*

In isolated cases it becomes apparent during the course of root canal treatment that despite thorough cleaning and antiseptic medication, periapical irritation persists. Thus, a purulent exudate may continue to drain through the pulp cavity or by way of a sinus, or the tooth may continue to cause pain. In these cases also, periapical surgery is the treatment of choice, and is performed with the object of eliminating any unfavourable factor which has previously escaped detection.

vii. ADJACENT ABNORMALITIES*

Occasionally surgery is necessary to eradicate some abnormality, such as a supernumerary tooth, in the immediate vicinity of the apex of a tooth requiring root canal treatment (*Fig.* 68). Assuming that it does not involve the removal of a gross amount of additional tissue, extension of the operation to include periapical surgery facilitates treatment of the diseased tooth and is indicated.

c. Comments on other conditions

The influence of certain other conditions on prognosis is less certain, whilst some conditions formerly regarded as indications for periapical surgery or extraction are now known to be treatable without these measures.

i. AGED PATIENT; ILL-HEALTH

Because of a supposedly low general resistance, aged persons are sometimes re-garded as bad risks for treatment. This also applies to people who, whilst not suffering from any definite systemic disease, are susceptible to minor illnesses.

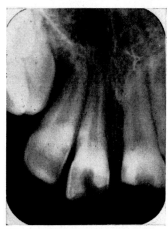

Fig. 67. The ends of two barbed broaches have been broken beyond the apex of |1 and need to be removed surgically.

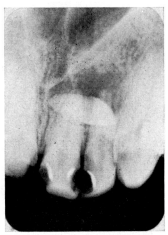

Fig. 68. The decision to remove a supernumerary tooth close to the root apices of |12 makes it expedient to include periapical surgery in the treatment of these teeth.

However, Strindberg (1956) could find no relation between either of these factors and the likelihood of success. It is feasible, however, that periapical repair may be slower in such patients.

ii. PRESENCE OF MANY ROOT-FILLED TEETH

It has been said that root canal treatment of a tooth is contraindicated where as many as 5 or 6 root-filled teeth are already present in the patient's mouth. The implication is that the patient's powers of resistance are being burdened by the root-filled teeth already present. In the absence of demonstrable changes in the periapical tissues, however, it would seem reasonable to suppose that no such burden exists, and therefore that there is no contraindication to the treatment of another tooth.

iii. PERIODONTAL DISEASE

At one time it was thought that treatment should not be undertaken where peri-odontal disease had led to extensive loss of alveolar bone with resultant tooth mobility. The rationale for this contention was that movements of the tooth lead to constant dissemination of micro-organisms from the periodontal pocket by way of the lymphatics. In consequence, the defensive and reparative capacities of the periapical tissues were thought to be diminished.

Provided effective periodontal treatment is possible, there is no contraindication to root canal treatment (*Fig.* 69).

iv. 'PERIAPICAL-CREVICULAR' SINUS

Where there is a definite breakdown of the periodontal membrane with the establishment of a communication between a periapical lesion and the gingival crevice —in other words, a 'periapical-crevicular' sinus (*Fig.* 70)—both the root canal and the gingival crevice may act as sources of irritation to the periapex. In such a case,

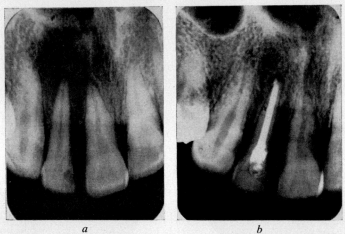

a   *b*

Fig. 69. 2|. *a*, Gross periodontal and periapical bone destruction is evident; *b*, Two years later there is almost complete periapical repair, except around the excess root-filling material.

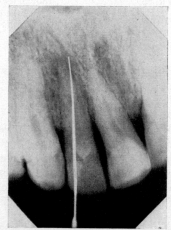

Fig. 70. Silver point inserted into 'periapical-crevicular' sinus involving 2|.

reattachment of the periodontal membrane to the root is necessary before irritation from the gingival crevice can be eliminated.

There is evidence that provided the periapical lesion has followed on pulpal disease and is in no way periodontal in origin, a successful result may sometimes be obtained by root canal treatment alone. In other instances, planing of the involved surface of the root, together with curettage of the gingival tissue if this is in direct contact with the root, is also necessary if the tooth is to be retained.

The treatment of this type of case is described in greater detail in Chapter 14.

v. INCOMPLETELY FORMED APEX IN CONJUNCTION WITH A NECROTIC PULP

Development of the root apex may be so far short of completion that the walls of the root canal diverge in a gingivo-apical direction, with the result that the apical region of the canal, which is the widest part, cannot be adequately filled (*Fig.* 71).

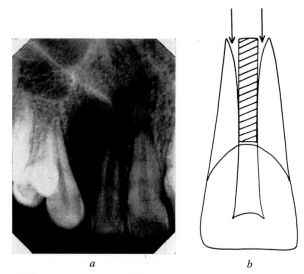

a   *b*

Fig. 71. *a,* Divergence of root canal 2| gingivo-apically prevents adequate treatment through the pulp chamber where the pulp is necrotic; *b,* The apical part of such a root canal cannot be adequately filled through the pulp chamber.

Formerly, periapical surgery was considered the treatment of choice for such teeth. However, it is now apparent that even though the pulp is necrotic, it is usually possible to induce closure of the apical foramen with calcific tissue, so facilitating root filling and obviating the need for surgical treatment (Chapter 13).

vi. TRANSVERSE ROOT FRACTURE WITH PULPAL NECROSIS

It was formerly believed that a transverse root fracture in conjunction with necrosis of the pulp was a contraindication to non-surgical treatment. Where the fracture was in the apical part of the root (*Fig.* 72), root canal treatment of the coronal part of the tooth with surgical removal of the apical fragment was considered advisable. With fractures of the middle or coronal one-third of the root (*Fig.* 73), extraction of both fragments was often performed because of inadequate alveolar support for the tooth.

There is now evidence that although the pulp in the coronal fragment may be necrotic, that in the apical fragment is usually vital, especially with fractures in the apical part of the root (Andreasen and Hjorting-Hansen, 1967). Unless the apical part of the root is associated with radiographic evidence of periapical disease, therefore, there seems no indication to remove it surgically. Following root canal treatment of the coronal part of the tooth, however, clinical and radiographic observation is indicated in case periapical disease does develop.

Where the fracture is situated further coronally and the periodontal attachment of the coronal part of the tooth is inadequate for its support, retention of the tooth may still be possible by the use of an endodontic stabilizer (Chapter 14).

vii. APICAL ROOT RESORPTION IN CONJUNCTION WITH PERIAPICAL RAREFACTION

Some authors formerly regarded resorption of the apex of the root in conjunction with periapical rarefaction as a contraindication to non-surgical treatment. However, it is now generally agreed that the prognosis for these cases is good (Steiner,

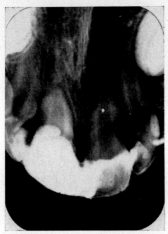

Fig. 72. Fractures of apical one-third of roots of 1|1. Although the pulp in the coronal part of each tooth became necrotic, that in the apical fragments will probably retain its vitality.

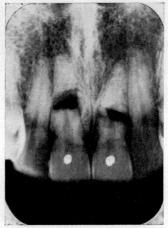

Fig. 73. Although the 1| has a fracture in the coronal one-half of the root, it could probably be retained with the aid of an endodontic stabilizer. The prognosis for |1 is dubious because of the proximity of the fracture line to the gingival crevice distally.

1969) and that surgical intervention is indicated only when postoperative observation shows non-surgical treatment to have failed. Often it does not (*Figs.* 74 and 75).

vi. LARGE PERIAPICAL LESIONS: CIRCUMSCRIBED PERIAPICAL LESIONS

In the past, periapical surgery was commonly advocated as part of the treatment of large periapical lesions. A large lesion was usually defined as one which appeared radiographically to involve more than one-third of the root length or to be more than one-third the root length in diameter.

This view was based on two beliefs. The first was that a large lesion would have been present for a considerable time, so that chronic inflammatory changes, especially fibrosis, would be more pronounced and would make repair less probable than with a smaller lesion. This belief is open to some doubt, if only because of the fact that the size of a lesion depends not only on its age, but also on its speed of growth, and this presumably varies according to the circumstances of the individual case.

The second belief was that a lesion which appears radiographically as a large or circumscribed area of radiolucency is considerably more likely to be cystic than one which is small or diffuse, and therefore needs surgical as well as root canal treatment. As was indicated in Chapter 1, however, within the size range of peri-apical lesions normally seen, the histopathological nature of such a lesion cannot be reliably assessed on the basis of radiographical criteria. Also, although until a few years ago resolution of a radicular cyst without surgical intervention was

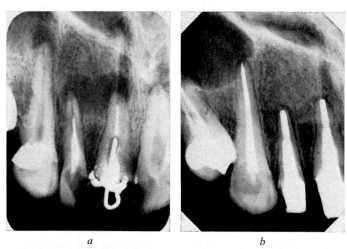

a   b

Fig. 74. 2|. *a*, Obvious root resorption apically; *b*, Two and a half years after non-surgical root canal treatment there is almost complete periapical repair.

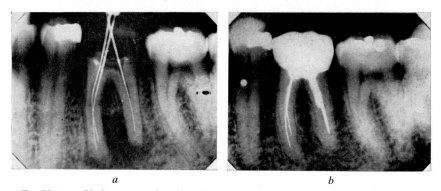

a   b

Fig. 75. |6. *a*, Obvious resorption of both root apices; *b*, Three years after non-surgical root canal treatment there is complete periapical repair.

thought unlikely, there is some evidence that this may not be so. Recent large-scale studies by Bhaskar (1966) and Lalonde and Luebke (1968) have reported that radicular cysts constitute more than 40 per cent of periapical lesions. Since the failure rate of non-surgical treatment of unselected periapical lesions is known to be considerably less than 40 per cent, the obvious implication is that cystic lesions may heal without surgical intervention. More direct evidence is provided by the report of Morse et al. (1975) on 17 periapical lesions diagnosed as cysts by poly-acrylamide-gel electrophoresis (*see* Chapter 1). Fourteen of the 17 lesions showed radiographic evidence of partial or virtually complete bone repair 4–21 months after non-surgical root canal treatment.

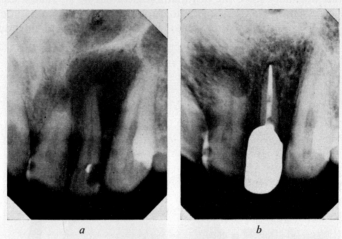

a   *b*

Fig. 76. |2. *a*, A large periapical lesion is present; *b*, Five and a half years after non-surgical root canal treatment, repair is virtually complete.

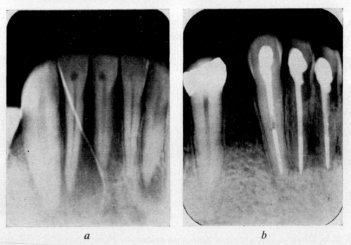

a   *b*

Fig. 77. 321|. *a*, A large diffuse periapical lesion is present; *b*, One year after non-surgical treatment, repair is complete.

The possible mode of healing of a cystic lesion following non-surgical treatment is debatable. Bhaskar (1967, 1972) suggests that acute periapical inflammation following instrumentation of the root canal leads to subepithelial haemorrhage and lysis of epithelial cells by polymorphonuclear leucocytes, and to this end suggests that a fine reamer or file be inserted about 1·0 mm beyond the root apex during treatment. On the other hand, Bender (1972) believes that root canal treatment facilitates drainage of fluid from the cyst cavity, leading to proliferation of fibroblasts and collagen deposition; the latter restricts the blood supply to the cyst lining, which in consequence degenerates.

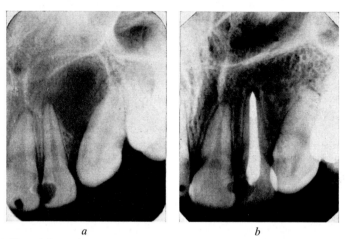

a   *b*

Fig. 78. |2. *a*, A large circumscribed periapical lesion is present; *b*, Five and a half years after non-surgical treatment, repair is virtually complete.

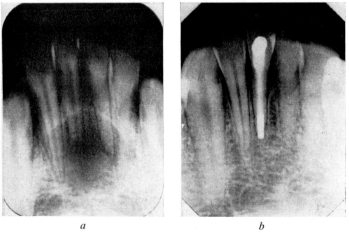

a   *b*

Fig. 79. ⊤|. *a*, A large circumscribed periapical lesion is present; *b*, Four and a half years after non-surgical treatment, repair is complete.

It seems fair to conclude, therefore, that surgical treatment is not indicated merely because a lesion is large or has the appearance radiographically of being circumscribed (*Figs.* 76, 77, 78 and 79). With lesions such as these, surgery is performed only when postoperative observation shows non-surgical treatment to have failed, or when the patient will not be able to attend for postoperative examination and is moving to an area without adequate dental facilities.

vii. ISOLATION OF TOOTH NOT POSSIBLE

Periapical surgery in addition to root canal treatment is often advocated for a tooth which, as a result of coronal fracture or extensive caries, cannot be satisfactorily isolated. However, such a tooth often cannot be adequately restored in any case. If restoration is thought possible then generally the tooth can be satisfactorily isolated, even though this may make necessary other procedures, such as a gingivectomy.

REFERENCES

Adenubi J. O. and Rule D. C. (1976) Success rate for root fillings in young patients: a retrospective analysis of treated cases. *Br. Dent. J.* **141**, 237.

Andreasen J. O. and Hjorting-Hansen E. (1967) Intraalveolar root fractures: radiographic and histologic study of 50 cases. *J. Oral Surg.* **25**, 414.

Andreasen J. O. and Rud J. (1972) A histobacteriologic study of dental and periapical structures after endodontic surgery. *Int. J. Oral Surg.* **1**, 272.

Avny W. Y., Heiman G. R., Madonia J. V., Wood N. K. and Smulson M. H. (1973) Autoradiographic studies of the intracanal diffusion of aqueous and camphorated parachlorphenol in endodontics. *Oral Surg.* **36**, 80.

Barker B. C. W. (1976) Examples of healing following partial root canal filling. *J. Br. Endodont. Soc.* **9**, 3.

Barrett M. T. (1925) The internal anatomy of the teeth with special reference to the pulp with its branches. *Dent. Cosmos* **67**, 581.

Bender I. B. (1972) A commentary on General Bhaskar's hypothesis. *Oral Surg.* **34**, 469.

Bender I. B., Seltzer S. and Freedland J. (1963) The relationship of systemic diseases to endodontic failures and treatment procedures. *Oral Surg.* **16**, 1102.

Bhaskar S. N. (1966) Oral Surgery–Oral Pathology Conference No. 17, Walter Reed Army Medical Center. Periapical lesions: types, incidence, and clinical features. *Oral Surg.* **21**, 657.

Bhaskar S. N. (1967) Bone lesions of endodontic origin. In *Dent. Clin. North Am.* **11**, pp. 521–33.

Bhaskar S. N. (1972) Nonsurgical resolution of radicular cysts. *Oral Surg.* **34**, 458.

Binnie W. H. and Rowe A. H. R. (1974) The incidence of epithelial rests, proliferations and apical periodontal cysts following root canal treatment in young dogs. *Br. Dent. J.* **137**, 56.

Burch J. G. and Hulen S. (1972) The relationship of the apical foramen to the anatomic apex of the tooth root. *Oral Surg.* **34**, 262.

Chirnside I. M. (1958) The bacteriological status of dentine around infected pulp canals. *N.Z. Dent. J.* **54**, 173.

Figg W. A., Hatton E. H. and Hewitt M. (1944) Bacterial distribution in infected pulps. (Abstract.) *J. Dent. Res.* **23**, 214.

Fish E. W. (1939) Bone infection. *J. Am. Dent. Assoc.* **26**, 691.

Furseth R. (1974) The structure of peripheral root dentin in young human premolars. *Scand. J. Dent. Res.* **82**, 557.

Goldman M. and Pearson A. H. (1965) A preliminary investigation of the 'hollow tube' theory in endodontics; studies with neo-tetrazolium. *J. Oral Therap. Pharmacol.* **1**, 618.

Grahnen H. and Hansson L. (1961) The prognosis of pulp and root canal therapy. A clinical and radiographic follow-up examination. *Odont. Revy* **12**, 146.

Green D. (1955) A stereo-binocular microscopic study of the root apices and surrounding areas of 100 mandibular molars. *Oral Surg.* **8**, 1298.

Green D. (1956) A stereomicroscopic study of the root apices of 400 maxillary and mandibular anterior teeth. *Oral Surg.* **9**, 1224.

Green D. (1973) Double canals in single roots. *Oral Surg.* **35**, 689.

Grossman L. I. (1959) Bacteriologic status of periapical tissue in 150 cases of infected pulpless teeth. *J. Dent. Res.* **38**, 101.

Harrison J. W. and Madonia J. V. (1971) The toxicity of parachlorphenol. *Oral Surg.* **32**, 90.

Harty F. J., Parkins B. J. and Wengraf A. M. (1970) Success rate in root canal therapy: a retrospective study of conventional cases. *Br. Dent. J.* **128**, 65.

Hedman W. J. (1951) An investigation into residual periapical infection after pulp canal therapy. *Oral Surg.* **4**, 1173.

Kuttler Y. (1955) Microscopic investigation of root apexes. *J. Am. Dent. Assoc.* **50**, 544.

Lalonde E. R. and Luebke R. G. (1968) The frequency and distribution of periapical cysts and granulomas: an evaluation of 800 specimens. *Oral Surg.* **25**, 861.

Martin H., Lasala A. and Michanowicz A. (1968) Permeability of the apical third of the root to drugs used in endodontic therapy: an *in vitro* study. *J. Oral Therap. Pharmacol.* **4**, 451.

Michanowicz A. E., Michanowicz J. P. and Abou-Rass M. (1971) Cementogenic repair of root fractures. *J. Am. Dent. Assoc.* **82**, 569.

Morse D. R., Wolfson E. and Schacterle G. R. (1975) Nonsurgical repair of electrophoretically diagnosed radicular cysts. *J. Endodontol.* **1**, 158.

Muruzabal M. and Erausquin J. (1973) The process of healing following endodontic treatment in the molar of the rat. In: Grossman L. I. (ed.), *Transactions of the 5th International Conference on Endodontics*. Philadelphia, University of Pennsylvania, pp. 126–54.

Nicholls E. (1961) An investigation into the factors which may influence the prognosis of root canal therapy. M.D.S. Thesis, University of London, p. 178.

Phillips J. M. (1967) Rat connective tissue response to hollow polyethylene tube implants. *J. Can. Dent. Assoc.* **33**, 59.

Pineda F. and Kuttler Y. (1972) Mesiodistal and buccolingual roentgenographic investigation of 7 275 root canals. *Oral Surg.* **33**, 101.

Rickert U. G. and Dixon C. M. (1931) The controlling of root surgery, *8° Congrès Dentaire Internationale. Fédération Dentaire Internationale*, Section IIIa, pp. 15–22.

Schilder H. and Amsterdam M. (1959) Inflammatory potential of root canal medicaments: a preliminary report including non-specific drugs. *Oral Surg.* **12**, 211.

Seltzer S., Bender I. B. and Turkenkopf S. (1963) Factors affecting successful repair after root canal therapy. *J. Am. Dent. Assoc.* **67**, 651.

Seltzer S., Soltanoff W. and Bender I. B. (1969) Epithelial proliferation in periapical lesions. *Oral Surg.* **27**, 111.

Seltzer S., Soltanoff W., Sinai I., Goldenberg A. and Bender I. B. (1968) Biologic aspects of endodontics. Part III. Periapical tissue reactions to root canal instrumentation. *Oral Surg.* **26**, 534.

Seltzer S., Soltanoff W. and Smith J. (1973) Biologic aspects of endodontics. V, Periapical tissue reactions to root canal instrumentation beyond the apex and root canal fillings short of and beyond the apex. *Oral Surg.* **36**, 725.

Selye H. (1959) Diaphragms for analysing the development of connective tissue. *Nature (Lond.)* **184**, 701.

Shindell E. (1961) A study of some periapical roentgenolucencies and their significance. *Oral Surg.* **14**, 1057,

Shovelton D. (1964) The presence and distribution of micro-organisms within non-vital teeth. *Br. Dent. J.* **117**, 101.

Stanley H. R., Conti A. J. and Graham C. (1975) Conservation of human research teeth by controlling cavity depth. *Oral Surg.* **39**, 151.

Steiner J. C. (1969) Guidelines for selecting teeth to be treated with endodontic therapy. *Dent. Clin. North Am.* **13**, 769–82.

Strindberg L. Z. (1956) The dependence of the results of pulp therapy on certain factors. *Acta Odont. Scand.* **14**, Suppl. 21, pp. 94, 100 and 101.

Thoma K. H. (1918) The histopathology of alveolar abscesses and diseased root-ends. *Dent. Cosmos* **60**, 13.

Torneck C. D. (1966) Reaction of rat connective tissue to polyethylene tube implants, Part 1. *Oral Surg.* **21**, 379.

von der Lehr W. N. and Marsh R. A. (1973) A radiographic study of the point of endodontic egress. *Oral Surg.* **35**, 105.

Wach E. C., Hauptfuehrer J. D. and Kesel R. G. (1955) Endodontic significance of the penetration of S[35]-labeled penicillin in extracted human teeth. *Oral Surg.* **8**, 639.

Chapter 4

Sterilization of instruments and materials

Sterilization denotes the destruction of all micro-organisms. Disinfection means the elimination of vegetative organisms likely to cause disease.

It has been argued that the instruments and materials used in endodontic treatment need only be disinfected. This attitude is unsound, for three reasons. First, the methods of disinfection used cannot be relied upon to eliminate all organisms which may cause disease. Secondly, organisms normally regarded as non-pathogenic may acquire the ability to produce disease should they gain access to necrotic or damaged tissue in the pulp cavity or periapical region. Thirdly, instruments which come into contact with body fluids are capable of transmitting serum hepatitis from one patient to another unless they are sterilized. Knighton (1961) states that as little as 0·0004 ml of infected blood is needed to transmit this disease.

Therefore, if treatment is to be performed in an aseptic manner, all instruments and materials introduced into the pulp cavity must be sterilized beforehand. Either an autoclave or a hot air oven may be used for sterilization. If a method which only disinfects, such as boiling water or a chemical antiseptic solution, has to be relied upon, it should be supplemented at the chairside by using a 'hot-salt sterilizer', an apparatus which will be described later in this chapter.

METHODS OF STERILIZATION
1. Steam under pressure: autoclave

An autoclave works on the same principle as a pressure cooker. Water is heated under pressure and so is made to boil and form steam at a temperature higher than its normal boiling point. At a pressure of 103·5 kPa in excess of atmospheric pressure, water boils at 121 °C; at this temperature, once all air has been displaced from the apparatus and replaced by steam, sterilization occurs in 15 minutes. Higher pressures lead to further raising of the boiling point and even shorter sterilization times. Several autoclaves designed for dental use are available in Great Britain (*Fig.* 80). Browne's sterilization tubes, Type 1, may be used to check that the requisite time–temperature relationship has been achieved.

The advantage of the autoclave is that sterilization is rapid. The major disadvantage is that instruments and other metallic objects which are not made of stainless steel may corrode, so that the edges of cutting instruments are blunted. MacCulloch and Smith (1964) report that this corrosion may be prevented by wrapping instruments in paper impregnated with a vapour-phase inhibitor, such as Shell VPI 260.

One of the major advantages of the autoclave is that it may be used for the sterilization of articles such as towels and swabs which would be burned by the higher temperatures used in a hot air oven.

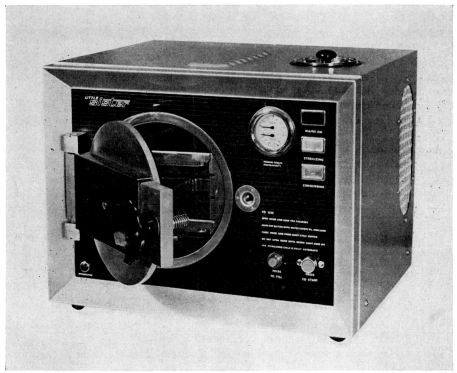

Fig. 80. An autoclave designed for dental use.

A form of sterilization somewhat similar to autoclaving is the Harvey Vapour Pressure method. In this method a mixture of alcohols, ketones, formaldehyde and water is used, so that instrument corrosion is reduced.

2. Dry heat: hot air oven

Sterilization by dry heat in a hot air oven is the method of choice for root canal instruments, since rusting of non-stainless steel articles does not occur. It has the advantage that a complete kit sufficient for one appointment, including reamers, files, broaches and spiral root fillers, together with burs, wool pledgets and cotton-wool rolls, may be packed in a metal tray and sterilized (*Fig.* 81). Provided the lid of the tray is a close fit and is not removed, the contents should remain sterile for at least 1 week, and probably appreciably longer if kept in a cabinet away from dust and draughts.

4

It is useful if kits containing a limited range of instruments are made up. These may be used for the emergency treatment of acute conditions, when relatively few instruments are needed. As a container for such a kit, a small metal box (*Fig.* 82) or a glass tube stoppered with non-absorbent cottonwool may be used. It is also

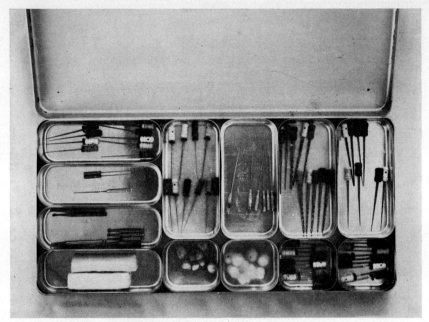

Fig. 81. A kit of root canal instruments, burs and absorbent materials.

convenient to sterilize and store individual sizes of absorbent paper points in used cartridge tubes stoppered with non-absorbent wool.

The larger hand instruments used in root canal treatment may also be assembled to form a kit and sterilized by hot air. The instruments are wrapped in a three-ply disposable paper towel and sterilized inside a metal box of suitable size. The disposable towel provides a sterile working surface on which the instruments are placed. A convenient kit consists of a mirror, probe, college tweezers, instrument holding forceps, excavator, flat plastic instrument, root canal spreader and root canal pluggers, together with a stainless steel mixing 'slab' and spatula, a dismantled glass–metal syringe and needle, and an instrument measuring device (*Fig.* 83). It should be verified that the cement joint of the glass–metal syringe will withstand the temperature of the hot air oven. Alternatively, a disposable, pre-sterilized syringe may be preferred. A cartridge syringe assembled ready for use may also be included in the kit. Individual articles may be placed in heat-resistant paper bags, which are sealed following sterilization. Handpieces to be sterilized by hot air are placed in metal tubes; their working parts are coated with a special heat-resisting oil, such as Shell Tellus Oil 27 (Johnston, 1961), preparatory to sterilization.

Owing to the poorer thermal conductivity of air and the greater susceptibility of micro-organisms in the moist state to destruction by heat, sterilization with a hot air oven takes longer and needs a higher temperature than with an autoclave. The objects to be sterilized must be dry, otherwise an even longer time will be needed. The lids of trays and containers are propped open to facilitate the free circulation of air. The articles are kept at a temperature of 160 °C for 1 hour. A period of 30 minutes is normally allowed after loading and switching on the oven for this

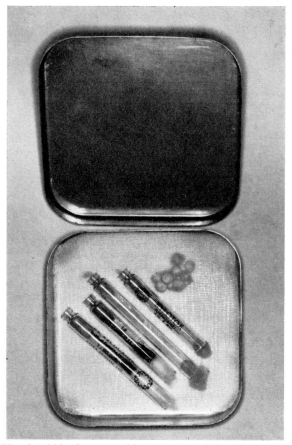

Fig. 82. An abbreviated kit of root canal instruments and absorbent materials in used cartridge tubes in a metal box. Such a kit is useful for the emergency treatment of acute conditions.

temperature to be attained. If the oven has been heavily loaded, a longer period of time, up to 1 hour even, may have to elapse before 160 °C is reached. The current is switched off after 1 hour at this temperature, and the articles are left inside until the oven has cooled. Immediately following their removal from the oven, the lids or covers of trays and other containers are pushed firmly into place.

Because of the lengthy nature of the process, the turnover of instruments is slow when using hot air for sterilization. In consequence, rather than loading the oven lightly and having to sterilize the objects in batches, the apparatus is generally loaded as fully as possible. A timing device with an automatic cut-out after the elapse of the required time is incorporated in most ovens, so allowing sterilization outside of normal surgery hours without supervision of the apparatus. Alternatively, to achieve a faster turnover, some workers advocate using a higher temperature for a shorter time. For example, depending on how heavily the oven is loaded, a period of between 12 and 30 minutes is used when the temperature is

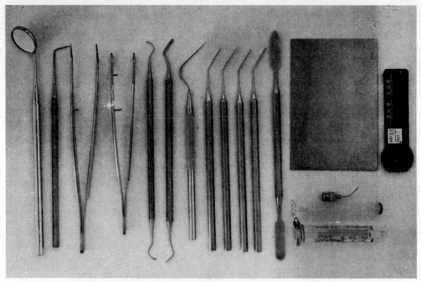

Fig. 83. Kit of larger hand instruments, comprising mirror, probe, college tweezers, instrument holding forceps, excavator, flat plastic instrument, root canal spreader and pluggers, stainless steel mixing 'slab' and spatula, dismantled syringe and needle, and instrument measuring device (Variegauge).

raised to 185 °C. For handpieces coated with Shell Tellus Oil 27, a temperature of 175 °C for 90 minutes is recommended (Johnston, 1961). However, it must be noted that at temperatures significantly above 160 °C, paper points, wool pledgets, paper towels and similar articles char and become brittle. Also, the solder joints of some instruments may melt.

Several patterns of electrically heated hot air ovens designed for dental use are available in Great Britain (*Fig.* 84). Alternatively, an oven designed for medical laboratory use may be employed. The efficacy of a hot air oven may be checked with the aid of Browne's sterilization tubes, Type 3.

3. Dry heat: flaming

The direct application of heat by a flame can only be relied upon to sterilize if the article becomes, literally, red hot. It must not be applied, therefore, to cutting instruments, since these would become brittle and be likely to break when in use within the root canal. It may be used for instruments in which loss of temper of the working ends does not matter, such as an old pair of tweezers used to remove articles from an instrument tray.

Apart from being a little quicker, it offers no real advantage over a hot-salt sterilizer, described presently.

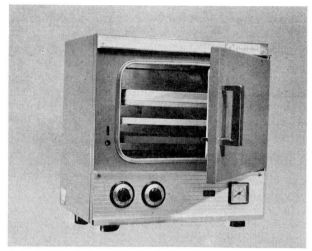

Fig. 84. A hot air sterilizer designed for dental use.

METHODS OF DISINFECTION

1. Boiling water

Immersion in boiling water for 10 minutes is commonly used for the 'sterilization' of dental instruments, but is not recognized as a method of sterilization. Whilst commonly employed for hand instruments, boiling water cannot be relied upon to eliminate the virus responsible for serum hepatitis unless used for a longer period of time than that normally employed. Like the autoclave, it results in the loss of fine edges from cutting instruments.

If boiling water has to be employed, its use should be restricted to large hand instruments, such as probes, excavators and plastics. With the exception of the mouth mirror, which need not touch the field of operation, all of these instruments are treated in a hot-salt sterilizer before contacting the field of operation or touching other objects which will contact this field.

2. Antiseptic solutions

Extravagant claims have been made for antiseptic solutions. The position regarding these solutions was summed up very well by Williams et al. (1966), who said: 'Sterilization by chemicals is an immensely more complex and difficult subject than sterilization by heat. It abounds in pitfalls, and much of the copious literature on it is of little value because the authors have fallen headlong into one of these. Many other papers are misleading because, of the almost infinitely variable conditions under which an experiment can be conducted, those have been chosen which will favour a particular germicide.'

Apart from this, chemical antiseptic solutions have a number of obvious drawbacks. Thus, they can be used only for solid, non-absorbent articles, such as those of metal or glass. Rusting of instruments may occur. Solutions which are caustic must be kept well away from the patient and must be removed before the articles are used by rinsing the latter in other liquids, such as alcohol. Chemical antiseptics are largely ineffective against the virus responsible for serum hepatitis, which it has been pointed out can be transmitted by extremely small inocula, such as could be left on a used reamer or file.

If an antiseptic solution is used, the container should be kept covered. In common with all methods of sterilization and disinfection, articles must be clean. They are therefore scrubbed with soap and water or placed in an ultrasonic cleaner, and then rinsed and dried before immersion. With chemicals, cleanliness of instruments is especially important, since adherent material will prevent contact between the antiseptic and the instrument. Also, substances of a protein nature may interfere with the action of the antiseptic. Objects must be thoroughly dried before immersion, otherwise dilution, and even inactivation, of the antiseptic may occur. With most antiseptic solutions, articles must be immersed for at least 30 minutes, and preferably considerably longer.

A moderately effective chemical antiseptic is a 0·5 per cent alcoholic solution of chlorhexidine. However, following immersion, instruments have to be rinsed before use. Less effective but probably more commonly used antiseptics are those of the quaternary ammonium group, such as benzalkonium chloride (0·1 per cent) and cetrimide (0·25 per cent). These have the advantage that no harm is done if a trace of the antiseptic is left on an instrument and accidentally contacts the patient. Sodium nitrite (0·5 per cent) is often added as an anti-rust agent to cetrimide. The quaternary ammonium compounds are inactivated by soap, which must therefore not be left on instruments. Rubber articles should not be immersed since, depending on the nature of the rubber, they may become softened. Besides metallic instruments and glass slabs, silver points can be stored in these solutions, separate containers being used for the different sizes. Before being used, points are dried and treated in a hot-salt sterilizer.

Since heat cannot be used for their sterilization, gutta percha points have to be treated with an antiseptic before use. They may be immersed in thiomersal solution (0·1 per cent) or in 60 per cent ethyl alcohol, and are dried prior to use. Silver points may be stored in these solutions, if so wished. A recent study indicates that gutta percha points may be sterilized by immersion in a 5·25 per cent solution of sodium hypochlorite for 60 seconds (Senia et al., 1975).

Either thiomersal solution or 60 per cent alcohol, or thiomersal followed by alcohol, may also be used in conjunction with sterile wool rolls to scrub a glass slab prior to mixing root canal cements. Dappens glasses may be treated in the same way. Alternatively, glassware may be wiped down with alcohol which is then ignited to destroy surface organisms.

'HOT-SALT STERILIZER'

A 'hot-salt sterilizer' consists essentially of a metal well which contains salt and is heated either electrically or by a flame. An electrically heated sterilizer incorporates a thermostat for maintaining the salt at the required temperature. Should a flame be relied upon as the heat source, a spirit lamp may be used (Nicholls, 1963), as shown in *Fig.* 85. Grossman described a sterilizer for attachment to the top of a bunsen burner several years ago (Grossman, 1940). The gas jet on the dental unit may also be employed.

The use of table salt in the sterilizer was suggested originally by Grossman (1956). Previous to that time, fusible alloy, glass beads and ball bearings had each

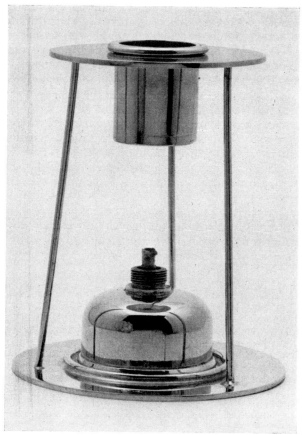

Fig. 85. A home-made hot-salt sterilizer heated by a spirit lamp.

been tried and found to have disadvantages. For example, fusible alloy oxidizes at its surface and by sticking to instruments was sometimes inadvertently transferred to the root canal, where it occasionally resulted in blockage. Beads also stick to objects if they are wet. Table salt does not suffer from these disadvantages, and since it is soluble in water, any which enters the root canal is easily removed by irrigation.

Differing conclusions have been reached on the temperature at which the contents of the well should be maintained and for how long objects should be inserted. The most comprehensive study is probably that of Findlay (1955). At a temperature of 271 °C, Findlay found that metallic instruments such as reamers and files were sterilized in 9 seconds. The physical qualities of the instruments treated in this way were not noticeably impaired. However, cottonwool pledgets and absorbent paper points needed a considerably longer period, at the end of which they were very brittle, and so liable to fragment in the root canal. Whilst satisfactory for metallic instruments and silver points, therefore, this method should not be used for wool pledgets and absorbent points.

The value of the hot-salt sterilizer lies in its simplicity as a rapid method of dry-heat sterilization of the working ends of instruments which previously have only been disinfected, or which were sterile initially but have been contaminated during treatment. However, as a routine method of sterilizing every instrument to be used during treatment it would obviously be far too time-consuming.

When first used, the temperature attained in the well should be checked with a thermometer, and the setting of the thermostat, or the height of the flame, adjusted accordingly and noted. Heating of the apparatus should be started about 10 minutes before the patient arrives, to allow time for the required temperature to be reached. It should be noted that a definite temperature gradient exists within the well, and that with glass beads or salt the temperature superficially is considerably less than that at deeper levels (Koehler and Hefferen, 1962; Windeler and Walter, 1975). The working ends of instruments should therefore be thrust deep into the contents of the well.

When table salt is used it has to be replaced every few weeks, since the deeper layers tend to form dense aggregates into which instruments cannot be inserted. Whatever substance is used within the well, instruments must not be left inserted for long periods, otherwise they may become brittle.

REFERENCES

Findlay J. (1955) A report on the efficacy of molten metal and ball bearings as media for sterilization. Br. Dent. J. 98, 318.
Grossman L. I. (1940) Root-canal Therapy. London, Kimpton, p. 103.
Grossman L. I. (1956) A hot-salt sterilizer. (Letter.) Br. Dent. J. 100, 283.
Johnston C. M. (1961) The sterilization of dental handpieces. Br. Dent. J. 110, 205.
Knighton H. T. (1961) Viral hepatitis in relation to dentistry. J. Am. Dent. Assoc. 63, 21.
Koehler H. M. and Hefferen J. J. (1962) Time-temperature relations of dental instruments heated in root-canal instrument sterilisers. J. Dent. Res. 41, 182.
MacCulloch W. T. and Smith D. C. (1964) Vapour-phase inhibition of corrosion in autoclaving. Br. Dent. J. 116, 78.
Nicholls E. (1963) A simple sterilizer for use in endodontic treatment. Br. Dent. J. 115, 15.
Senia E. S., Marraro R. V., Mitchell J. L., Lewis A. G. and Thomas L. (1975) Rapid sterilization of gutta-percha cones with 5·25% sodium hypochlorite. J. Endodontol. 1, 136.
Williams R. E. O., Blowers R., Garrod L. P. and Shooter R. A. (1966) Hospital Infection. Causes and Prevention., 2nd. ed. London, Lloyd-Luke, p. 311.
Windeler A. S. and Walter R. G. (1975) The sporicidal activity of glass bead sterilizers. J. Endodontol. 1, 273.

FURTHER READING

Crawford J. J. (1975) New light on the transmissibility of viral hepatitis in dental practice and its control. J. Am. Dent. Assoc. 91, 829.
MacFarlane T. W. (1976) Cross infection and sterilisation in dental practice. Br. Dent. J. 141, 213.
McLundie A. C., Kennedy G. D. C., Stephen K. W. and Kennedy T. F. (1968) Sterilization in general dental practice. Br. Dent. J. 124, 214.
Torneck C. D. (1967) An aseptic approach to endodontic practice. Dent. Clin. North Am. 11, 567–78.

Chapter 5

Preparation of teeth for root canal treatment—anaesthesia, isolation, surface sterilization

ANAESTHESIA

Profound anaesthesia is needed for the removal of vital pulp tissue; unless it is obtained the result is not only a distressed patient but also an inadequately performed operation. Considerable attention must therefore be paid to this aspect of treatment, for which local anaesthesia is normally used. Although a local anaesthetic may have been given already for the removal of caries, if more than a few minutes have since elapsed, another injection is given immediately before the rubber dam is applied.

Sometimes anaesthesia is needed when treating teeth which have necrotic pulps but which show no periapical changes radiographically. This may be because of the persistence of vital tissue in the extreme apical part of a canal, or it may conceivably arise from pressure on the apical periodontal membrane due to the 'piston' effect of instruments in a very narrow root canal. Whatever the cause, it is well worth using local anaesthesia routinely where obvious periapical destruction is not visible radiographically. Even where periapical bone destruction is apparent radiographically, local anaesthesia is occasionally necessary, since some vital tissue, including nerves, may still be present in the root canal (Langeland, 1967).

In the maxilla, although submucous infiltration is usually effective for cavity preparation, it is often inadequate for removal of pulpal tissue. Subperiosteal injection, however, is almost invariably effective provided it is correctly used. The preoperative radiographs are studied not only for root length but also for mesio-distal root curvature and inclination of the tooth, and the injection site is planned accordingly (*Fig.* 86). After depositing a few drops of anaesthetic solution under the mucous membrane to anaesthetize the superficial tissues, the needle is advanced at such an angle that its bevelled surface contacts bone at the required level. Considerable pressure has to be used to force solution through the needle while it is maintained close to the bone surface. With maxillary premolar teeth, subperiosteal injections are given 2·0–3·0 mm mesial and distal to the root apex as well as directly over it. Although buccal injections will normally produce complete anaesthesia of a maxillary molar, a palatal injection is occasionally needed to eliminate residual sensitivity in the palatal root.

With mandibular teeth, a nerve block injection is given routinely. With both premolar and anterior teeth, this is supplemented by a subperiosteal infiltration injection. Whilst a mental injection is usually satisfactory for the anterior teeth and the first premolar, an inferior dental block is preferable and should be used routinely for the second premolars. When giving an inferior dental injection, it is advisable to deposit solution a few millimetres anterior and posterior to the usual site, as well as in the normal position, to cover deviations from the typical anatomy.

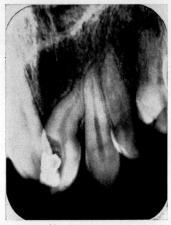

Fig. 86. The curvature of the root of |1 will influence the site at which anaesthetic solution is injected.

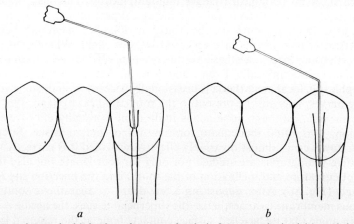

a   *b*

Fig. 87. In intrapulpal injection, the coronal pulp is first anaesthetized (*a*), and then the radicular pulp (*b*).

If after an inferior dental injection the onset of lip anaesthesia has not occurred within 60 seconds, pulpal anaesthesia will probably be incomplete, and a second injection should be given immediately. In conjunction with an inferior dental nerve block, Goldman (1974) recommends the injection of a few drops of anaesthetic solution lingually at the base of the interdental papilla immediately distal to the tooth under treatment, and coronal to the mental foramen buccally; the object is to anaesthetize any fibres of the mylohyoid nerve and the ascending branch of the transverse cutaneous colli which may contribute to pulpal innervation.

Although it is not uncommon to encounter slight sensitivity when the pulp chamber of a mandibular molar is penetrated, it rarely occurs with premolar and anterior teeth provided proper care has been taken during injection. Should slight pulpal sensitivity persist, three courses of action are open.

First, an intraosseous injection may be given. This has the disadvantage that the rubber dam has to be removed for the injection to be given properly.

Secondly, anaesthetic solution may be injected directly into a vital pulp. This procedure, known as intrapulpal injection, gives immediate anaesthesia when correctly carried out (*Fig.* 87). The study of Birchfield and Rosenberg (1975) suggests that anaesthesia may result from the pressure developed within the pulp rather than the anaesthetic component of the solution. The cut surface of the pulp is first irrigated with an antiseptic solution, such as sodium hypochlorite, to remove debris and micro-organisms, and is then dried with wool pledgets. The needle of the syringe is gently insinuated into the pulp chamber and a few drops of anaesthetic solution injected. Although much of the solution flows back and escapes through the occlusal or lingual opening, anaesthesia of the coronal pulp should result. The latter is removed with excavators and burs and the pulp chamber irrigated with hypochlorite and dried. The needle of the syringe is now inserted for 1·0 or 2·0 mm into the pulp in each root canal and one or two more drops of anaesthetic solution injected. When the root canal is appreciably wider than the needle, gutta percha may be packed into the pulp chamber to reduce the backflow of solution.

Because of the risk of periapical infection, intrapulpal injection must not be used where there is evidence of pulpal necrosis. For these cases a third course of action is followed, namely to insert a sedative dressing, as described in Chapter 10.

ISOLATION

Isolation from saliva is essential if the tooth is to be treated in an aseptic manner. Whenever possible the rubber dam is applied, since this provides the only completely satisfactory method of isolation. Wool rolls are only used where application of a dam is not possible and where treatment will occupy a short time. They are not reliable for the isolation of teeth other than maxillary incisors and canines, even for relatively short periods.

Isolation by a rubber dam has many advantages besides excluding saliva from the field of operation. The most important of these is that it prevents the inhalation or ingestion of a small root canal instrument accidentally dropped in the mouth. Where a rubber dam is not used, some device attached to the instrument, such as a safety chain (*Fig.* 88), is essential to obviate this risk. Other advantages of the rubber dam are that it eliminates interference from the tongue, improves vision, protects the soft tissues from injury from burs or irritation from irrigating agents, facilitates the removal of debris by high-velocity aspiration and, as a consequence of these benefits, shortens treatment time.

All instruments and materials used prior to and during application of the rubber dam are kept separate from those to be used during the succeeding stages of treatment. This is necessary for the maintenance of asepsis, besides being more conducive to an orderly manner of treatment.

1. Preparatory procedures

Before the rubber dam is applied, all carious cavities in the tooth to be treated are cleaned. Where the pulp is vital and is to be removed at the same visit, heat is

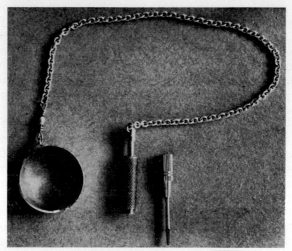

Fig. 88. A safety chain for attachment to root canal instruments.

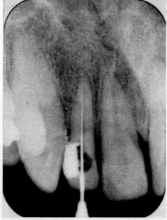

Fig. 89. The distal dressing in 2| has been shaped to make a broad area of contact with 3|, and will so help to retain a rubber dam.

used to cauterize any exposure present. If, on the other hand, it is more convenient to defer vital pulpectomy to a subsequent visit, the pulp is capped.

A fast-setting zinc oxide–eugenol compound provides a superior seal to other cements and is used for dressing cavities. Leaky fillings suspected of communicating with the pulp chamber are also replaced by this material. The mesial or distal surface of each dressing is shaped to make a broad area of contact with the adjacent tooth, since this helps to retain the rubber dam (*Fig.* 89).

Mesial and distal fillings in each tooth to be isolated are checked, and any sharp margins likely to tear the rubber are eliminated. Calculus and plaque are removed, since these may prevent application or close adaptation of the rubber to the tooth;

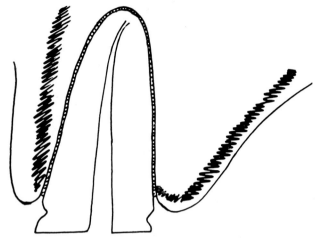

Fig. 90. Showing in buccolingual section the slots which may be cut to help retain a rubber dam on a tooth which is to be restored later with a post crown.

also, calculus may be dislodged and driven into the periodontal membrane when clamps are applied to the teeth. The tooth under treatment should be cleaned by polishing, since there is evidence that this facilitates sterilization of the enamel surface later (Melville and Birch, 1961).

The contact areas of each tooth to be isolated are tested with dental floss so that the operator is aware beforehand whether the passage of rubber to the gingival region is likely to be difficult. Each tooth which is to be clamped is inspected, and the clamp applied to check its stability. Where clamps are to be applied to adjacent teeth, a check is made that the presence of one clamp does not impede the application of another.

These preliminary procedures may indicate that care will be needed not to dislodge the rubber dam during treatment. In such cases, the bulk of the cavity which is to provide access to the pulp chamber is prepared before the dam is applied, a thin layer of dentine being left over the coronal pulp. Thus, when the dam is in position, the major cause of its dislodgement, namely movement of a handpiece, is largely eliminated. Where the tooth is to be restored with a post crown immediately after the completion of root canal treatment, the stability of a clamp may be increased considerably by cutting slots or grooves in the cervical region of the buccal and lingual enamel surfaces (*Fig.* 90). These slots receive the gripping edges of the clamp. This procedure can be useful where the crown of a partly erupted incisor has been fractured.

Where measures such as these do not retain a rubber dam, the cementation of a metal band or steel tube is indicated, and this will be described presently. Where, as a result of caries or fracture, part of the root has been lost, gingival surgery is indicated.

Since the mouth has to be kept open after the dam has been applied, the patient's lips are coated liberally with face cream if they have a tendency to cracking.

2. General principles of isolation by rubber dam

Application of the rubber dam for endodontic treatment differs in two important respects from its use for restorative dentistry. First, unless the inclusion of other

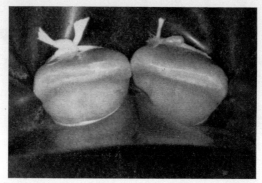

Fig. 91. Ligatures used for the isolation of 1|1 do not hold the rubber as far away from the teeth palatally as do clamps (*see Fig.* 92).

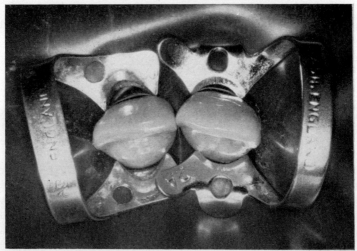

Fig. 92. Clamps used for the isolation of 1|1 hold the rubber farther away from the teeth palatally than do ligatures (*see Fig.* 91).

teeth is necessary for adequate access or for retention of the dam, only the tooth to be treated is isolated. The fewer the number of teeth isolated, the less is the risk of leakage and the quicker is the application of the dam. Secondly, clamps are preferable to floss or tape ligatures for retaining the dam, since they hold the rubber farther from the tooth under treatment, so providing more access to the lingual surface of an anterior tooth (*Figs.* 91 and 92). They are also quicker to apply.

Sometimes it is advantageous to use both methods of retention. For example, if three adjacent anterior teeth are being treated, the application of a ligature to the middle of the three teeth and a clamp to the tooth on either side provides satisfactory access and retention (*Fig. 93*). Similarly, when the rubber cannot be effectively retained on an incisor, it is useful to clamp a posterior tooth on either side to retain the dam, and to apply a ligature to the incisor; the punching of holes in

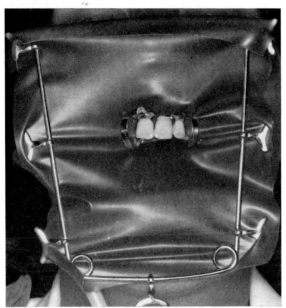

Fig. 93. Retention of a rubber dam by clamps on 1|2 and a ligature on |1. A rubber dam frame has been used to stretch the rubber clear of the field of operation.

the rubber for the posterior teeth is generally unnecessary (*Fig. 94*). The insertion interdentally of wooden wedges or strips of rubber on either side of the tooth further stabilizes the rubber.

Occasionally it is advisable to clamp additional teeth, not for the retention they give, but for the extra access they provide. The choice of teeth depends on the reasons why greater access is needed. For example, in using reamers on mandibular molar teeth, it is sometimes found that the fingers rub against the dam lingually. Here the rubber is clamped to a posterior tooth on the opposite side. By contrast, where it is anticipated that the placing of an X-ray film on the palatal aspect of a maxillary first molar may cause the patient to retch, the inclusion of the adjoining premolar teeth will facilitate positioning of the film.

3. Technique

a. Clamps
The range of clamps illustrated in *Fig. 95* is suitable for most cases. The Ivory No. 2A and the Ash No. 27 clamps are used mainly for maxillary central incisors and canines, maxillary and mandibular premolars, and mandibular canines, the Ivory No. 00 clamp for mandibular incisors and maxillary lateral incisors, and the Ivory

No. 7A and the Ash No. 26A clamps for molar teeth. Each of these five clamps is placed so that its bow reduces access as little as possible. Thus, in treating a maxillary left central incisor, the clamp is applied so that the bow is opposite the distal surface of the tooth, assuming the operator to be right-handed.

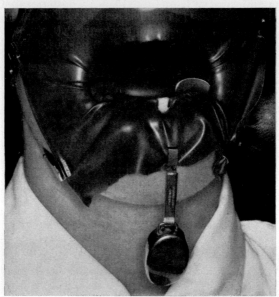

Fig. 94. Retention of a rubber dam on ⊓ by clamps on 5|5, for which holes have not been punched, and a ligature on ⊓. The rubber is stretched clear of the operative field by a rubber dam strap and a rubber dam weight has been applied anteriorly to hold the dam down.

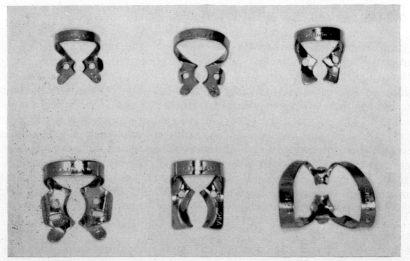

Fig. 95. A range of clamps suitable for most cases. From left to right: top row—Ivory No. 00, Ivory No. 2A and Ash No. 27; bottom row—Ivory No. 7A, Ash No. 26A and Ivory No. 9.

The Ivory No. 9 clamp is occasionally necessary for an anterior tooth. However, it is avoided whenever possible, since owing to its large bow it restricts access more than the other clamps. A useful alternative to this clamp is the S. S. White No. 212 (Ferrier) clamp.

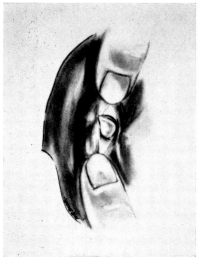

Fig. 96. When being applied, the rubber on either side of the hole is held parallel to the long axis of the tooth and stretched buccolingually, and then slipped past the contact areas to the gingival sulcus.

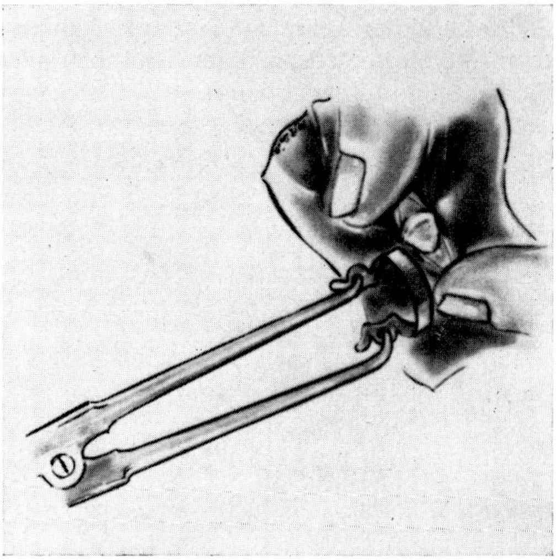

Fig. 97. When applying a clamp, the rubber is stretched buccolingually so that the gingival region may be seen.

b. *Application of rubber*
The rubber should cover the major parts of both upper and lower lips, otherwise saliva tends not only to creep on to the rubber dam but also to contact the fingers of the operator. The unstretched sheet of rubber should therefore measure not less than 15 × 15 cm, and the holes punched in the rubber should be carefully placed. To ensure that the interdental gingivae are completely covered, the holes for adjacent teeth are normally made at least 5·0 mm apart.

Various thicknesses of rubber dam are available, in both dark grey and light yellow colours. For root canal treatment 'medium weight' dam is preferred. Leakage of saliva is more obvious when a dark grey rubber is used.

For anterior and premolar teeth, the rubber dam is generally placed over the tooth before the clamp is applied. The rubber on either side of the hole is held parallel to the long axis of the tooth and stretched in a buccolingual direction, and is then slipped with a sawing motion past the contact areas into the gingival sulcus (*Fig.* 96). Should application prove difficult, attention is concentrated first on one side of the tooth and then on the other. It is useful to lubricate the rubber around the hole with shaving cream. When applying the clamp, the rubber is again stretched in a buccolingual direction so that the gingival region may be seen and the clamp applied in the correct position (*Fig.* 97).

Owing to the limited access, this method is often difficult to employ at the back of the mouth. In consequence, for molar teeth one of the following three methods is used.

The method generally used is to hold the clamp in clamp forceps over the hole in the stretched sheet of rubber, which is then allowed to close on the projecting wings of the clamp. In the mouth the clamp is opened by the forceps, so allowing the tooth under treatment to be seen, and is placed on the tooth (*Fig.* 98). After removing the forceps, a blunt hand instrument is used to release the rubber from the buccal and lingual wings.

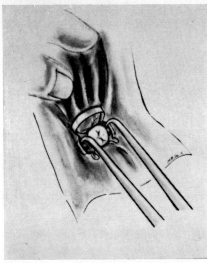

Fig. 98. One method of applying a rubber dam to a molar tooth is first to place the rubber over the wings of the clamp and then to apply the clamp to the tooth. The rubber is then released from the buccal and lingual wings and worked past each contact area.

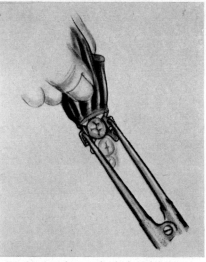

Fig. 99. Another method of applying a rubber dam to a molar tooth is to place the rubber round the base of the bow of the clamp and then to apply the clamp to the tooth. The rubber is then stretched over the remainder of the clamp and worked past each contact area.

The second method is to allow the hole in the rubber to close, not on the wings, but around the base of the bow of the clamp. By holding the rubber away from the line of vision, the crown of the tooth can be seen in its entirety whilst the clamp is being placed (*Fig.* 99). The rubber is then stretched over the remainder of the clamp and on to the tooth, first buccally and then lingually.

In the third method, the clamp and the rubber are applied separately. The clamp is first placed on the tooth, after which the hole in the rubber is stretched first over the bow and then over the buccal and lingual parts of the clamp (*Fig.* 100). This method is occasionally useful, typically when maximum visibility and access are needed in placing the clamp. There is a risk, however, that the clamp may be dislodged and swallowed before the rubber is applied (Alexander and Delhom, 1971). If this method is used, therefore, it is advisable to tie a length of dental floss to either side of the clamp and to drape the floss from the mouth.

With each of these three methods, the rubber, although brought into contact with the buccal and lingual surfaces of the tooth, will not normally have passed to the gingival region mesially and distally. It is therefore necessary to work the rubber past each contact area and into the gingival sulcus with the aid of dental tape or floss, which is then withdrawn in a buccal or lingual direction.

c. Application of rubber dam strap or frame

Two devices are available for stretching the rubber and so allowing access to the field of operation. One is a strap which extends behind the head and holds the rubber taut against the lips and cheeks (*Fig.* 94). The other is a metal or plastic

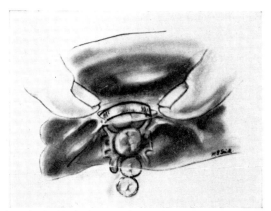

Fig. 100. A third method of isolating a molar tooth by a rubber dam is first to apply the clamp to the tooth and then to stretch the rubber over the clamp and work it past each contact area.

circular or U-shaped frame with small projections along its sides, by means of which the rubber is stretched from side to side (*Fig.* 93). Although a rubber dam strap often provides better access, a frame is more comfortable for the patient and permits the rubber to cover the nose without impeding breathing. The patient's breath may therefore be deflected farther from the field of operation. In using a frame, the rubber is stretched in the direction least likely to displace any clamps which have been applied, that is from side to side rather than from top to bottom.

A rubber dam on a mandibular anterior tooth occasionally tends to be displaced only after the strap or frame has been applied. This usually results from tension exerted on the rubber in a gingivo-incisal direction by an active lower lip. In such cases it is helpful to attach one or more weights to the lower border of the rubber (*Fig.* 94).

The use of a saliva ejector is frequently unnecessary. Where an ejector is used and the operator is right-handed, it is generally more convenient when treating an anterior tooth to have the ejector, which is out of sight under the rubber, over the left side of the lower lip, since then it is less likely to be pressed into the floor of the mouth. A thin layer of absorbent material, such as a napkin, may be placed between the rubber and the surface of each lip to absorb perspiration and any saliva which creeps over the lips.

4. Aids to retention of rubber dam

Besides those already mentioned, two other major aids to retention of a rubber dam are available. These are copper or stainless-steel bands, and steel tubes. Dentine pins may be used in conjunction with bands.

a. Copper and stainless-steel bands

There are three main indications for the cementation of a copper or stainless-steel band to a tooth preparatory to endodontic treatment. The first is the need to support a large dressing which might otherwise collapse during treatment or between

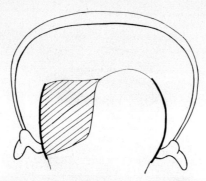

Fig. 101. When applying a clamp to a banded tooth, the gripping edges of the clamp should contact only the band.

appointments. The second is the existence of one or more weakened cusps which without adequate support might fracture before a coronal restoration is placed. The third is the absence of sufficient coronal structure to retain a dam.

Although bands are used for the anterior teeth of children, their unsightly appearance limits their use in adults to the posterior teeth. A copper band is used in the unannealed state to ensure sufficient rigidity when a clamp is applied.

To avoid leverage and possible dislodgement of the band by a clamp, the gripping edges of the latter should contact only the band and not the tooth (*Fig.* 101). The band is therefore made to extend just into the gingival sulcus around the entire periphery of the tooth. The contacts which the fitted band makes with adjacent teeth must not be so tight as to hinder later the passage of the rubber to the gingival region. With anterior teeth especially, correct contouring of the band, making its mesiodistal width greater incisally than gingivally, will enhance the retention of the dam.

When the band has been cleared of the occlusion, its occlusal or incisal rim will be found to stand away from the buccal and lingual surfaces of the crown. If left in this form, the adjacent parts of the tongue and cheek, or lip, will be abraded. With posterior teeth this is prevented by contouring the band to the tooth surface with suitable pliers. Alternatively, with a copper band vertical cuts about 1·0 mm long and the same distance apart are made in the occlusal rim of the band, and then, with the band on the tooth, the 'flaps' of copper between the cuts are adapted to the surface of the enamel with amalgam pluggers (*Fig.* 102). The surface of the band is then stoned smooth and coated with low-fusing solder. By following this procedure not only for the buccal and lingual aspects but also for the mesial and distal surfaces, sharp edges which might otherwise catch the rubber during its application are removed. With an anterior tooth, one long vertical cut is made in the lingual part of the band, so enabling one flap of copper to be folded over the other (*Fig.* 103). The band is then burnished against the tooth surface and soldered.

Where there is very little of the crown remaining, one or more dentine pins may be inserted in the tooth; these later become embedded in the material used to cement the band, and so help to retain it (*Fig.* 104). After treatment has been completed, the pins are either ground flush with the adjacent dentine or are used

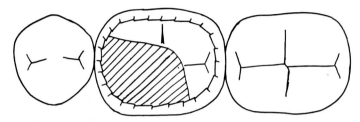

Fig. 102. One method of preventing the occlusal rim of a band on a posterior tooth from abrading the tongue or cheek is to make vertical cuts in the rim and to adapt the 'flaps' of metal between the cuts to the enamel surface. The flaps are then coated with low-fusing solder.

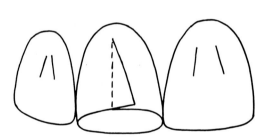

Fig. 103. To prevent the incisal rim of a band on an anterior tooth from abrading the tongue or lip, one long vertical cut is made in the band lingually, and the metal then adapted to the enamel surface.

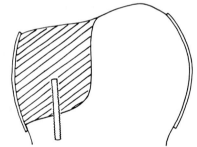

Fig. 104. A dentine pin is sometimes useful in retaining a band on a very broken down tooth.

to assist retention of the coronal restoration. Under some circumstances, described presently, the use of pins to retain a temporary crown may be preferable to cementing a tube in the root canal.

If the pulp cavity is open to the mouth, or if an occlusal cavity is present, a cottonwool pledget is inserted in the crown before the band is cemented, so facilitating opening of the pulp cavity later. The size of the pledget is carefully chosen, since one which is too large will prove difficult to remove without seriously weakening the cement, whilst one which is too small will not serve its purpose. Before the band is cemented, the wool is moistened with alcohol to prevent the cement adhering to it.

A fast-setting zinc oxide–eugenol compound is used to cement the band. Enough cement is mixed to coat the cervical region of the tooth and to fill the band, the latter then being seated in position with one finger held partly over the open end. The fit of the occlusal rim of the band against the tooth facilitates localization. The excess cement which exudes interproximally is not removed until it has set.

Where the stability of the clamp is at all suspect, it is advisable to ligate the banded tooth and to place a clamp on an adjoining tooth when applying the rubber dam.

b. Steel tubes

Where little or none of the crown of an anterior tooth remains, it is sometimes possible to cement a section of stainless-steel tube in the coronal part of the root canal. This tube provides access to the canal and serves to retain a temporary crown (*Fig.* 105), over which is placed the rubber dam. To avoid unnecessary stress

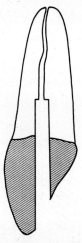

Fig. 105. Where little or none of the crown of a single-rooted tooth remains, a stainless-steel tube may be cemented in the root and used to retain a temporary acrylic crown or a metal band.

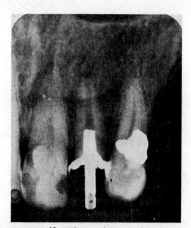

Fig. 106. |2. When using a stainless-steel tube as an aid to retention of a rubber dam, it should extend about 4·0 mm into the root.

on the temporary crown, a ligature is applied to the tooth under treatment and a clamp to a neighbouring tooth. When the tooth is root filled, only the canal, and not the tube itself, is filled.

Whilst the tube must not be so wide as seriously to weaken the root, its internal diameter must be at least as great as the diameter of the shank of the largest reamer or file which will be used to prepare the canal. Tubes of from 1·0 to 1·5 mm internal diameter are used. These calibres are approximately equivalent to external diameters of 1·3 and 2·2 mm respectively.

The tube should extend about 4·0 mm into the root (*Fig.* 106). A shorter distance is insufficient for retention, whilst a longer one unduly weakens the root. Burs or engine reamers of appropriate width are used to drill a hole to this depth. The part of the tube which projects into the mouth should be long enough to reach the surface of the temporary crown. To improve retention, shallow notches may be cut on the outer aspect of that part of the tube within the root.

A temporary crown may be made either from a stock acrylic tooth or from autopolymerizing resin in a preformed crown. If a stock tooth is to be used, it is fitted to the root face and adjusted as necessary mesially, distally and incisally. With the tube in position in the root, a hole is cut through the acrylic crown from its base to the incisal edge lingually to accommodate the tube. The surplus metal is removed so that the rim of the tube follows the surface of the acrylic (*Fig.* 105). If an autopolymerizing crown is planned instead, the preformed crown is fitted at this stage and the length of the tube adjusted as necessary.

In cementing the tube, care has to be taken that neither the root canal nor the tube becomes blocked by cement. To this end a length of wire of the same diameter as the calibre of the tube is trimmed to a pointed end and is wedged into the orifice

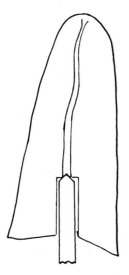

Fig. 107. When cementing a stainless-steel tube into a root, a wire with a pointed end is wedged into the coronal orifice of the canal. This prevents blockage of the canal or the tube by cement.

of the canal at the base of the hole which has been drilled (*Fig.* 107). The walls of this hole and the outer surface of the tube are coated with fast-setting zinc oxide–eugenol cement and the tube inserted into position with its inclined opening facing lingually.

Following cementation, the surplus cement is removed, the wire withdrawn and a plug of cottonwool packed firmly into the coronal end of the tube. A crown made from a stock tooth is now cemented with fast-setting zinc oxide–eugenol cement. If an autopolymerizing crown is planned instead, petroleum jelly is applied to the outer surface of the tube and to the root face, and the previously fitted crown form filled with resin and seated in position. When polymerization is well advanced, the crown is removed and its polymerization completed in warm water. The crown is trimmed as necessary and is then cemented with zinc oxide–eugenol cement, after which the wool pledget is withdrawn from the tube.

Based on the technique described by McGibbon (1956), a kit of 1·5 mm calibre tubes and matching wires, together with an engine reamer corresponding to the outer diameter of the tubes, is available commercially.

Whilst the technique described is very useful, it is not readily applicable to roots which are slender, such as those of mandibular incisors, nor to canals which are very wide buccolingually, such as those of single-rooted premolars. Furthermore, where there is obvious curvature of the root canal, deflection of the cutting edges of instruments against the opposite side of the tube may hinder cleaning of the canal. In cases such as these, instead of using a steel tube, it is usually possible to retain a temporary crown by means of dentine pins inserted in the root-face.

SURFACE STERILIZATION

After the tooth has been isolated, its surface is scrubbed for at least 60 seconds with a wool pledget moistened with a chemical antiseptic, the object being to sterilize it preparatory to opening the pulp cavity. Of the various preparations which they tested, both Birch and Melville (1961) and Moller (1966) found tincture of iodine to be the most effective for this purpose.

A disadvantage of tincture of iodine B.P. (weak iodine solution) is that some staining of plastic restorations may occur. However, this seems mainly superficial, and can usually be eliminated with a polishing agent after the dam is removed. Probably the most effective non-staining antiseptic is a 0·5 per cent alcoholic solution of chlorhexidine. Other preparations which may be used are 60–70 per cent alcohol, and non-staining iodine compounds such as povidone–iodine (Betadine). The latter has been shown by Baumgartner and Machen (1975) to be as effective as isopropyl alcohol.

During root canal treatment, instruments may inadvertently touch the rubber in the vicinity of the tooth, sometimes without the operator's knowledge. The surface of the rubber immediately adjoining and opposite the tooth is therefore usually sterilized also.

REFERENCES

Alexander R. E. and Delhom J. J. (1971) Rubber dam clamp ingestion, an operative risk; report of a case. *J. Am. Dent. Assoc.* **82**, 1387.
Baumgartner J. C. and Machen J. B. (1975) Povidone-iodine and isopropyl alcohol as disinfectants in preparation for endodontics. *J. Endodontol.* **1**, 276.
Birch R. H. and Melville T. H. (1961) Preliminary sterilisation of the endodontic field: comparison of antiseptics. *Br. Dent. J.* **111**, 362.
Birchfield J. and Rosenberg P. A. (1975) Role of the anesthetic solution in intrapulpal anaesthesia. *J. Endodontol.* **1**, 26.
Goldman M. (1974) Root-end closure techniques including apexification. *Dent. Clin. North Am.* **18**, 297–308.
Langeland K. (1967) The histopathologic basis in endodontic treatment. *Dent. Clin. North Am.* **11**, pp. 491–520.
McGibbon D. M. (1956) Stainless-steel tubing as an aid in the treatment of crownless upper anterior teeth. *Dent. Practnr Dent. Rec.* **6**, 338.
Melville T. H. and Birch R. H. (1961) Preliminary sterilisation of the endodontic field. *Br. Dent. J.* **110**, 313.
Moller A. J. R. (1966) *Microbiological Examination of Root Canals and Periapical Tissues of Human Teeth. Methodological Studies.* Goteborg, Akademiforlaget, p. 63.

FURTHER READING

Elderton R. J. (1971) A modern approach to the use of rubber dam. *Dent. Practnr. Dent. Rec.* **21**, 187, 226, 267–73.

Chapter 6

Cleaning the pulp cavity

Cleaning the pulp cavity, and in particular the root canal, is one of the most important stages of treatment. It is also one of the most difficult, and a number of studies have demonstrated that even in cleaning extracted teeth some areas of the root canal wall may be untouched by instruments, and in consequence necrotic material may well remain (Haga, 1968; Vyzantiadou and Nicholls, 1969; Davis et al., 1972; Moodnik et al., 1976).

Nonetheless, despite the shortcomings of currently used techniques, there is considerable evidence that the majority of contaminated root canals yield negative bacteriological specimens after thorough cleaning (Auerbach, 1953; Stewart, 1955; Nicholls, 1962; Stewart et al., 1969). Whilst such a specimen does not necessarily indicate a sterile canal, it does imply that the number of micro-organisms originally present has been drastically reduced, so facilitating the elimination by antiseptic drugs of any which remain. Cleaning not only eliminates micro-organisms and the necrotic material in which they exist, but also removes irregularities along the walls of the root canal and so leads to better contact between antiseptic drugs and these walls. Moreover, by enlarging and suitably shaping the root canal, it facilitates root filling.

For purposes of description, cleaning the pulp cavity may be divided into four stages:

Opening and cleaning the pulp chamber;
Removing vital radicular pulp;
Assessing the working length;
Preparing the root canal.

The following account, apart from purely general considerations such as the requirements of the opening into the pulp cavity, deals only with anterior and premolar teeth with completely formed roots. The cleaning of the pulp cavities of teeth with incompletely formed roots and of molar teeth, together with other aspects of the root canal treatment of these teeth, is dealt with separately in Chapters 12 and 13 respectively. It is assumed that the root canal, although not necessarily straight, shows no more than a slight curvature. The treatment of canals which do not fulfil this description is based on the same principles as those followed in cleaning the finer canals of molar teeth.

The reader is reminded that the expression 'apical limit' is used to denote the level to which the root canal is prepared and filled. Wherever possible the apical limit will be about 1·0–1·5 mm short of the root apex, irrespective of the pulpal status.

113

OPENING AND CLEANING THE PULP CHAMBER

The opening made into the pulp chamber should be large enough to allow the apical part of the root canal to be reached without unnecessary risk of instrument breakage. Ideally, an instrument inserted to the vicinity of the apical foramen should contact only the walls of the apical part of the canal. In a mesiodistal plane this is normally easy to achieve provided the roof of the pulp chamber is removed in its entirety, and it is only when access is mistakenly attempted through a mesial or distal cavity that there is a risk of instrument breakage or root perforation (*Fig.* 108).

In the buccolingual plane, however, the long axis of the root canal of an anterior tooth is typically in line with the incisal edge of the crown, or even slightly towards the labial aspect (*see Figs.* 125 and 126). Thus, to obtain truly straight-line access o the apical region of such a canal would entail opening the pulp chamber throught the incisal edge. Since this is undesirable from the aesthetic viewpoint, access in anterior teeth is normally gained through the lingual aspect of the crown, with the result that a slight bending of instruments is unavoidable. As will be seen presently, this bending is reduced to a minimum by the removal of dentine on the lingual aspect of the canal coronally.

The size, shape and position of the opening into the pulp chamber should also be such that the crown is not unnecessarily weakened. Thus, the form of the opening depends not only on the long axis of the root canal, but also on the form of the pulp chamber. In consequence, after the initial penetration of the pulp chamber, preparation of the opening is carried out mainly from within the tooth outwards.

1. Preparation of opening

There are three main stages in preparing the opening into the pulp chamber, namely penetration of the enamel, penetration of the roof of the pulp chamber and removal of this roof (*Fig.* 109). Although the initial penetration of enamel may be achieved with an air-turbine drill, the subsequent stages are best carried out with a slow-speed handpiece. After dentine has been exposed, a round bur, directed as far as possible in line with the long axis of the canal, is used to penetrate the roof of the pulp chamber. The third and final stage is to remove the roof of the chamber and enlarge the opening until the cavity permits ready access to the apical part of the canal. This also is accomplished with round burs, cutting from within the pulp chamber outwards to remove the overhanging tissue. Following the completion of the outline form of the cavity in an anterior tooth, it is necessary to remove dentine linguocervically to improve access to the apical part of the canal (*Fig.* 109, X).

The form of the opening into the pulp chamber varies with individual teeth according to the anatomy of the pulp cavity. The preoperative radiographs should be studied to assess the latter.

a. Anterior teeth

The opening into the pulp chamber of an anterior tooth is normally confined to the lingual surface of the crown, and the initial penetration of enamel is at the centre of this surface, midway between both the mesial and distal borders and the cervix and the incisal edge. Should the mesiodistal width of the chamber be greater incisally than cervically, as in maxillary central incisor teeth, the opening is extended mesio-incisally and disto-incisally, so resulting in a roughly triangular-shaped cavity (*Fig.* 110*a*).

If the chamber is relatively uniform in width mesiodistally, as in canine teeth and in the maxillary incisor teeth of older patients following continued dentine

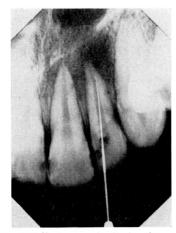

Fig. 108. |2. As a result of using the mesial cavity to provide access to the pulp cavity, the distal wall of the canal is in danger of being perforated.

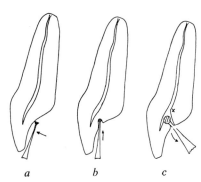

a   *b*   *c*

Fig. 109. The three stages in preparing the opening into the pulp chamber: *a*, penetrating the enamel; *b*, Penetrating the pulp chamber roof; and *c*, Removing the pulp chamber roof. In an anterior tooth, it is necessary after completing the opening to remove dentine linguocervically at X.

formation, the cavity outline tends to be roughly ovoid (*Fig.* 110*b*). Where the pulp chamber has been obliterated completely by calcification, the opening is smaller than usual, but must still be sufficiently large to admit the shanks of the largest hand instruments which will be needed to prepare the root canal. If an appreciable part of the crown has been lost incisally and the tooth is to be restored by a post crown, true straight-line access may be achieved by cutting the opening between the labial and lingual enamel plates.

b. Premolar teeth

With maxillary premolar teeth, the initial penetration of enamel is in the occlusal fissure, midway between the mesial and distal surfaces. The bur is directed along the general long axis of the tooth to penetrate the roof of the pulp chamber. Irrespective of the number of root canals, the width of the pulp chamber bucco-palatally is considerable. The anatomy of the radicular part of the pulp cavity is such, however, that in extending the opening buccally and palatally it is not usually necessary to encroach upon the cusp tips (*Fig.* 110*c*). Owing to the ribbon shape of the pulp chamber in cross-section, the final opening is relatively narrow mesio-distally, and is elliptical in outline (*Fig.* 111).

Mandibular premolar teeth normally possess only one major root canal, and although the pulp chamber is definitely ribbon-shaped in cross-section, the difference between the buccolingual and mesiodistal widths is less than in maxillary premolar teeth. In consequence, there is less disparity between the mesiodistal and buccolingual dimensions of the outline form of the opening cut into the pulp

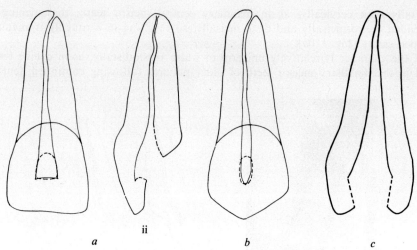

ii

a   *b*   *c*

Fig. 110. *a,* Where the mesiodistal width of the pulp chamber of an anterior tooth is greater incisally than cervically, the opening is extended accordingly; i and ii show mesiodistal and labiolingual sections respectively of the completed opening.
b, Where the mesiodistal width of the pulp chamber of an anterior tooth is relatively uniform, the opening into the chamber has an ovoid outline.
c, Buccopalatal section of opening into pulp chamber of maxillary premolar.

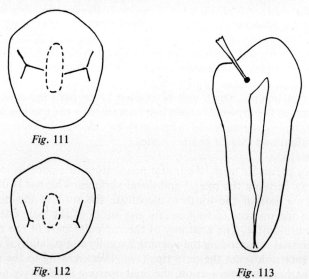

Fig. 111

Fig. 112   *Fig.* 113

Fig. 111. Occlusal view of opening into pulp chamber of maxillary premolar, showing its elliptical outline.

Fig. 112. Occlusal view of opening into pulp chamber of mandibular premolar. Compare with *Fig.* 111.

Fig. 113. In opening the pulp chamber of a mandibular first premolar tooth through the occlusal fissure, the bur is directed buccally.

chamber (*Fig.* 112). With mandibular first premolar teeth, the buccolingual centre of the pulp chamber tends to be in line with the buccal cusp and not with the occlusal fissure of the tooth. In opening the pulp chamber of this tooth, therefore, the head of the bur is directed towards the buccal aspect (*Fig.* 113). This also applies to the second premolar tooth, although not to the same extent.

2. Elimination of remnants of coronal pulp

Even though the bulk of the coronal pulp is removed in preparing the opening into the pulp cavity, remnants on the side walls of the pulp chamber will still be present. These must be removed, otherwise they may later cause discoloration of the crown. Although they may be eliminated now, time is saved if they are removed later during treatment, namely whilst the radiograph which has to be taken presently to assess the level of the apical limit is being processed. To facilitate description, however, the procedure will now be discussed.

Whilst most of the pulpal remnants may be eliminated with excavators, small round burs are usually necessary to remove the pulp horns. The walls of the pulp chamber are wiped free of remaining fragments of pulp and dentine with wool pledgets moistened with sodium hypochlorite solution. Where debris is particularly resistant to removal, or where there has been bleeding from a vital pulp into the chamber, hydrogen peroxide (10 vol.) may be used; this is followed by sodium hypochlorite to eliminate traces of peroxide.

REMOVING VITAL RADICULAR PULP

The removal of a vital pulp to the vicinity of the apical foramen is known as 'total pulpectomy'. This term is not strictly accurate, since normally the extreme apical part of the pulp is left. The expression 'partial pulpectomy' is reserved for that procedure where a vital pulp is removed to a level well short of the apical foramen, so that the pulp in the apical one-third of the root remains. This form of treatment, although advocated by a few workers as a routine procedure when removing a vital pulp, is only adopted when some factor, such as a sharply curved root canal, prevents further penetration.

Most operators remove the radicular part of a vital pulp immediately after the pulp chamber has been opened and the coronal pulp removed. The following technique is used. The exposed area of the pulp at the entrance to the root canal is cauterized with a hot instrument, so reducing the risk of transmitting organisms in an apical direction when the radicular pulp is removed. The patency of the canal is then confirmed by inserting a fine reamer or smooth broach (*Fig.* 123) to a level about 1·0–2·0 mm short of the probable level of the apical limit, as judged from the preoperative radiograph. This also creates a pathway for a barbed broach (*Fig.* 123), which is now inserted to the same level, rotated around its long axis through 360° to catch up the pulp on its barbs and then withdrawn from the canal with the pulp entwined around it. This procedure is called 'pulp extirpation'.

The shanks of both smooth and barbed broaches may be held either in a handle incorporating a chuck or directly in the fingers. Barbed broaches are fairly delicate instruments and must not be inserted farther apically, or rotated, once resistance from dentine is felt. Instead, the instrument is withdrawn until it can be rotated without difficulty. Barbed broaches are not used in narrow root canals, such as those of adult maxillary premolar teeth, or where previous introduction of a reamer or smooth broach has revealed a partial obstruction of the canal, due, for example, to a localized calcification of the pulp. Instead, the pulp is removed piecemeal with reamers and files, following which loose shreds of tissue remaining within the root canal are eliminated by irrigation. The techniques of reaming, filing and irrigation are discussed later in this chapter.

There are two objections to extirpating a pulp with a barbed broach. One is that the level at which the pulp is severed cannot be accurately controlled; even though the broach remains within the root canal, tearing of the periodontal membrane may occur. This drawback may be overcome by using reamers and files, as described previously. A refinement is to use a Hedstroem file with its pointed tip ground flat (*Fig.* 114). A file of approximately the same width as the apical part of

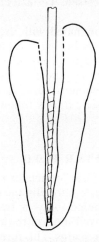

Fig. 114. A Hedstroem file with its pointed end ground flat may be used for pulpectomy.

the canal is selected. Upon insertion to the appropriate level, this should 'bite' into the root canal walls when rotated, so severing the pulp.

The second objection is that, whatever instruments are used, until the level of the apical limit has been assessed, it is uncertain if the level to which the pulp has been removed is correct. Thus, even though damage to the periapical tissues may be avoided by deliberately keeping instrument tips coronal to the apical limit, an appreciable length of apical pulp may be left as a result. The significance of this objection depends on the anatomy of the root canal, on the instruments which are used for pulp removal, and on the scheme of treatment which is being followed.

When pulpectomy is performed as an emergency treatment and, owing to time being limited, it is planned to prepare the root canal at a subsequent visit, retention of pulp coronal to the apical limit is an unavoidable hazard. Local anaesthesia will therefore be needed at the next visit. If the canal is curved, the use of reamers and files for pulp removal to a level coronal to the apical limit may result in the formation of ledges, and these may later hinder preparation of the canal farther apically; in such cases, it is better to use a barbed broach instead. Where the canal is straight, however, this hazard does not apply, and reamers and files may be used.

When the pulp is removed as a planned rather than an emergency procedure, the root canal is usually prepared at the same visit. Thus, if reamers and files are used to remove the pulp, provided the root canal is straight it is of little consequence whether pulp removal is begun before the level of the apical limit has been assessed by radiographic examination or is deferred till after this assessment.

Whatever procedure is followed, the radiographic examination for assessing the level of the apical limit is made as soon as all debris in the vicinity of the pulpal wound at the base of the pulp chamber has been removed, provided access to the root canal has been completed. Particular care should be taken to ensure that a second root canal has not been overlooked. This applies not only to maxillary premolar teeth but also to mandibular incisors, of which a significant proportion have two canals, although these generally join to share a common apical foramen (Rankine-Wilson and Henry, 1965; Ainamo and Löe, 1968; Laws, 1971; Benjamin and Dowson, 1974).

Whilst the film is being processed, cleaning of the pulp chamber is completed. Haemorrhage from the pulpal wound apically is controlled by inserting an absorbent point to the same level as that to which the pulp was removed, and leaving it in this position for 1–2 minutes.

ASSESSING THE WORKING LENGTH

The level of the apical limit was defined in Chapter 3 as 1·0–1·5 mm short of the root apex. Its distance from some easily accessible point from which to measure must now be assessed. Failure to do this before any serious attempt is made to prepare the root canal is likely to result in the passage of instruments beyond the apical foramen or the creation of a ledge in the wall of the canal some distance from the desired level. The penalties of the first type of accident were discussed in Chapter 3. Although correction of the second type of accident is usually possible, it may prove very difficult if the canal is curved.

1. Definition of 'working length'

For convenience of description, the term 'working length' will be used to denote the distance between the apical limit to instrumentation and the point from which measurement is to be made coronally.

With anterior teeth, the working length is measured from the incisal edge. Since this is not typically at right-angles to the long axis of the canal, the length recorded varies according to which part of the edge is used. Normally, the most convenient is that directly labial to the shank of an instrument inserted into the canal. Where the crown has been fractured, measurement is facilitated if the central portion of the incisal edge is ground at right-angles to the canal; this also obviates fracture and loss of enamel during treatment, with consequent loss of the measuring point.

With single-rooted premolar teeth, the most convenient measuring point is normally the tip of the buccal cusp. With a maxillary first premolar with splayed roots, it is often more convenient to measure the working length of the buccal canal from the palatal cusp tip, and vice versa. Where the crown of the tooth has been restored temporarily with a copper band and cement, it is sometimes more satisfactory to measure from the rim of the band than from the tip of a cusp.

2. Assessment of working length

The level at which pain is elicited by an instrument in the root canal is not a reliable guide in assessing the working length. Where there is a periapical lesion, an instrument can sometimes be thrust beyond the apical foramen without the patient feeling pain (*Fig.* 115). Conversely, where the canal is narrow in calibre, pain is sometimes felt a few millimetres short of the apex, even though the pulp is to all intents and purposes necrotic and a periapical lesion is present. It was pointed out

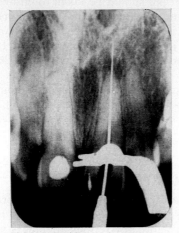

Fig. 115. Pushing an instrument into the periapical lesion associated with |1 did not cause pain.

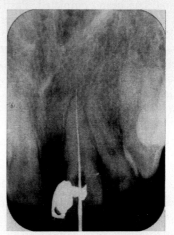

Fig. 116. Pushing an instrument into the periapical region of |1 did not cause pain. Local anaesthesia had not been used.

in Chapter 5 that this may result from pressure on the periapical tissues owing to the instrument acting as a piston, or from the presence of vital tissue in the apical part of the canal.

A tooth from which a vital pulp was removed at a previous visit may also give pain when the tip of an instrument is still some distance short of the apical limit, owing to the presence of remnants of vital pulp. Occasionally, an instrument may be thrust beyond the apical foramen into radiographically intact periapical bone without any sign of pain from the patient (*Fig.* 116).

Assessment of the working length entails radiographic examination after inserting an instrument to the vicinity of the apical limit. To the distance from the occlusal measuring point to the instrument tip is added the radiographic length by which the instrument tip is short of the apical limit (*Fig.* 117). Where the instrument has inadvertently been inserted too far and has passed beyond the apical limit, the corresponding radiographic length is subtracted from the known distance to the measuring point.

a. Guides in assessing working length

Various guides are available in deciding how far to insert an instrument preparatory to radiographic examination.

i. PREOPERATIVE RADIOGRAPH

A carefully taken preoperative radiograph provides a reasonably accurate guide to the working length. Comparison of the radiographic and clinical lengths of the crown of the tooth helps in evaluating the preoperative radiograph in this respect. Where the working length of an adjacent root-filled tooth was noted at the time of its treatment, the radiographic working length of this tooth may be compared with that previously recorded.

ii. AVERAGE TOOTH LENGTHS

In assessing working length, it is useful to know the average length of the tooth under treatment. Since this is measured from the incisal edge, or the occlusal

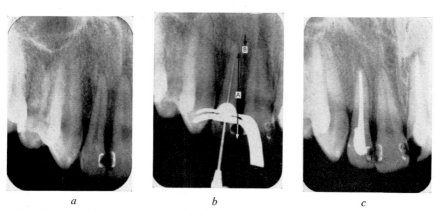

Fig. 117. Assessing the working length of 2|: *a*, Preoperative view of tooth provides guide to working length; *b*, A reamer has been inserted to a level about 1·0 mm short of the probable level of the apical limit. The distance A is known. The distance B is measured on the radiograph and added to A to give the working length; *c*, The completed root filling, terminating about 1·0 mm short of the root apex.

margin, to the root apex, 1·0–1·5 mm is subtracted to obtain the corresponding working length.

The average working lengths of anterior and premolar teeth are as follows:

1|1	..	19·0 mm
4|4	..	19·0 mm
2|2	..	19·5 mm
4|4	..	20·0 mm
5|5	..	20·0 mm
2|2	..	20·5 mm
1|1	..	21·0 mm
5|5	..	21·0 mm
3|3	..	24·0 mm
3|3	..	25·0 mm

In the same individual, corresponding teeth in the same arch are usually of similar length.

iii. USE OF INSTRUMENTS

The width of the terminal 2·0 or 3·0 mm of the instrument inserted into the tooth should correspond roughly to the mesiodistal width of the apical part of the canal, as judged from the preoperative radiograph. Thus, the resistance encountered gives the operator some idea when the apical part of the canal has been reached.

5

A sudden narrowing or curvature of the root canal may also be a useful guide (*Fig.* 118). Its distance from the apical limit will be known fairly accurately from the preoperative film. Its level in the root may usually be detected by an instrument of suitable width, and this may then be advanced by the appropriate distance.

b. Technique in assessing working length

It has already been pointed out that the delay incurred during processing of the X-ray film may be largely avoided by performing the radiographic examination as soon as access to the apical part of the canal is satisfactory. Whilst the film is being

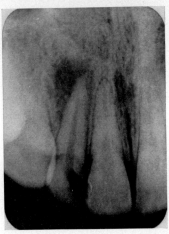

Fig. 118. The sudden narrowing of the root canal of 2| apically will provide a useful guide to position when an instrument is inserted preparatory to taking a radiograph and assessing the working length.

processed, cleaning of the pulp chamber may be completed. Where the pulp cavity is to be left open to the mouth for drainage of an acute periapical abscess, it saves time at the next visit if at this stage the necessary radiographic examination can be made.

It is important that necrotic pulpal tissue, which is probably infected, is not thrust in an apical direction. Before assessing the working length, therefore, a drop of sodium hypochlorite is introduced into the pulp chamber; gross debris is then removed carefully from the canal with barbed broaches. In the narrower canals of premolar teeth, reamers and files may have to be used instead of broaches. As in removing a vital pulp, instruments are not allowed to approach the probable level of the apical limit closer than 1·0–2·0 mm, otherwise the periapical tissues may be injured. Where treatment has previously been started by some other operator, the canal is carefully explored for the presence of radiolucent materials, such as cotton-wool or a section of absorbent paper point.

The instrument to be inserted into the canal must be straight, otherwise measurement is difficult; a reamer is preferred. As explained presently, the inaccuracy involved in determining the working length increases the farther the tip of the reamer is from the apical limit. The aim, therefore, is to insert the instrument to the vicinity of this level, but not to inflict trauma on the periapical tissues. Thus, a level 1·0–2·0 mm coronal of the probable level of the apical limit is aimed at

radiograph gives a two-dimensional picture only (*Fig.* 122). Where the instrument is radiographically short of the apical limit and its shape upon withdrawal from the canal indicates a buccolingual curvature, therefore, a further radiograph with the instrument tip actually at the apical limit is necessary to verify its relation to the root apex.

4. Electronic methods of assessing working length

Two other methods of assessing the working length are available. Each relies on registering the level of the apical periodontal membrane, from which the working

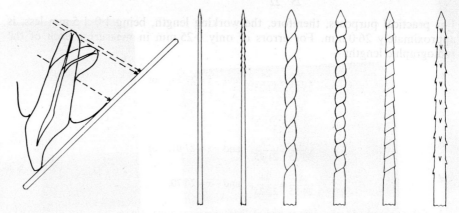

Fig. 122. A buccolingual curvature of the apical part of the root canal leads to an error in assessing the working length, since it results in foreshortening of the image of this part of the canal.

Fig. 123. Instruments which may be used during root canal preparation. From left to right: Smooth broach, barbed broach, reamer, K-type file, Hedstroem file, rat-tail file.

length may be computed. One, the Endometer, is based on the finding of Sunada (1962) that when the tip of a reamer reaches the apical periodontal membrane, the electrical resistance between the instrument and the oral mucosa is virtually the same whatever the tooth. The apparatus is calibrated to give a reading of 40 when the instrument inserted in the canal has reached the periodontal membrane apically. The other device, the Sono-explorer (Inoue, 1972), relies on sonic measurements. As the root canal is penetrated by the instrument, two distinct sounds are heard, but these synchronize once the apical periodontal membrane is reached.

Although the report of Blank et al. (1975) indicates that the two devices give acceptable results in 85–90 per cent of teeth, Seidberg et al. (1975) found that the Sono-explorer was less reliable in determining the position of the apical limit than the use of digital-tactile sensation with a reamer in the canal.

PREPARING THE ROOT CANAL

1. Instruments

Apart from those necessary for irrigation, three types of instruments are used during cleaning, namely broaches, reamers and files (*Fig.* 123).

a. Broaches

Two patterns of broaches are available, smooth or plain-sided, and barbed.

Smooth broaches may be round, pentagonal or square in cross-section and have a pointed end. They may be used not only to determine the patency of narrow canals but also to create a pathway for barbed broaches, which, because of their irregular surfaces, might otherwise force contaminated pulpal tissue in an apical direction.

Barbed broaches are used to remove pulpal tissue and dressing materials from root canals.

b. Reamers

A reamer is a twist drill having a fairly wide flute. Reamers cut by being rotated, either by hand or by means of a dental handpiece.

Numerous patterns of engine-driven reamers are available, both for straight and right-angle handpieces. All share two major disadvantages. First, they do not readily follow the course of a curved canal, and may therefore perforate the root. Secondly, owing to their speed of rotation, they are likely to break in the event of suddenly binding in a narrow or curved canal. In consequence, few experienced operators use these instruments to any extent. If one should be used, the engine cord should be slackened to allow for sudden binding and stopping of the instrument.

c. Files

Files are of three patterns, Hedstroem, K-type and rat-tail. All are used in the same manner; the file is held firmly against one side of the root canal whilst being withdrawn towards the operator. The Hedstroem and K-type instruments may be slightly rotated so as to 'bite' into the dentine before being withdrawn. The rat-tail file has the drawback that only a relatively small part of its surface area actually cuts dentine.

For the same length and width of instrument, the cutting edge of both a Hedstroem and a K-type file is longer than that of a reamer, the spiral being a closer one. There is evidence that Hedstroem files produce a relatively rough surface to the root canal compared with reamers and other patterns of file (Fromme and Riedel, 1972). It is feasible that a rough surface may hinder the adaptation of root-filling material.

d. Other instruments

Special forms of engine-driven instruments, other than engine reamers, are available. Although they can be used on anterior and premolar teeth, these instruments find their greatest application in the treatment of molars, and are therefore described in Chapter 12.

2. Instrument calibration

Depending on the manufacturer, broaches are generally available in five to twelve different widths. The instruments may be numbered in the same way as reamers and files, or their sizes may be indicated by such descriptions as 'XX fine', 'X fine', 'fine', 'medium', 'coarse' and 'extra coarse'.

Reamers and files are generally available in seventeen to twenty different widths. The sizes of the instruments are marked on the handles, and were formerly indicated by the numbers 00, 0 and 1 to 18 inclusive. Some manufacturers use handles of different colours or engrave rings on the handles to indicate the sizes. Both reamers and files are made in various lengths from 19·0 to 31·0 mm, excluding the length of the handle, which may be fixed or adjustable in position.

As a result of suggestions made by Ingle and LeVine (1958), a system of calibrating reamers and files was introduced which permits canals to be enlarged more gradually and with less risk of instrument breakage or root perforation. The number of each instrument indicates, in one-hundredths of a millimetre, the diameter at the apical end of the blades, just behind the instrument tip (*Fig.* 124 A). Instruments are numbered 8, 10, 15, 20, 25, 30, 35, 40, 45, 50, 55, 60, 70, 80, 90, 100 and 110. Some manufacturers provide three additional sizes, giving a total of

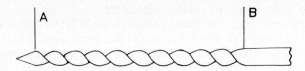

Fig. 124. The system of calibrating reamers and files. Each instrument is numbered according to its diameter in one-hundredths of a millimetre at A. The diameter of each instrument at A is 0·3 mm less than at B. The distance from A to B is 16·0 mm.

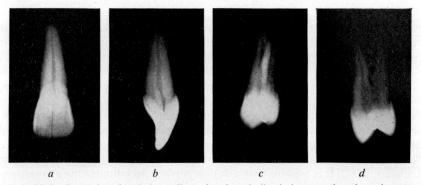

Fig. 125. Radiographs taken in buccolingual and mesiodistal planes to show how the root canals of maxillary central incisors and two-rooted maxillary first premolars tend to be roughly circular in cross-section for most of their length. *a* and *b*, Maxillary central incisor; *c* and *d*, Maxillary first premolar.

twenty instruments. All instruments have the same taper, the diameter at the apical end of the blades being 0·3 mm less than that 16·0 mm nearer the handle (*Fig.* 124 B).

Root canal instruments may be made of carbon steel or stainless steel. Carbon steel instruments are susceptible to corrosion. Although stainless-steel reamers and files are more likely to be deformed under stress, they are more resistant to breakage than carbon-steel instruments (Craig and Peyton, 1963).

3. Influence of root canal anatomy on preparation

The root canals of anterior and premolar teeth are generally narrower mesiodistally than buccolingually. With some teeth, for example maxillary central incisors and two-rooted premolars, the difference is relatively small, or even non-existent; in consequence, the canal tends to be roughly circular in cross-section for much of its length (*Fig.* 125). With other teeth, especially canines, mandibular incisors and single-rooted premolars, the difference is considerable (*Fig.* 126). In these teeth it is only in the apical part of the root that the canal is likely to be circular in outline; elsewhere, it is broad buccolingually and narrow mesiodistally. Whatever the tooth, most canals taper gingivo-apically.

In reaming, dentine is only cut where during rotation the instrument contacts at least two opposing aspects of the canal wall (*Fig.* 127). Wherever the canal is wider than the reamer, dentine is not cut. Thus, the apical part of the canal, being roughly circular in outline, may be prepared quickly with reamers. However, the coronal part of the root canal, being wider and non-circular in shape, could only be prepared with reamers if large instruments were used. If this were done, much dentine would be removed unnecessarily, especially apically.

It is for this reason that files are used. Because of the construction and mode of use of these instruments, each aspect of the root canal wall—buccal, lingual, mesial and distal—may be cleaned and prepared separately. Thus, the operator may be selective in the removal of dentine, and in consequence less root structure need be removed, and therefore less time spent during preparation.

In using files, more dentine tends to be removed coronally than apically. In *Fig.* 128, with the instrument inserted to the apical limit, level B is crossed by a greater length of instrument, and therefore a longer cutting edge, than is level A when the instrument is withdrawn from the canal. In consequence, files increase the taper of the root canal; this applies not only buccolingually but also mesiodistally.

There is evidence that in anterior root canals the use of reamers, or of files with a rotary action, usually leads to a preparation which is circular in cross-section, whereas files used with a filing action produce a non-circular shape (Vessey, 1969).

4. Length control during preparation

To ensure that the root canal is reamed and filed as far as the apical limit, but not beyond, some form of measuring device has to be used. The devices available fall into four main categories, namely disk markers, sliding metal markers, test handles and direct measurement with a ruler (*Fig.* 129).

In the absence of some form of one of the marker-setting devices described presently, a 0·5 mm graduated steel ruler is probably the simplest and quickest form of measurement. Each instrument is inserted until the length protruding beyond the occlusal measuring point equals the difference between the instrument length and the working length. A ruler that has been deliberately shortened may have to be used for premolar and mandibular incisor teeth, since their position and inclination are often such that the ruler would otherwise impinge on the opposing teeth. For greater convenience, the section of ruler may be soldered to a suitable handle (*Fig.* 130).

With each of the other three devices, a marker is placed on the shank of the instrument at a distance from the tip corresponding to the working length. With disc markers, a piece of rubber dam, or a disc of heat-resistant silicone rubber or thin metal foil, is pierced with the instrument and slid into position. Other types of sliding metal marker besides that illustrated in *Fig.* 129 are available. For example, the one described by Krueger (1935) consists of a split metal sleeve,

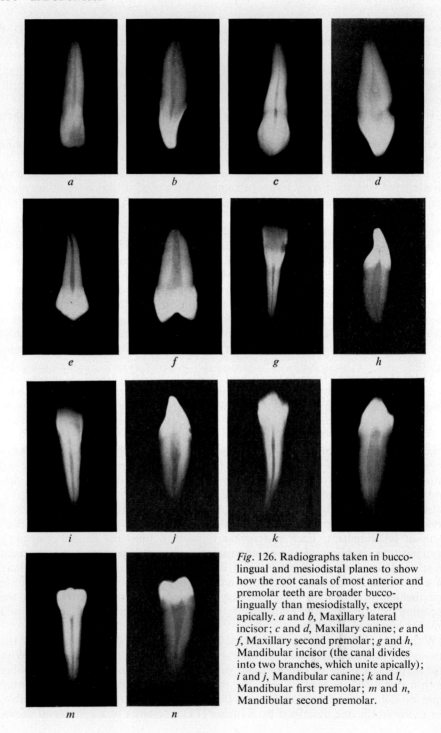

Fig. 126. Radiographs taken in bucco-lingual and mesiodistal planes to show how the root canals of most anterior and premolar teeth are broader bucco-lingually than mesiodistally, except apically. *a* and *b*, Maxillary lateral incisor; *c* and *d*, Maxillary canine; *e* and *f*, Maxillary second premolar; *g* and *h*, Mandibular incisor (the canal divides into two branches, which unite apically); *i* and *j*, Mandibular canine; *k* and *l*, Mandibular first premolar; *m* and *n*, Mandibular second premolar.

which grips the instrument handle, and a projecting portion, the end of which encircles the shank of the instrument. Similar devices made of heat-resistant plastic material and known as 'Endomatic stops' are described by Saunders (1970). These are available in different lengths, so enabling instruments of standardized length to be set at the appropriate measurement.

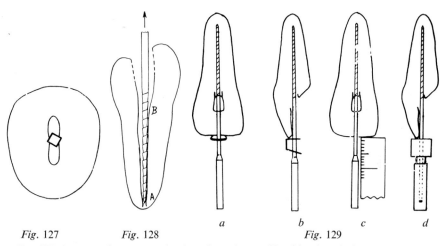

Fig. 127   Fig. 128   Fig. 129

Fig. 127. A reamer does not cut dentine where the canal is wider than the instrument itself; a cross-section of a reamer in the coronal part of a root.

Fig. 128. In filing, level B is crossed by a longer cutting edge than level A, with the result that the taper of the canal is increased.

Fig. 129. Measuring devices for instruments used to prepare root canals. From left to right: *a*, Disc marker; *b*, sliding metal marker; *c*, steel ruler; *d*, test handle.

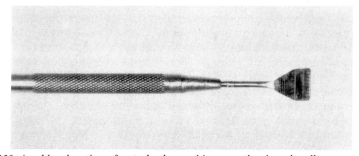

Fig. 130. A soldered section of a steel ruler used in a mouth-mirror handle.

Calibrated test handles are manufactured separately from the instruments with which they are used (*Fig.* 131). Each instrument has a right-angle bend at its wider, coronal end, and is movable in a chuck within the handle. By aligning the bend with the appropriate marking on the handle, the length of instrument projecting from the handle is made to correspond to the working length. The chuck is then tightened by a nut incorporated in the handle, so locking the instrument in position.

Contact between the handle and the incisal or occlusal margin of the tooth prevents the instrument penetrating beyond the apical limit.

5. Marker-setting devices

Apart from test handles and endomatic stops, positioning of a marker on the instrument shank formerly had to be done by direct measurement with a ruler.

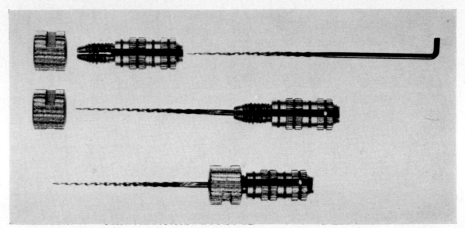

Fig. 131. The assembly of an instrument and its test handle. The bend at the coronal end of the instrument is aligned with the appropriate engraved ring on the handle.

Recently, however, various setting devices have been introduced which simplify the positioning of a sliding rubber or metal marker at the appropriate working length (*Fig.* 132).

One such device consists of a series of clear plastic rods, each with a longitudinal hole of known length. After the working length has been assessed, each instrument in turn is inserted into the appropriate rod so that its tip contacts the base of the hole; the marker is then moved to the top of the rod, so setting it at the working length. After use, the rods are sterilized by immersion in a chemical antiseptic. This device is known as the Endicator (*Fig.* 132 *a*) and is based on the publications of Guldener and Imobergsteg (1972) and Rowe and Forrest (1973).

A more complex method is described by Barnard (1974). Two circular parallel plates are joined at their centres by a vertical calibrated rod. The upper plate is perforated by a series of holes and is movable along the calibrated rod; it is adjusted in height so that its distance from the lower plate corresponds to the working length. Each instrument is inserted through a hole in the upper plate so that its tip rests against the lower plate. The marker is then moved to contact the top of the upper plate. This device is available commercially as the K.D. Endogauge (*Fig.* 132 *b*).

Probably the simplest setting device is the Variegauge (*Fig.* 132 *c*). This consists essentially of a plastic ruler with a handle at one end and a slot at the other. The instrument is positioned so that the marker is located in the slot, and is then moved until its tip is opposite the appropriate calibration on the ruler. Small metal markers are supplied for use with the Variegauge. If larger silicone rubber markers are preferred, the slot may need to be enlarged to accommodate them. Similarly, a depression adjoining the slot which accommodates the handle of the instrument may have to be enlarged to receive the handles of some patterns of reamers and files. The Variegauge can be sterilized in a hot air oven and is sufficiently small to be included in a root canal kit.

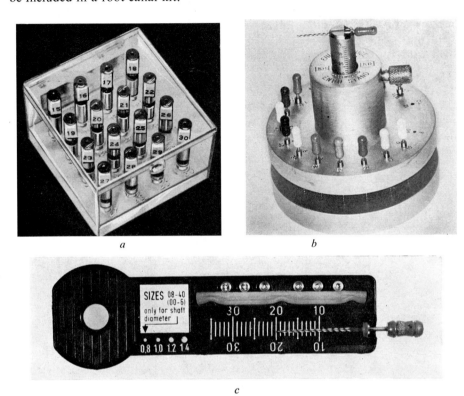

Fig. 132. Marker-setting devices: *a*, The Endicator; *b*, The K.D. Endogauge; *c*, The Variegauge.

6. Technique of instrumentation

The study of Chapman (1971) has shown that in both reaming and filing there is a pronounced risk of forcing micro-organisms through the apical foramen. Considerable care should therefore be taken during preparation of the root canal to minimize the risk of driving necrotic material and micro-organisms in an apical direction. It has already been pointed out that with a necrotic pulp the canal is first carefully explored with broaches to remove as much debris as possible. During this procedure the canal is flooded with a mild antiseptic solution such as sodium hypochlorite. These precautions are especially advisable where the pulp cavity has previously been left open to the mouth for drainage, and in consequence almost certainly contains food debris.

Reamers are used before files, since their wide flutes provide more space for the collection of necrotic material. Reaming and filing are performed with an antiseptic solution or a chelating agent in the root canal. These enhance the cutting action of instruments by virtue of their wetting action. Also, an antiseptic solution helps to eliminate micro-organisms and, in the case of sodium hypochlorite, has a solvent effect on necrotic material. The use of chelating agents and antiseptic solutions is discussed further when describing irrigation of the canal.

The first size of reamer selected for use should not meet obvious resistance before it reaches the close vicinity of the apical limit. Instruments are employed in strict numerical sequence; no size should be omitted. Each reamer is given no more than a 180° turn after contacting the root canal wall apically. The instrument is then

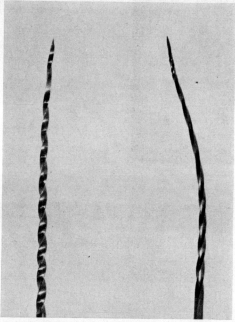

Fig. 133. Instruments with widening (left) and narrowing (right) of the apical end of the flute, both should be discarded. The instrument on the right also shows widening of the flute 'coronal' to the distorted 'apical' end.

removed and its flute wiped clear of material, using, for example, a wool roll. Before reinsertion into the canal, the instrument is examined to ensure that its flute is still of even width. Evidence of widening or narrowing of the flute indicates deformation, with the risk of instrument breakage (*Fig.* 133); such an instrument should be discarded and replaced.

This process is repeated until the reamer passes freely to the apical limit, when the next size of instrument is used. Sometimes difficulty is encountered because of an excessive difference in width between successive sizes. Where this occurs, the smaller instrument which has already been used is ground to remove its tip, and is then used again. This in effect creates an instrument of intermediate size and enables the larger instrument to reach the apical limit. Reaming is continued until the apical part of the canal is clean, as judged by the removal of dentine of normal colour and consistency. At the completion of reaming, a 'stop' conforming in shape to the tip of the largest reamer used will have been formed at the apical limit (*Figs.* 134 and 135).

Each aspect of the coronal and middle parts of the root canal is now filed. To avoid forcing material apically from these parts of the canal, which have not yet been cleaned, each file which is used should fit loosely within the canal. In consequence, the first file selected is three to four sizes smaller than the largest reamer used.

Filing is continued until shavings of clean dentine are removed from all parts of the canal. Since particles of zinc oxide–eugenol cement from an adjacent dressing

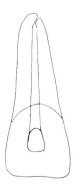

Fig. 134. At the completion of reaming, a 'stop' should have been formed at the apical limit.

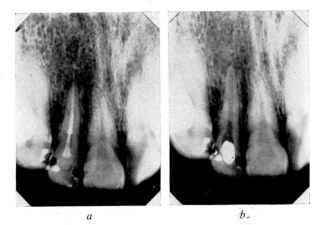

a   *b*

Fig. 135. 2|. Radiographs *a*, before and *b*, after root canal preparation, showing the formation of an apical 'stop'.

may be confused with dentine shavings, such a dressing should be trimmed well clear of the path followed by instruments. Owing to the construction and action of a file, shavings of dentine do not collect on the instrument, but instead tend to remain within the canal, and in consequence are likely to be packed in an apical direction when an instrument is next inserted. To avoid this, periodic irrigation and reaming are necessary.

Some operators use reamers and files alternately during preparation. Thus, the sequence might be a no. 25 reamer, a no. 15 file, a no. 30 reamer, a no. 20 file and so on. This technique, although lengthier, is useful where the root canal is curved, since filing increases its taper and so tends to make the curvature more gradual.

Negotiation of a curved canal may be facilitated by gently bending the instrument a few millimetres from its tip. Rounding the pointed tip of the instrument with a sandpaper disc is also helpful, and makes the formation of a ledge in the region of the curvature less likely. Alternatively, instruments manufactured with rounded ends (Batt instruments) may be used. In difficult cases, a chelating agent is particularly useful. Where failure to negotiate a canal has led to the formation of a ledge in the wall of the canal, however, such an agent should not be used, since its softening action will facilitate deepening of the ledge upon subsequent instrumentation.

7. Removal of existing root fillings

Sometimes during root canal treatment it is necessary to remove an existing root filling.

Where the bulk of the filling is of gutta percha, its removal, although sometimes time-consuming, is usually quite straightforward. As soon as the pulp chamber has been cleared of filling material, the coronal end of the root filling is inspected. Sometimes there is evidence that instead of a root canal cement, which sets, a root canal paste, which does not set, has been used. Alternatively, obvious voids, sometimes radiographically apparent also, may be visible (*Fig.* 135). In cases such as

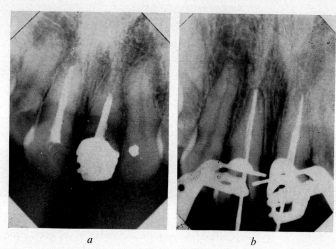

a   *b*

Fig. 136. 1|1. *a*, Before treatment; *b*, Radiographic examination for assessing the working lengths, performed immediately after penetrating the existing root fillings and reaching the probable levels of the apical limits.

these it may be possible to insert a reamer or file alongside the filling and to pull it out. After this it is a simple matter to remove the remaining material.

Where a filling of gutta percha and cement has been well condensed and cannot be pulled out, the root filling is first softened with a heated probe and the pulp chamber then flooded with chloroform. This dissolves and softens not only gutta percha but also some root canal cements. If it is necessary to seal a solvent within the pulp cavity for a few days to obtain a more prolonged action, eucalyptol, being less volatile, is preferable; it is inserted on a wool pledget.

Small reamers are used to penetrate the softened gutta percha and are gradually worked in an apical direction. From time to time more chloroform is added. Where possible a slightly larger instrument is used once a few millimetres' progress has been made, since a fine instrument can easily be broken when surrounded by a mass of filling material. Directly the vicinity of the probable apical limit has been reached, the radiographic examination necessary for assessing the working length is made (*Fig.* 136). After this has been done, the remaining part of the root filling is removed with progressively larger instruments. This should be done carefully, otherwise root-filling material may be driven into the periapical tissues (*Fig.* 137).

Where the entire length of the root canal was filled, of course, instrumentation must extend as far as the apical foramen. Once the desired level has been reached, progressively larger reamers, followed by files, are used to remove the remaining material and to prepare the canal.

A silver point is generally more difficult to remove than gutta percha, especially if the root has been properly filled. A point which protrudes into the pulp chamber of a posterior tooth can sometimes be grasped with a pair of pliers and loosened by rotation, following which it may be withdrawn and the remainder of the filling material removed with reamers and files. Where a point has been severed flush with

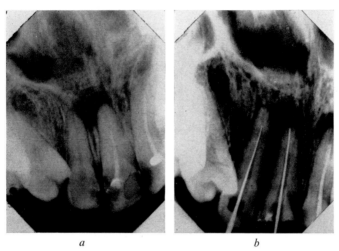

a   *b*

Fig. 137. 1|. *a*, Before treatment; *b*, Root-filling material has been driven into the periapical region by careless instrumentation.

the base of the pulp chamber, it may sometimes be prised from the canal with an excavator, especially if the surrounding cement can first be softened with chloroform and instruments worked alongside the point.

Where a section of silver point has been used to fill just the apical part of the canal, it is hardly ever possible to remove it by way of the pulp chamber unless it is of the type with a threaded extension at its coronal end (Chapter 8). If such a threaded extension is present, cement in the vicinity of the extension is first removed with the aid of a solvent, such as chloroform. A hollow cylindrical handle, used to insert this form of point at the time of root filling, is then introduced into the canal and an attempt made to screw it onto the extension. On the occasions when this is successful, it may be possible to withdraw the point from the canal.

Root fillings are occasionally encountered which apparently consist entirely of zinc phosphate cement. Such fillings are virtually impossible to remove, partly because of their hardness and partly because their colours are often such that in the depths of a root canal they cannot be distinguished from the adjoining dentine. In cases such as these and others where the filling cannot be removed, surgical treatment, in the form of periapical surgery or extraction, is necessary.

8. Irrigation

The debris produced by reamers and files but incompletely removed by these instruments would, if left, impede antiseptic medication of the canal and might hinder its filling. Also, there is evidence that reaming and filing produce a layer of 'smeared' dentine on the walls of the root canal, somewhat similar to that produced by cutting instruments in coronal preparations (McComb and Smith, 1975). The object of irrigation, both during and after the completion of instrumentation, is to remove both debris and, if possible, smeared dentine.

Complex devices relying on pumps for the aspiration of irrigating solutions introduced into the root canal have been described, but these are used infrequently. Instead, a glass–metal pattern of syringe (*Fig.* 138) or a disposable, presterilized

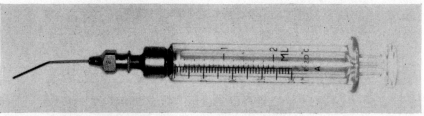

Fig. 138. A glass–metal syringe for irrigating root canals.

syringe is generally employed. The bevelled point of the syringe needle is ground flat to prevent it catching on the root canal wall. Irrigating solutions must not be forced into the periapical region but must be allowed to escape coronally. The needle of the syringe should therefore fit loosely within the canal and the solution should be injected slowly.

At the completion of instrumentation and irrigation, the pulp cavity should be dried thoroughly to prevent residual solution diluting, and possibly inactivating, the antiseptic dressing sealed in the tooth. Preliminary drying of the pulp cavity may be achieved with a high velocity aspirator or by retracting the plunger of the syringe and so sucking fluid back into the barrel. Absorbent paper points are used to remove any residual solution. Compressed air should not be used within the pulp cavity, since this carries a risk of surgical emphysema (Shovelton, 1957). A possible case of death from this cause has been reported (Rickles and Joshi, 1963).

9. Irrigating solutions

Of the many solutions which have been advocated for irrigation, hydrogen peroxide (10 vol. strength), sodium hypochlorite (1–6 per cent) and chelating agents are probably the most popular.

Formerly, 5 per cent sodium hypochlorite was widely used, but Spangberg (1973) has demonstrated that, at this strength, vital tissue is broken down, and in consequence periapical irritation could result. The use of more dilute preparations is probably advisable, therefore; one such preparation is 'Milton', which is a 1 per cent solution of electrolytic sodium hypochlorite. It should be noted that sodium hypochlorite solutions lead to a gradual corrosion of carbon steel instruments. Also, if left within a root canal syringe they crystallize and cause jamming of the plunger within the barrel; after use with such a solution, therefore, the syringe should be dismantled and washed without undue delay.

Sodium hypochlorite solution may be used alone or in conjunction with hydrogen peroxide. In the latter procedure, separate syringes are used to irrigate the canal alternately with the two solutions. This leads to effervesence, with the release of nascent oxygen and the resultant dislodgement of debris. Where peroxide is used, it must be eliminated from the pulp cavity before the crown is sealed, otherwise oxygen may be evolved afterwards as a result of contact with blood or tissue fluid. Besides causing pressure within the periapical region, this could force debris and micro-organisms into these tissues. This is prevented by irrigating with hypochlorite to eliminate any residual peroxide. Since there is evidence that hypochlorite may crystallize on the root canal walls and so interfere with later adaptation of the root filling (Gutiérrez and Garcia, 1968), the canal should be irrigated finally with sterile water.

Chelating agents combine with calcium ions, so decalcifying the dentinal walls of a root canal and facilitating its preparation. The chelating agent recommended by Nygaard-Ostby (1957) is ethylene diamine tetra-acetic acid (EDTA), made up as follows:

Disodium salt of EDTA	17·0 g
Distilled water	100·0 ml
5 N sodium hydroxide	9·25 ml

An antiseptic of the quaternary ammonium group such as cetrimide may be added to the solution as a precaution against extraneous contamination.

There seems little doubt about the efficacy of EDTA as an aid in root canal preparation. Thus, von de Fehr and Nygaard-Ostby (1963) found that EDTA produced a partial demineralization of dentine to a depth of 20–30 μ within a few minutes, whilst Patterson (1963) demonstrated a significant softening of the dentine bordering the root canal from its use. However, recent work by Fraser (1974) suggests that the softening action is confined to the coronal and middle parts of the canal, with the apical dentine remaining unaffected.

When used to facilitate root canal preparation by its decalcifying action, EDTA solution may be applied either by using it to moisten instruments or with the aid of a root canal syringe. Alternatively, a cream preparation recommended by Stewart et al. (1969) may be used. This is known as R.C.Prep. and consists of disodium EDTA and urea peroxide in a water-soluble base. Instruments coated with the cream are used to prepare the canal. Periodically the canal is irrigated with sodium hypochlorite solution, which reacts with the urea peroxide and leads to effervescence, with the release of oxygen and the dislodgement of debris.

Solutions of EDTA may also be used to advantage as irrigating agents. Both Gutiérrez and Garcia (1968) and McComb and Smith (1975) found that irrigation with EDTA solution produces a smoother canal than that resulting from the use of sodium hypochlorite solutions. There is also evidence that irrigation with such a solution removes much of the smeared dentine from the canal (McComb and Smith, 1975; McComb et al., 1976).

Preparations of EDTA may be neutralized by the use of calcium or sodium hypochlorite solutions. Since they may damage periapical bone they should not be sealed within the root canal.

REFERENCES

Ainamo J. and Löe H. (1968) A stereomicroscopic investigation of the anatomy of the root apices of 910 maxillary and mandibular teeth. *Odontol. Tidskr.* **76**, 417.

Auerbach M. B. (1953) Antibiotics vs. instrumentation in endodontics. *N.Y. St. Dent. J.* **19**, 225.

Barnard D. (1974) The Carousel endometer. *J. Br. Endodontic Soc.* **7**, 28.

Benjamin K. A. and Dowson J. (1974) Incidence of two root canals in human mandibular incisor teeth. *Oral Surg.* **38**, 122.

Blank L. W., Tenca J. I. and Pelleu G. B. (1975) Reliability of electronic measuring devices in endodontic therapy. *J. Endodontol.* **1**, 141.

Chapman C. E. (1971) The correlation between apical infection and instrumentation in endodontics. *J. Br. Endodontic Soc.* **5**, 76.

Craig R. G. and Peyton F. A. (1963) Physical properties of stainless steel endodontic files and reamers. *Oral Surg.* **16**, 206.

Davis S. R., Brayton S. M. and Goldman M. (1972) The morphology of the prepared root canal: a study utilizing injectable silicone. *Oral Surg.* **34**, 642.

Fraser J. G. (1974) Chelating agents: their softening effect on root canal dentin. *Oral Surg.* **37**, 803.

Fromme H. G. and Riedel H. (1972) Treatment of dental root canals and the marginal contact between filling material and tooth, studied by scanning electronic microscopy. *J. Br. Endodontic Soc.* **6**, 17.

Guldener P. H. and Imobersteg C. (1972) New method of measuring the exact length of root canal instruments. *J. Br. Endodontic Soc.* **6**, 51.

Gutiérrez J. H. and Garcia J. (1968) Microscopic and macroscopic investigation on results of mechanical preparation of root canals. *Oral Surg.* **25**, 108.

Haga C. S. (1968) Microscopic measurements of root canal preparations following instrumentation. *J. Br. Endodontic Soc.* **2**, 41.

Heling B. and Karmon A. (1976) Determining tooth length with bisecting angle radiographs. *J. Br. Endodontic Soc.* **9**, 75.

Inoue N. (1972) Dental 'stethoscope' measures root canal. *Dent. Surv.* **48**, 38.

Ingle J. I. and LeVine M. (1958) The need for uniformity of endodontic instruments, equipment and filling materials. In: Grossman, L. I. (ed.), *Transactions of the 2nd International Conference on Endodontics.* Philadelphia, University of Pennsylvania, pp. 123–43.

Krueger L. F. (1935) Root canal therapy and root canal filling. *J. Can. Dent. Assoc.* **1**, 533.

Laws A. J. (1971) Prevalence of canal irregularities in mandibular incisors: a radiographic study. *N.Z. Dent. J.* **67**, 181.

McComb D. and Smith D. C. (1975) A preliminary scanning electron microscopic study of root canals after endodontic procedures. *J. Endodontol.* **1**, 238.

McComb D., Smith D. C. and Beagrie G. S. (1976) The results of *in vivo* endodontic chemo-mechanical instrumentation—a scanning electron microscopic study. *J. Br. Endodontic Soc.* **9**, 11.

Moodnik R. M., Dorn S. O., Feldman M. J., Levey M. and Borden B. G. (1976) Efficacy of biomechanical instrumentation: a scanning electron microscopic study. *J. Endodontol.* **2**, 261.

Nicholls E. (1962) The efficacy of cleansing of the root canal. *Br. Dent. J.* **112**, 167.

Nygaard-Ostby B. (1957) Chelation in root canal therapy. *Odontol. Tidskr.* **65**, 3.

Patterson S. S. (1963) *In vivo* and *in vitro* studies of the effect of the disodium salt of ethylene-diamine tetra-acetate on human dentine and its endodontic implications. *Oral Surg.* **16**, 83.

Rankine-Wilson R. W. and Henry P. (1965) The bifurcated root canal in lower anterior teeth. *J. Am. Dent. Assoc.* **70**, 1162.

Rickles N. H. and Joshi B. A. (1963) A possible case in a human and an investigation in dogs of death from air embolism during root canal therapy. *J. Am. Dent. Assoc.* **67**, 397.

Rowe A. H. R. and Forrest J. O. (1973) The endo-meter: a new method for adjusting the length of root canal instruments. *Br. Dent. J.* **134**, 437.

Saunders M. (1970) Length control of root canal instruments: an improved system. *Br. Dent. J.* **129**, 337.

Seidberg B. H., Alibrandi B. V., Fine H. and Logue B. (1975) Clinical investigation of measuring working lengths of root canals with an electronic device and with digital-tactile sense. *J. Am. Dent. Assoc.* **90**, 379.

Shovelton D. S. (1957) Surgical emphysema as a complication of dental operations. *Br. Dent. J.* **102**, 125.

Spangberg L. (1973) Cellular reaction to intracanal medicaments. In: Grossman L. I. (ed.), *Transactions of the 5th International Conference on Endodontics.* Philadelphia, University of Pennsylvania, pp. 108–23.

Stewart G. G. (1955) The importance of chemomechanical preparation of the root canal. *Oral Surg.* **8**, 993.

Stewart G. G., Kapsimalis P. and Rappaport H. (1969) EDTA and urea peroxide for root canal preparation. *J. Am. Dent. Assoc.* **78**, 335.

Sunada I. (1962) New method for measuring the length of the root canal. *J. Dent. Res.* **41**, 375.

Vessey R. A. (1969) The effect of filing versus reaming on the shape of the prepared root canal. *Oral Surg.* **27**, 543.

von de Fehr F. R. and Nygaard-Ostby B. (1963) Effect of EDTAC and sulfuric acid on root canal dentine. *Oral Surg.* **16**, 199.

Vyzantiadou A. and Nicholls E. (1969) Root canal morphology following instrumentation. *Acta Stomatol. Greek Dent. Assoc.* **13**, 174.

FURTHER READING

Craig R. G., McIlwain E. D. and Peyton F. A. (1968) Bending and torsion properties of endodontic instruments. *Oral Surg.* **25**, 239.

Gurncy B. F. (1974) Clinical pharmacology in endodontics and intracanal medicaments. *Dent. Clin. North Am.* **18**, 257–68.

Levin H. J. (1967) Access cavities. *Dent. Clin. North Am.* **11**, 701–10.

Chapter 7

Antiseptic medication

The term 'antiseptic medication' denotes the application of an antiseptic agent to the walls of the pulp cavity with the object of eliminating micro-organisms still present after cleaning.

The antiseptic agent which is used should be capable of eliminating all species of micro-organisms liable to be present. Furthermore, since tissue exudate may enter by way of the apical foramen, the agent should be active in the presence of protein derivatives and should not limit its own diffusion by precipitation of albumin. To reach organisms located in minor irregularities of the canal, it should also be freely diffusible. This obviously implies diffusion of the agent in an apical direction. Another highly desirable property, therefore, is that whilst being lethal to micro-organisms, it is not irritant to pulpal or periapical tissue. Finally, it should not stain the tooth, nor should it interfere with bacteriological examination of the canal when this form of examination is to be used. Unfortunately, no single agent fulfils all these requirements.

MICROBIAL FLORA OF INFECTED ROOT CANALS

As would be expected, most species of organisms present in the mouth have also been isolated from infected root canals. Although studies differ in the frequencies which they report for individual species of organisms, they agree in certain broad aspects. The large majority—from 80 to 90 per cent—of organisms isolated are Gram-positive; most of these are streptococci, predominantly of the viridans variety. Gram-negative organisms, particularly rods, are isolated from roughly 5–10 per cent of canals, whilst yeast forms, mainly *Candida albicans*, are present in up to 10 per cent of cases. Generally, the infecting organisms are isolated in pure culture, but up to 40 per cent of canals yield mixed cultures of two or more species.

Attempts to isolate viruses from cases of pulpal and periapical disease have been unsuccessful. The isolation of pleuropneumonia-like organisms (mycoplasma) from human root canals has been reported by Serene and Anderson (1967).

METHODS OF ANTISEPTIC MEDICATION

There are three main methods of antiseptic medication:
1. Topical application of chemical antiseptics.
2. Electromedication.
3. Topical application of antibiotics.

142

Medication with the sulphonamide group of drugs will not be discussed, since there is evidence that these drugs are, at best, no more effective than chemical antiseptics, no doubt because they are bacteriostatic rather than bactericidal in the concentrations in which they may be used.

1. Topical application of chemical antiseptics

Most of the chemical antiseptics used in the past fall far short of the requirements which have just been discussed, and will not be considered. Into this category fall such drugs as phenol, formalin, cresol and formalin in combination, the essential oils, silver nitrate and various dyes.

The following chemicals are regarded by most authorities as acceptable and effective agents: camphorated paramonochlorphenol, beechwood creosote and cresatin.

Camphorated paramonochlorphenol (CMCP) is made by mixing crystals of paramonochlorphenol with camphor, when liquefaction occurs spontaneously. Various proportions of the two constituents are advocated, the most common being 7 parts of camphor to 3 parts of paramonochlorphenol. Whilst CMCP is a more powerful bactericidal agent than phenol, it is much less irritant and does not coagulate albumin. It is compatible with penicillin and, as described later, has been used in conjunction with it.

Recently, attention has been directed to the efficacy of more dilute forms of paramonochlorphenol. It has been demonstrated both by Avny et al. (1973) and by Taylor et al. (1976) that a 2·0 per cent aqueous solution of this drug showed a much deeper penetration of root canal dentine than CMCP. A 1·0 per cent aqueous solution of paramonochlorphenol has been shown *in vitro* to be effective against a variety of micro-organisms encountered in infected root canals (Harrison and Madonia, 1970), and to be appreciably less toxic in experimental animals than CMCP (Harrison and Madonia, 1971).

Although beechwood creosote is an effective antiseptic, it is also a moderately severe irritant, occupying in this respect a position between phenol and CMCP. Like the latter drug, it also has been combined with penicillin as a root canal dressing.

Cresatin, or metacresylacetate, is favoured particularly by American workers. It is stated to have a low surface tension and to cause little irritation. It has an anodyne action on periapical tissue and residual pulpal tissue. The antiseptic efficiency of cresatin has been found by Grossman (1972) to be less than that of other phenolic derivatives, and for this reason it is sometimes used in combination with paramonochlorphenol.

Sullivan and Jolly (1955) suggested a mixture of aminoacridine, cetrimide, methyl parahydroxybenzoate and propyl parahydroxybenzoate, whilst Atkinson and Hampson (1964) reported encouraging clinical results following the use of such a mixture with the addition of chlorhexidine. On the basis of cytotoxic studies, Spangberg (1973) has recommended an aqueous solution of 2·0 per cent iodine and 4·0 per cent potassium iodide.

Each of the preparations described is in the form of a liquid. Formerly, such preparations were applied directly to the root canal by the insertion of an absorbent paper point moistened with the drug. However, in view of the diffusibility of the chemical antiseptics commonly used, this is now generally considered unnecessary.

Instead, a wool pledget moistened with the drug is sealed in the pulp chamber, leaving the root canal empty. Wantulok and Brown (1972) have demonstrated that following such treatment both CMCP and cresatin diffuse to the apical foramen.

If an absorbent point is used it should not impinge upon periapical tissue. The point should not fit the canal tightly, since entry of periapical exudate into the canal will cause it to swell and may make its removal difficult. The butt end of the point should project for a short distance into the pulp chamber so that it may be easily removed at the next visit (*Fig.* 139). In a wide root canal the point may be

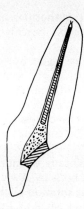

Fig. 139. A point used to apply an antiseptic preparation to the root canal walls should not fit the canal tightly. Between the cement seal and the coronal end of the point is a layer of cottonwool or gutta percha.

moistened with antiseptic before it is introduced. However, in a narrow canal a moistened point is likely to buckle during insertion. In these cases, therefore, the point is introduced first and is then moistened with the antiseptic, either with the aid of forceps or by moistening the wool pledget placed in the tooth before the pulp cavity is sealed.

Certain of the organisms initially present in the pulp cavity may be resistant to a particular chemical. Thus, it is feasible that the repeated application of this chemical may eventually lead to a pure growth of resistant organisms. For this reason it has been advocated that at each visit a different chemical be used to dress the canal. This is known as 'rotation of medication'.

Besides being applied in liquid form, chemical antiseptics may also be incorporated in a cream base. Thus, Stewart and Gautieri (1962) reported very good results using a mixture of CMCP, thymol and hexachlorophene in a base of Xylocaine (lignocaine) ointment.

2. Electromedication

Electromedication is also known as 'electrolytic medication', 'electrosterilization', 'ionic medication' and 'ionization'. Although fairly popular in the past, it is now used relatively infrequently.

In electromedication, an electric current is passed through an electrolyte within the pulp cavity, one electrode being placed in the root canal and the other in the patient's hand. This results not only in an increase in ionization, but also in the migration of ions towards their respective electrodes. Ions reaching the electrode in the root canal regain molecular form, and the molecules are discharged in the nascent state. In this state they have a greater bactericidal effect. The claim that there is greater penetration of the drug into the periapical tissues does not seem to have been substantiated.

There is no convincing evidence that electromedication is significantly superior to medication with chemical antiseptics sealed within the pulp cavity. Despite the claims which have been made, sterilization of the canal after one treatment by this technique cannot be relied upon. Also, whereas antiseptic drugs sealed within the tooth act during the interval between visits, electromedication does not. For these reasons, only a brief account of electromedication will be given.

a. Electrolyte

Of a variety of electrolytes which have been advocated, the one found to be the most effective by Grossman and Appleton (1931), and probably the most popular, is a zinc iodide–iodine solution, made up as follows:

Zinc iodide	15·0 g
Iodine crystals	0·6 g
Distilled water	50·0 ml

This solution ionizes into Zn^+ (cations) and I^- (anions). It may occasionally stain dentine.

b. Apparatus

The apparatus consists of an electrolyser and two electrodes. The electrolyser supplies a current of up to about 5 mA. There is evidence that placing the positive electrode, or anode, within the root canal and the other in the patient's hand gives a greater antibacterial effect than the reverse arrangement (Grossman and Appleton, 1931). The electrode placed within the canal is a thin iridioplatinum wire.

c. Technique

The tooth should be isolated by a rubber dam, since less current will be tolerated if the electrolyte contacts adjacent soft tissue or other teeth. Metallic articles such as rings are removed from the patient's hand, otherwise a short circuit may result. The electrode held by the patient must make a broad area of contact with the skin, otherwise the latter may be burned; it may be wrapped in a damp cloth.

The prepared root canal is flooded with the electrolyte and the other electrode inserted so that its tip is just short of the apical limit. The current is turned on and gradually increased until the patient is just aware of sensitivity; it is then reduced slightly and left at this level. During electromedication the electrolyte within the pulp cavity has to be replenished periodically to replace that lost by evaporation and diffusion.

The length of time for which current is passed depends on the level of current which the patient tolerates. It is generally accepted that a total of 30 mA-minutes is sufficient for any one appointment. Thus, if the patient tolerates no more than 3 mA, current is passed for 10 minutes. Before the electrode is removed from the tooth, the current must be switched off, otherwise pain will be felt. It is usually advocated that the drug used as the electrolyte is also employed to dress the pulp cavity until the next appointment.

Electromedication with high-frequency current

The use of a high-frequency current for electromedication has from time to time been advocated. The object of this form of treatment is to raise the temperature of the electrolyte and the neighbouring periapical region sufficiently to destroy micro-organisms but not to burn the periapical tissues. It is doubtful if this technique has any significant advantage (Nicholls, 1962).

3. Topical application of antibiotics

Certain selected antibiotics, such as penicillin, satisfy many of the requirements of a root canal antiseptic, in that they are active in the presence of tissue fluid, do not stain the tooth and are virtually non-irritant to tissue cells. Since they are non-irritant, very high concentrations of antibiotic may be used, and so a bactericidal effect achieved. At present, however, there is no single antibiotic effective against all micro-organisms liable to be present in contaminated root canals. A combination of antibiotics, or of one or more antibiotics with a chemical antiseptic, is therefore necessary.

Since preparations containing very high concentrations of antibiotics may be used, it might be supposed that significantly fewer applications of such a preparation would be needed for eradication of organisms than with accepted chemical antiseptics. Whilst this is the experience of Grossman (1951), neither Ostrander (1958) nor Ingle and Zeldow (1958) have found it so. From this aspect, therefore, the choice between antibiotic preparations and chemicals for antiseptic medication of the pulp cavity is largely a matter of personal preference. However, where the pulp is still vital at the beginning of treatment and the pulp cavity presumably only lightly contaminated, it would certainly seem unnecessary to use antibiotic preparations.

a. Possible objections to antibiotics

Four main criticisms have been made concerning the use of antibiotics as root canal antiseptics.

First, it has been suggested that resistant strains of micro-organisms may develop. If at a later date these organisms were to cause disease elsewhere in the body, treatment could be handicapped by their resistance to the drugs already used. The development of resistance would result from using an inadequate concentration of the particular antibiotic within the root canal. However, if the canal is filled almost completely with the preparation, the concentration of antibiotic in the canal should virtually correspond to that in the original preparation. Thus, so long as the vehicle permits a high concentration of antibiotic, and provided the pulp cavity has been thoroughly cleaned beforehand, the possibility of organisms becoming resistant appears remote. To date, there seems no evidence that the use of antibiotics in this way has led to resistant strains of organisms.

The second possibility is that an allergic response may be elicited in a patient already sensitive to an antibiotic; this hazard applies particularly to penicillin. Grossman (1974) states that in his experience this has occurred only once amongst 'several thousand cases' treated with polyantibiotic pastes containing penicillin since 1949. Fox and Moodnik (1964) record a case of sensitivity to a polyantibiotic paste containing penicillin, whilst Bender and Seltzer (1954) cite two known instances of an allergic response to penicillin in 2500 cases. Stewart (1954) also reports two instances of an allergic reaction to root canal dressings containing penicillin, although it is not stated whether the patients were known to be allergic to the drug. Also, an allergic reaction following the use of a neomycin–bacitracin preparation in root canal treatment has been recorded (Pirila and Rantanen, 1960).

The third possibility is that a person who was previously insensitive to an anti-biotic may become sensitized following its use in the root canal. The failure of Grossman (1967) to demonstrate the presence of penicillin in blood samples following the use of a penicillin-containing polyantibiotic paste in root canal treatment suggests that this is unlikely. Nonetheless, the possibility does exist. Thus, Schmidt (1956) published a case report which strongly suggested the development of sensitivity to one of the constituents of a polyantibiotic preparation. Also, the passage of tetracycline from the pulp cavity into the circulatory system has been demonstrated in experimental animals (Page et al., 1973).

Finally, where treatment is being controlled by bacteriological examinations of the pulp cavity, it is possible that the growth of organisms transferred from the latter to the culture medium may be inhibited by remnants of antibiotic transferred at the same time. This implies that the dressing has had a bacteriostatic and not a bactericidal effect. The study of Grossman et al. (1957) shows that this disadvantage may be partly overcome, at least with the polyantibiotic preparation devised by Grossman (1951), by removing the preparation mechanically with absorbent paper points before examining the canal. Furthermore, any penicillin transferred from the canal may be inactivated by including penicillinase in the culture medium. Some antibiotics, for example streptomycin, are in any case inactivated by the constituents normally incorporated in the liquid culture media used.

b. Antibiotic preparations available

Three forms of antibiotic preparations have been used: aqueous solutions, impregnated absorbent points and pastes. The use of aqueous solutions for injection into periapical lesions or for irrigation of root canals is now obsolete. The former procedure is irrational, since most periapical lesions are sterile, whilst the latter form of treatment is of relatively little value, since the length of time for which a solution is in contact with the infecting organisms is very short, and in any case aqueous solutions of some antibiotics, including penicillin, lose potency relatively quickly. It is for the second reason that impregnated absorbent points have not become popular, since liberation of the antibiotics depends on their passage into aqueous solution in the root canal. For this reason, the paste form of preparation is generally used.

Many different antibiotic pastes have been advocated. Probably the best known is that devised by Grossman (1951) and known as 'Grossman's paste', or, from the initials of its constituents, 'PBSC'. The formula of this is:

Potassium penicillin G	1 000 000 units
Bacitracin	10 000 units
Streptomycin sulphate	1·0 g
Sodium caprylate	1·0 g
Silicone fluid, 3–30 centistokes	3·0 ml

Silicone fluid is used as the vehicle since its relative immiscibility with water prevents rapid loss of potency of the antibiotics. The low surface tension of the silicone fluid used facilitates diffusion of the preparation. The remainder of the compound is formulated with the object of being bactericidal against the entire range of organisms found in contaminated root canals. Gram-positive organisms are eliminated by penicillin, Gram-negative organisms by streptomycin and yeast forms by the chemical, sodium caprylate. Bacitracin is included for its action against penicillin-resistant organisms, such as enterococci and certain staphylococci.

Instead of sodium caprylate, 10 000 units of nystatin, an antifungal antibiotic, may be used.

Bender and Seltzer (1952) reported on a preparation consisting of penicillin, streptomycin, chloramphenicol and sodium caprylate, in a base of silicone fluid, with the addition of barium sulphate to make the preparation radio-opaque. Stewart (1953) has recommended a paste consisting of penicillin, chloramphenicol and chlorcyclizine hydrochloride in a base of Xylocaine ointment. Chlorcyclizine hydrochloride is an antihistamine and is added for its antifungal effect. Sommer et al. (1961) described a mixture of CMCP and penicillin; one drop of CMCP is spatulated with one tablet containing 50 000 units of penicillin to form a paste. Instead of CMCP, beechwood creosote may be used.

To avoid the use of penicillin, Curson (1966) has recommended the following preparation:

Neomycin sulphate	5·0 g
Bacitracin	100 000 units
Polymyxin B sulphate	2·0 mega units
Nystatin	1·5 mega units
White soft paraffin	8·5 g
Silicone MS200/1000cs.	8·5 g

A similar preparation, but with a polyethylene glycol instead of a silicone base, is described by Winter (1966).

Antibiotic–corticosteroid pastes also have been advocated for use in root canal treatment, mainly with the object of preventing an acute periapical inflammation following instrumentation within the root canal, or of eliminating such a condition when it already exists. There seems no published evidence that they are any more effective for this purpose than other preparations. Also, potentially serious sequelae could arise in the event of spread of resistant organisms periapically following suppression of the defence mechanism of the periapical tissues. If such pastes are used, therefore, particular care should be taken to ensure they are confined to the root canal, since deliberate forcing of the paste beyond the apical foramen may well result in inoculating the periapical tissues with residual micro-organisms from the pulp cavity.

c. Indications for using polyantibiotic pastes: selection of paste
Although there is generally little or no clinical advantage in employing a poly-antibiotic paste in preference to a chemical antiseptic, instances do arise when their use is justified. For example, in a small minority of cases evidence of root canal infection and periapical irritation persist despite apparently thorough cleaning of the pulp cavity and treatment with chemical antiseptics; in such teeth, the use of a polyantibiotic paste is usually effective. Since antibiotics are in general less irritant to periapical tissues than chemical antiseptics, there is an argument for using such a paste where the apical foramen has been inadvertently widened by over-instru-mentation and in immature teeth with wide apical foramina. Also, there is evidence that chemical antiseptics lose potency within a root canal more rapidly than poly-antibiotic preparations (Uchin and Parris, 1963). Thus, if the interval between the penultimate visit and that at which the tooth is root filled is longer than 14 days, the use of a polyantibiotic preparation is advantageous.

The patient should be questioned about sensitivity to antibiotics before poly-antibiotic preparations are used. In view of the potential dangers of an allergic reaction, an antibiotic to which a patient is known to be sensitive must not be used. Because of the risk, albeit remote, of sensitizing a patient to a particular antibiotic, pastes containing antibiotics which are commonly administered systemically, especially penicillin, are best avoided. A preparation comprising as far as possible antibiotics reserved for topical use, such as that described by Curson (1966), is preferable.

d. Technique of using antibiotic pastes

For the maximum antiseptic effect to be obtained, more care is needed in handling antibiotic preparations than chemical antiseptics.

To avoid dilution of the paste, or inactivation of one or more of its constituents, an absorbent point is first inserted into the canal to check that the solutions used

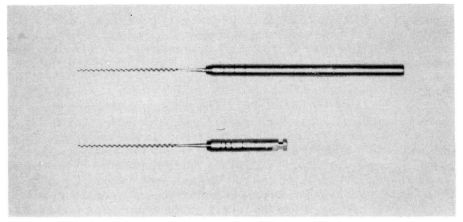

Fig. 140. Straight and right-angle Lentulo spirals (spiral root fillers).

for irrigation have been removed. The instruments used to handle the paste should be sterile and dry; they should not be hot, since some antibiotics are destroyed by heat. To avoid unnecessary risk of sensitization, the paste should not be allowed to contact the soft tissues of either the patient or the operator.

To obtain the maximum concentration of paste and so ensure a bactericidal rather than a bacteriostatic effect, the root canal is filled with paste. With some proprietary preparations, a syringe is used to inject the paste; in this technique the needle of the syringe is introduced into the canal as far as possible without binding, and then withdrawn slightly before injecting the paste whilst slowly removing the needle from the canal.

An alternative method of application, which is also used when the preparation is dispensed in some other form of container, is to transfer paste to the pulp chamber and then to propel this apically along the root canal by means of a Lentulo spiral (*Fig.* 140). This pattern of instrument, also known as a 'spiral root filler' or a 'rotary paste filler', is made in up to eight different widths and may be used in conjunction with a right-angle or a straight handpiece. Rotating the spiral in reverse propels paste out of the canal instead of into it. These instruments are relatively fragile and easily break if introduced so far into the canal that they bind.

Some operators insert an absorbent point into the canal to bring the preparation into close contact with the root dentine. This inevitably reduces the amount of paste which may be used. So long as the base of the compound is freely diffusible, it would seem more rational to omit the absorbent point and to fill the extra space in the canal with paste. Whichever method is followed, care must be taken that the paste is not driven into the periapical region, since apart from possible chemical irritation and conceivably a greater risk of sensitizing the patient, this causes pressure with resultant periapical inflammation. The patient is asked to warn the operator immediately if discomfort is felt during the insertion of paste.

SEALING THE PULP CAVITY

Considerable care should be taken in sealing the pulp cavity to prevent recontamination from leakage of the seal before the next appointment. A zinc oxide–eugenol mixture is used, since it has been shown by Grossman (1939) to give a seal superior to other materials. To prevent possible deformation from mastication prior to setting, a fast-setting mixture is usually advocated. Proprietary zinc oxide pastes, such as Cavit, give as effective a seal as a cement mixed at the chairside (Parris et al., 1964).

Before inserting the seal, excess medicament as far as the coronal orifice of the root canal is removed, and the walls of the pulp chamber and the coronal opening in the crown dried. Unless the pulp cavity has been dressed with a wool pledget moistened with a chemical antiseptic, a layer of cottonwool or gutta percha is placed in the pulp chamber to prevent cement entering the root canal during insertion of the seal and when the pulp cavity is next opened (*Fig.* 139). The remainder of the cavity is now sealed with cement, which is moulded flush with the margins of the opening. Before the patient is dismissed, the seal is checked to ensure it is clear of the opposing teeth.

When the antiseptic dressing is in the form of a paste, particular care has to be taken to ensure that the pressure used in placing the seal does not force paste into the periapical region. The patient is asked to warn the operator immediately should discomfort be felt during insertion of the seal. The pressure used to consolidate the cement is as light as possible and is exerted against the walls of the cavity rather than in an apical direction. Exacerbation following treatment can occur if these precautions are ignored.

REFERENCES

Atkinson A. M. and Hampson E. L. (1964) Sterilisation of root canals: an evaluation of mixtures containing aminoacridine, cetrimide and chlorhexidine. *Br. Dent. J.* **117**, 526.
Avny W. Y., Heiman G. R., Madonia J. V., Wood N. K. and Smulson M. H. (1973) Autoradiographic studies of the intracanal diffusion of aqueous and camphorated parachlorphenol in endodontics. *Oral Surg.* **36**, 80.
Bender I. B. and Seltzer S. (1952) Combination of antibiotics and fungicides used in treatment of the infected pulpless tooth. *J. Am. Dent. Assoc.* **45**, 293.
Bender I. B. and Seltzer S. (1954) The advantages and disadvantages of the use of antibiotics in endodontics. *Oral Surg.* **7**, 993.
Curson I. (1966) Endodontic techniques. 2, Diagnosis and assessment. *Br. Dent. J.* **121**, 90.
Fox J. and Moodnik R. (1964) Systemic reaction to polyantibiotic root canal dressing. *N.Y. St. Dent. J.* **30**, 282.
Grossman L. I. (1939) A study of temporary fillings as hermetic sealing agents. *J. Dent. Res.* **18**, 67.

Grossman L. I. (1951) Polyantibiotic treatment of pulpless teeth. *J. Am. Dent. Assoc.* **43**, 265.

Grossman L. I. (1967) Evaluation of penicillemia after medication of root canals with a poly-antibiotic. *J. Dent. Res.* **46**, 400.

Grossman L. I. (1972) Sterilization of infected root canals. *J. Am. Dent. Assoc.* **85**, 900.

Grossman L. I. (1974) *Endodontic Practice*, 8th ed. London, Kimpton, p. 257.

Grossman L. I. and Appleton J. L. T. (1931) Experimental and applied studies in electro-sterilization (Part 1). *Dent. Cosmos.* **73**, 147.

Grossman L. I., Parris L. and Cobe H. (1957) Antibacterial effect of residual bacitracin during culturing from root canal. *Oral Surg.* **10**, 426.

Harrison J. W. and Madonia J. V. (1970) Antimicrobial effectiveness of parachlorphenol. *Oral Surg.* **30**, 267.

Harrison J. W. and Madonia J. V. (1971) The toxicity of parachlorphenol. *Oral Surg.* **32**, 90.

Ingle J. I. and Zeldow B. J. (1958) A clinical-laboratory evaluation of three intra-canal antibacterial agents. In: Grossman L. I. (ed.), *Transactions of the 2nd International Conference on Endodontics.* Philadelphia, University of Pennsylvania, pp. 81–95.

Nicholls E. (1962) The efficacy of high-frequency current for root-canal sterilization. *Dent. Practnr Dent. Rec.* **12**, 229.

Ostrander F. D. (1958) The development of antiseptics and antibiotics for use in endodontics. In: Grossman L. I. (ed.), *Transactions of the 2nd International Conference on Endodontics.* Philadelphia, University of Pennsylvania Press, pp. 64–80.

Page D. O., Trump G. N. and Schaeffer L. D. (1973) Pulpal studies. I, Passage of ^{3}H-tetracycline into circulatory system through rat molar pulps. *Oral Surg.* **35**, 555.

Parris L., Kapsimalis P., Cobe H. H. and Evans R. (1964) The effect of temperature change on the sealing properties of temporary filling materials, Part II. *Oral Surg.* **17**, 771.

Pirila V and Rantanen A. V. (1960) Root canal treatment with bacitracin-neomycin as cause of flare-up of allergic eczema. *Oral Surg.* **13**, 589.

Schmidt G. (1956) Penicillin reaction in endodontic treatment (cases and comments). *J. Am. Dent. Assoc.* **52**, 196.

Serene T. P. and Anderson D. L. (1967) Isolation of mycoplasma from human root canals. *J. Dent. Res.* **46**, 395.

Sommer R. F., Ostrander F. D. and Crowley M. C. (1961) *Clinical Endodontics*, 2nd ed. London, Saunders, p. 366.

Spangberg L. (1973) Cellular reaction to intracanal medicaments. In: Grossman L. I. (ed.), *Transactions of the 5th International Conference on Endodontics.* Philadelphia, University of Pennsylvania, pp. 108–123.

Stewart G. G. (1953) An antihistamine-antibiotic compound for root canal medication. *Oral Surg.* **6**, 1338.

Stewart G. G. (1954) An improved antibiotic-antihistamine compound for root canal medication (D.C.P.). *J. Dent. Med.* **9**, 174.

Stewart G. G. and Gautieri R. F. (1962) Reduced inflammatory root canal medication. *Oral Surg.* **15**, 715.

Sullivan H. R. and Jolly M. (1955) Sterilization of pulp canals. *Oral Surg.* **8**, 414.

Taylor G. N., Madonia J. V., Wood N. K. and Heuer M. A. (1976) In vivo autoradiographic study of relative penetrating abilities of aqueous 2% parachlorophenol and camphorated 35% parachlorophenol. *J. Endodontol.* **2**, 81.

Uchin R. A. and Parris L. (1963) Antibacterial activity of endodontic medications after varying time intervals within the root canal. *Oral Surg.* **16**, 608.

Wantulok J. C. and Brown J. I. (1972) An in vitro study of the diffusibility of camphorated parachlorophenol and metacresylacetate in the root canal. *Oral Surg.* **34**, 653.

Winter G. B. (1966) The root treatment of infected permanent incisors in children. *Br. Dent. J.* **120**, 11.

FURTHER READING

Gurney B. F. (1974) Clinical pharmacology in endodontics and intracanal medicaments. *Dent. Clin. North Am.* **18**, 257–68.

Slack G. L. (1958) The microbiology of the pulp and periapical tissues. In: Grossman L. I. (ed.), *Transactions of the 2nd International Conference on Endodontics.* Philadelphia, University of Pennsylvania Press, pp. 39–52.

Chapter 8

Root canal filling

The criteria governing the time at which the root canal is filled are discussed in Chapter 9.

MATERIALS

The prime requirement of a root filling is that it completely obliterate the canal as far as the apical limit, but that it does not extend into the periapical region. To satisfy this requirement the bulk of the canal is filled with a solid material, such as gutta percha or silver, and the remaining gaps with an adaptable substance in the form of a cement. Since all cements are resorbable, the minimum amount of cement should be exposed to the remaining pulp or to the periapical tissues (Langeland, 1974). The silver or gutta percha point which is used should therefore fit as closely as possible against the walls of the prepared canal apically. Both gutta percha and silver are used in the form of points of various sizes, calibrated in width to conform approximately to the different sizes of hand instruments.

1. Advantages and disadvantages of silver and gutta percha points

There seems no firm clinical evidence that the prognosis of root canal treatment is influenced by the choice of gutta percha or silver for root filling. Implantation into bone in experimental animals has shown that both materials are reasonably well tolerated (Hunter, 1957; Spangberg, 1969). Although both Marshall and Massler (1961) and Cooke et al. (1976) found that a gutta percha point and cement sealed the apical part of a root canal more effectively than a silver point and the same cement, the results of Neagley (1969) and Ainley (1970) indicate that the seal using silver is at least as effective as that obtained with gutta percha.

The choice between gutta percha and silver, therefore, depends partly upon personal preference and partly on the circumstances of the individual case.

Compared with gutta percha, silver points are more accurately calibrated, especially in the smaller sizes, can be easily and rapidly sterilized by dry heat using a hot salt sterilizer, and are easier to use in conjunction with a sectional technique when only the apical part of the root canal is to be filled. Also, because they are more rigid, especially in their finer sizes, they are easier to use than gutta percha in the filling of narrow root canals.

Although many of the advantages of gutta percha relate especially to molar teeth, on occasions they apply also to anterior and premolar teeth. One of the main advantages of gutta percha is that by the use of suitable filling techniques it can be adapted closely to the walls of the root canal; thus, where the apical part of the prepared canal deviates from a circular outline, as is often the case with the finer canals of molar teeth (Chapter 12), effective sealing of the apical part of the canal is more likely with gutta percha than silver.

Where the entire length of the root canal is filled with a gutta percha point, excess gutta percha in the pulp chamber is easily removed with a hot instrument. A silver point, on the other hand, has either to be cut with a rotary instrument, which is more difficult, or embedded in cement in the base of the pulp chamber, which in a broken-down tooth decreases the retention available for the coronal restoration. Should removal of some of the root filling be necessary to provide room for a post, gutta percha is easier to cut away than silver; also, cutting of a silver point may disturb the cement seal and lead to renewed periapical irritation. Where only the apical part of the root has been filled with silver and evidence of periapical disease develops, removal of the silver by way of the pulp chamber is generally not possible.

In view of these considerations, silver should only be used where the prepared root canal is relatively straight and roughly circular in cross-section apically; it is unlikely that a silver point will fit accurately the apical part of a curved canal. A sectional technique to fill just the apical part of the canal with silver is useful where post crown construction is necessary. Unless necessary for post crown construction, however, the use of a sectional silver point technique in a posterior tooth which will not be amenable to periapical surgery in the event of failure is contraindicated, since retreatment by way of the pulp chamber will not be possible. Also, there is evidence that prolonged exposure of a silver point to tissue fluid can lead to corrosion with the formation of silver compounds which are highly cytotoxic (Seltzer et al., 1972; Brady and del Rio, 1975). The use of silver would therefore seem contraindicated in an immature tooth with a wide apical foramen, or where the apical foramen has been inadvertently widened during root canal preparation.

2. Root canal cements

Numerous cements specifically formulated for root filling have been devised.

a. Composition

Many root canal cements are based on zinc oxide–eugenol, which is known to provide a good seal. The following alphabetical list, whilst not exhaustive, includes the better known preparations:

i. '*AH26*': This is an epoxy resin, recommended by Schroeder (1954) as a root canal cement. Feldmann and Nyborg (1964) give the following composition:

Powder	*Liquid*
Bismuth oxide, 60·0%	Bisphenol diglycidyl ether
Hexamethylenetetramine, 25·0%	
Silver powder, 10·0%	
Titanium oxide, 5·0%	

ii. '*Diaket*': According to Stewart (1958), Diaket is a polyketone with 0·5 per cent dihydroxydichlorodiphenyl-methane. The introduction of Diaket as a root canal cement is attributed to Scheufele (1952).

6

iii. '*Endomethasone*': The manufacturer (Spécialités Septodont) states the formula of this preparation to be:

Powder	Liquid
Di-iodothymol, 25·00 g	Eugenol
Trioxymethylene (paraformaldehyde), 2·20 g	
Hydrocortisone acetate, 1·00 g	
Dexamethasone, 0·01 g	
Excipient, 71·79 g	

The excipient is not named, but is presumably zinc oxide.

iv. *Grossman's Sealer*: The sealer devised by Grossman (1958) consists of:

Powder	Liquid
Zinc oxide, 40 parts	Eugenol, 5 parts
Staybelite resin, 30 parts	Oil of sweet almond, 1 part
Bismuth subcarbonate, 15 parts	
Barium sulphate, 15 parts	

A later publication (Grossman, 1974) indicates that the formula has been changed by the omission of oil of sweet almond from the liquid, and the addition of anhydrous sodium borate to the powder.

v. '*Kerr Root Canal Sealer*': This is based on the cement described by Dixon and Rickert (1938):

Powder	Liquid
Zinc oxide, 41·21 parts	Oil of cloves, 78 parts
Precipitated silver, 30·00 parts	Canada balsam, 22 parts
White resin, 16·00 parts	
Thymol iodide, 12·79 parts	

vi. '*Kerr Tubli-Seal*': This preparation is supplied in the form of base and accelerator pastes. The manufacturer (Kerr Sybron Corporation) states that the composition of the mixed pastes is approximately:

Zinc oxide, 57·40%
Oleo resins, 21·25%
Bismuth trioxide, 7·50%
Oils, 7·50%
Thymol iodide, 3·75%
Modifier, 2·60%

vii. '*Kloropercha N-O*': This preparation, although not strictly a cement, is included under this heading since it 'sets' to a relatively firm state. The formula given by Nyborg and Tullin (1965) is:

Powder	Liquid
Zinc oxide, 49·0 parts	Chloroform
White gutta percha, 19·6 parts	
Canada balsam, 19·6 parts	
Colophony resin, 11·8 parts	

A mixture of gutta percha and chloroform is known simply as 'chloropercha'.

viii. '*N2 Permanent*': Various formulae have been given for this cement, probably due in part to a change in composition from time to time. A recent formula

(Sargenti, 1973) is:

Powder	Liquid
Zinc oxide, 69·00%	Eugenol
Lead tetroxide, 12·00%	
Paraformaldehyde, 6·50%	
Bismuth subcarbonate, 5·00%	
Bismuth subnitrate, 2·00%	
Titanium dioxide, 2·00%	
Barium sulphate, 2·00%	
Hydrocortisone, 1·20%	
Prednisolone, 0·21%	
Phenylmercuric borate, 0·09%	

This material will be considered in greater detail in Chapter 15.

ix. *Wach's Cement*: According to Wach et al. (1955), this consists of:

Powder	Liquid
Zinc oxide, 10·0 g	Canada balsam, 20·0 ml
Tricalcium phosphate, 2·0 g	Oil of cloves, 6·0 ml
Bismuth subnitrate, 3·5 g	Eucalyptol, 0·5 ml
Bismuth subiodide, 0·3 g	Beechwood creosote, 0·5 ml
Heavy magnesium oxide, 0·5 g	

In a later publication (McElroy and Wach, 1958) eucalyptol and beechwood creosote are omitted from the liquid.

In addition, many preparations used in restorative dentistry, such as zinc oxide–eugenol materials and polycarboxylate cements, have been suggested for use as root canal cements.

b. Properties

Numerous properties are desirable in a root canal cement. Amongst the more important are that it should effectively seal the apical end of the canal, be non-irritant to the periapical tissues, allow adequate working time during root filling, be dimensionally stable and insoluble in tissue fluid, and have adequate strength and adhesion to dentine to resist disruption of the apical seal during post hole preparation. In addition it should be radio-opaque and easy to mix, and should not stain the tooth.

Numerous studies have been carried out on these various properties, and no one cement has them all. Amongst the readily available cements that can be recommended for routine use are AH26, Diaket and Kerr Root Canal Sealer. AH26 has good adhesion to dentine (Grossman, 1976; McComb and Smith, 1976), but is exceptionally slow-setting; if an amalgam restoration is to be inserted immediately after root filling, a base of phosphate cement should first be inserted to prevent extrusion of root canal cement periapically during condensation of the amalgam. Kerr Sealer tends to stain dentine, largely because of the inclusion of precipitated silver; any surplus of this cement in the crown of an anterior tooth should therefore be removed immediately after root filling. Diaket is rather more difficult to manipulate than the other cements; although it adheres well to dentine (Grossman, 1976), it is more soluble than other cements (McComb and Smith, 1976). Also, there is some evidence that it has a relatively low rate of flow, which presumably would result in a thicker layer of cement between the gutta percha or silver point and the root canal walls apically (Weisman, 1970).

Tubli-Seal, on the other hand, has a high rate of flow, giving a thinner film (Weisman, 1970). However, there is evidence that it is more irritant than other root canal cements (Guttuso, 1963). It may be used where a shorter setting time is required, as, for example, where root filling is to be followed immediately by apicectomy.

Klöropercha N-O has been shown to be associated with a greater degree of leakage than other materials (Higginbotham, 1967). McElroy (1955) states that a 7·5 per cent shrinkage in volume occurs with chloropercha. Such materials are useful, though, where the apical part of a root canal is inaccessible. For example, the canal may divide in the apical part of the root into two major branches. Although both branches may be accessible to instrumentation, filling of one severely restricts access to the other. In such a tooth chloropercha may be forced beyond the level of division into the unfilled canal (*Fig.* 141). Similarly, chloropercha is useful

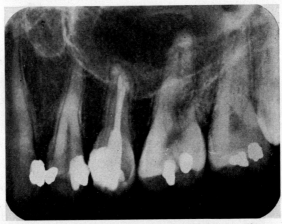

Fig. 141. |5. Division of root canal apically, filled with chloropercha.

where the creation of a ledge in the root canal wall during instrumentation prevents the insertion of a point to the apical limit.

In general, the cements used in restorative dentistry are unsatisfactory for use in the root canal. Polycarboxylate cements have been shown to give a relatively poor seal (Sanders and Dooley, 1974; Barry and Fried, 1975) and to be associated with severe periapical inflammation when used as root fillings in experimental animals (Seltzer et al., 1976). The speed of set and viscous nature of some proprietary zinc oxide–eugenol cements may make their manipulation within a root canal difficult.

TECHNIQUE

1. Preparation for filling

Unless Batt-ended instruments have been used, the extreme apical end of the prepared root canal will be cone-shaped, corresponding to the cone-shaped tip of the largest reamer used during preparation. Since the ends of both gutta percha and silver points tend to be rounded, a point which matches in width the largest instrument used to prepare the canal will stop slightly short of the apical limit (*Fig.* 142).

This discrepancy may easily be overcome with most sizes of silver points by trimming their apical ends with sandpaper disks. However, with silver points smaller than No. 40 this is not possible, and the gap has to be filled with cement. With the larger sizes of gutta percha point, it is possible to soften the extreme end of the point by immersion in chloroform and then to mould this to the required shape by inserting the point into the canal and exerting gentle pressure in an apical direction. Sometimes, especially with gutta percha, a point of the same size as the largest reamer used during preparation stops well short of the apical limit, and a narrower point, often about two sizes smaller, has to be used.

The point eventually selected should be a snug fit in the apical part of the canal. Just as the cementing agent is not expected to compensate for a poorly fitting gold inlay in the crown of a tooth, so a root canal cement should not be expected to compensate for a loose-fitting gutta percha or silver point.

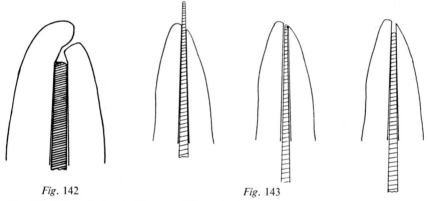

Fig. 142   *Fig.* 143

Fig. 142. If the apical end of the root-filling point is rounded, it will stop slightly short of the apical limit.

Fig. 143. Where instrumentation has extended beyond the apical foramen, a matched point is often a slack fit apically (*centre*). The apical end of the point should be removed section by section by the amount shown (*left*). A larger point generally binds before it reaches the apical foramen and is unsatisfactory (*right*).

When a suitable point has been fitted, the length projecting beyond the occlusal measuring point should correspond to the difference between the total length of the point and the working length. This is checked by direct measurement. The point may also be marked at a distance from its tip equal to the working length. With silver, a carborundum disk is used to do this; with gutta percha, a warmed plastic instrument is employed. Alternatively, the butt end of the point may be cut off so that the part which remains is equal to the working length. The larger sizes of silver points are cut with a disk, whilst gutta percha and the smaller sizes of silver points are cut with scissors. Whatever method is used, a slight reduction in measurement (0·5 mm or so) has to be made where it has not been possible to shape the point to conform to the apical end of the canal.

When a point has been fitted to the canal, it is desirable that a radiograph be taken to confirm its position in relation to the root apex. This is especially so where an error was made in assessing the working length and instrumentation has extended beyond the apical foramen. It is usually easy to tell when this has occurred, since there is no apical 'stop', and haemorrhage into the canal occurs very easily. To avoid overfilling in such a case, it is especially important that the point fits the apical part of the root canal closely. Usually the rounded apical end of the point conforms to the outline of the root apex. It may be found that a point the same size as the largest reamer used is a slack fit when inserted for the necessary distance (*Fig.* 143). This may be rectified by removing the apical end of the point section by section until a tight fit is obtained. Generally a larger point binds before the apical foramen is reached, and is therefore unsatisfactory (*Fig.* 143).

Immediately before insertion of the filling, the canal is thoroughly dried to ensure close adaptation of the cement to the root dentine. Absorbent paper points are inserted as far as the apical limit to instrumentation, but not beyond this level, otherwise haemorrhage will occur. Whereas each of the preceding stages of treatment has included the application of an antiseptic dressing, that at which the tooth is root filled does not. Special care should therefore be taken to maintain asepsis at this visit.

Following the completion of root filling, a radiograph is taken to check that it is satisfactory. In case overfilling has occurred, the film is examined before the patient leaves.

2. Methods of root filling

Following preparation, the apical part of the root canal should be roughly circular in cross-section, and a filling point which matches in width the largest reamer used during preparation should fit reasonably closely in this region. However, the middle and coronal parts of the canal vary in their cross-sectional shapes and in the taper they form, partly according to the original outlines and taper and partly according to the instruments used during preparation. The method used to root fill the tooth depends on the final anatomy of these parts of the root canal. Four methods are available—the single-point method, the lateral condensation method, the vertical condensation method and the sectional method.

a. Single-point method

The single-point method is used for canals which were originally narrow both mesiodistally and buccolingually, such as those of two-rooted maxillary premolars and of teeth with considerable dentine deposition along the root canal. Since it is possible to prepare this type of canal almost entirely with reamers, a point of the same width and taper as the largest reamer used should fit fairly closely for most of its length. Thus, only small spaces are left to be filled by the cement.

Merely coating the point with cement and inserting it into position does not usually produce a satisfactory root filling, since much of the cement is left at the entrance to the canal when the point is inserted (*Fig.* 144*a*). Moreover, most cement is lost from that part of the point which has to be inserted farthest, namely the apical end, where a seal is most important (*Fig.* 144*b*). Cement therefore has to be placed within the canal before the point is introduced. This cement has to be confined to the periphery of the canal and should not occupy its lumen, otherwise it may be driven into the periapical region when the point is inserted.

The technique of filling by the single-point method varies slightly with gutta percha and silver.

i. TECHNIQUE WITH GUTTA PERCHA (*Fig.* 145)

Where the single-point method is employed and it is thought the tooth may need a post crown later, gutta percha is used, since this material is much easier to cut away than silver.

After the selection of a suitable point, the walls of the prepared canal are coated with cement. A reamer one size smaller than the largest instrument used to prepare

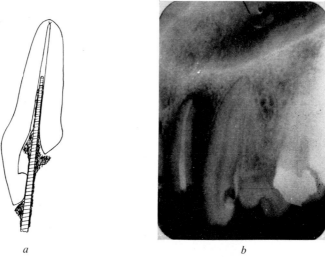

a   *b*

Fig. 144. *a*, Most of the cement used to coat a point is left at the entrance to the root canal when the point is inserted. *b*, In such a case, most cement is lost from the apical end of the point. Unless the canal is also coated with cement, the apical part of the root filling will contain voids, as in |2.

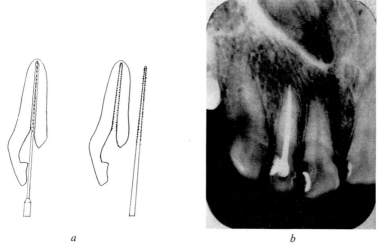

a   *b*

Fig. 145. *a*, Technique of filling by the single-point method. *Left*, Insertion of cement; *Right*, Coated point ready for insertion into canal. *b*, 2|, Root filled by single-point method, using gutta percha.

the apical part of the canal is coated with cement, inserted to the apical limit and then withdrawn with a counterclockwise movement. This procedure is repeated.

The selected gutta percha point is now coated with cement and inserted to the determined length. This is done slowly so as to allow the displacement of air. Whilst the point must be completely coated, there should not be excess cement projecting beyond its tip, otherwise this may be forced into the periapical region when the point is seated. The excess cement on the sides of the point is of no consequence, since it is left on the walls of the canal and displaced coronally as the point is advanced. The gutta percha protruding into the pulp chamber is now severed with a warmed plastic instrument. This is done in a mesiodistal rather than an apicogingival direction to avoid dragging the point from the canal.

ii. TECHNIQUE WITH SILVER

The use of silver points is generally confined to the finer root canals of two-rooted maxillary premolar teeth (*Fig.* 146). The filling is inserted in the same way as with

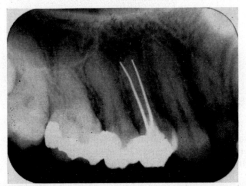

Fig. 146. 4|. Root filled by single-point method, using silver.

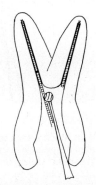

Fig. 147. The use of a large round bur to sever a silver point.

gutta percha. The part of the point protruding from the orifice of the root canal is cut as close to the base of the pulp chamber as possible with a pair of fine scissors, and that which still projects then bent over towards the floor of the pulp chamber. Alternatively, phosphate cement may be packed into the base of the cavity around the point, which is then severed flush with the cement using an inverted cone bur.

Instead of following this technique, a fast-setting cement may be used. Thus, the setting time of a zinc oxide–eugenol type of cement such as Kerr Root Canal Sealer may be accelerated by incorporating one or two crystals of zinc acetate in the mix. The decreased setting time enables the projecting point to be cut flush with the orifice of the canal after the cement has set. As much as possible of the excess point is first removed with scissors. The remainder is then severed with a large round bur or diamond instrument. The head of the bur is held alongside the point close to the entrance to the canal and is stabilized by resting the shank of the bur against the opposite cusp (*Fig.* 147). Considerable care has to be taken in doing this, otherwise the point may be twisted in the canal and the cement seal broken.

b. Lateral condensation method

Where the root canal is initially ovoid in cross-section or tapers appreciably, a matched point which fits the apical part of the canal closely will fit loosely elsewhere (*Fig.* 148). The use of the single-point method to fill this type of canal results in incomplete obliteration, since the cement in the middle and coronal parts of the canal cannot be adequately condensed owing to the loose fit of the point in these regions. For these cases, the lateral condensation method (*Fig.* 149) is one way of ensuring complete obliteration. Gutta percha is generally used in this method, although silver can be employed.

The initial stages of selecting a point and coating the canal with cement correspond to those of the single-point method. However, to ensure that the root canal is completely coated with cement, the reamer is withdrawn obliquely against the divergent walls. The gutta percha point is cut to correspond to the working length. This not only acts as a guide during its insertion but also provides a check that it

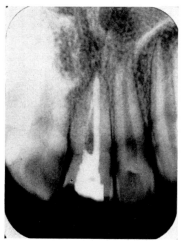

Fig. 148. The root canal of |1 has an appreciable taper, so that it is only apically that a matched point fits closely.

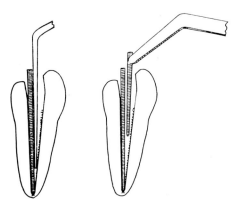

Fig. 149. Technique of filling by the lateral condensation method. *Left*, Compression of point against one side of canal; *Right*, Insertion of additional points one by one.

does not move during the later stages of filling. This 'master' point is coated with cement and is seated in position.

The spaces alongside the master point are now obliterated by packing additional gutta percha points into the canal. These points are shorter and stiffer than the master point. A root canal spreader (*Fig.* 150) is inserted as far as possible between the master point and one wall of the root canal and is swung from side to side to compress the gutta percha against the opposite wall of the canal. It is of no consequence which wall of the root canal the point is presssed against, although if the canal is ribbon-shaped in cross-section it must obviously be the buccal or lingual. In compressing the point, slight pressure in an apical direction is exerted, so ensuring that the point is not dragged coronally. The spreader is withdrawn, rotating it to and fro around its long axis to avoid pulling the point coronally. A short gutta percha point coated with a thin mix of cement is inserted immediately into the space which is left and is pushed apically as far as possible. The spreader is again inserted and thrust towards the root apex. It is then withdrawn and another point packed into the space created. The procedure is repeated until the spreader

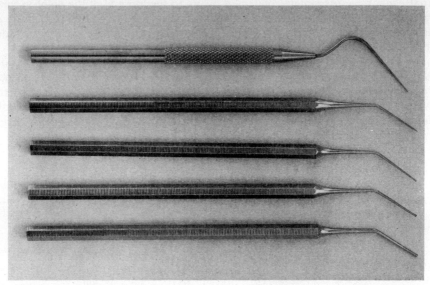

Fig. 150. Root canal spreader (*above*) and pluggers (*below*).

can no longer be inserted. Where the canal is ribbon-shaped in cross-section, only the buccal and lingual aspects will have to be attended to.

Properly used, the lateral condensation method results in a densely packed root filling (*Fig.* 151). However, the packing of a large number of additional points cannot influence the quality of the apical part of the root filling (*Fig.* 152). In consequence, the master point must fit this part of the canal closely. In using a root canal spreader, care has to be taken that the master point is not dragged coronally; the relationship between the coronal end of the gutta percha and the occlusal measuring point provides a check on this. Provided coronal movement of the master point is prevented, and so long as this fits the apical part of the canal closely, extrusion of filling material into the periapical region is unlikely.

Sommer et al. (1961) follow a similar technique, but use a master point of silver instead of gutta percha. Although cutting away the coronal part of the silver may be troublesome should a post crown have to be constructed later, the technique is useful where the canal is ribbon-shaped in cross-section and is very narrow mesiodistally, as with the mesial roots of some mandibular molar teeth. In these cases the rigidity of the silver master point prevents buckling when it is inserted.

c. Vertical condensation method

Schilder (1967) recommends a technique in which gutta percha is condensed in an apical, or vertical, direction, rather than laterally. The advantage claimed for this technique is that it leads to a more complete obliteration of the prepared canal by a largely homogeneous mass of gutta percha, often with the filling of lateral and accessory canals (*Fig.* 153).

A gutta percha point which is slightly wider than the apical end of the prepared canal, and which therefore binds 2·0–3·0 mm short of the apical limit, is selected. The canal is coated with the minimum amount of cement. The sides of the gutta percha point are coated with cement only at its apical end.

After insertion of the point, excess gutta percha coronally is removed with a hot plastic instrument. The coronal end of the point is softened by inserting a heated

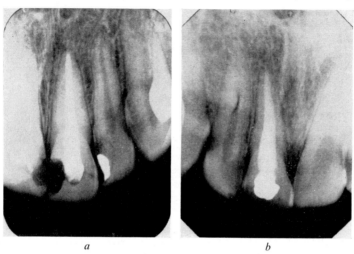

a   *b*

Fig. 151. *a*, |1 and *b*, 1|, each filled with gutta percha and cement by lateral condensation method.

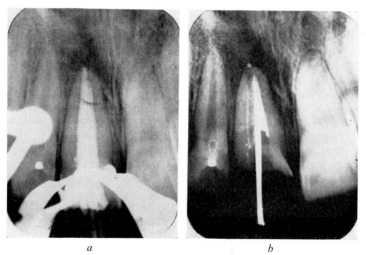

a   *b*

Fig. 152. 1|. *a*, After filling by lateral condensation method. The packing of additional gutta percha points into the coronal and middle parts of the canal has not eliminated the voids which are apparent apically. *b*, The presence of voids apically resulted in the master point being dragged from the canal during post crown preparation.

root canal spreader 2·0–3·0 mm into the canal. A root canal plugger of appropriate width (*Fig.* 150) is then forced through the softened gutta percha in an apical direction. This is repeated several times, with the heated spreader gradually being inserted deeper into the canal until the apical part of the point is softened and forced to the apical limit.

During this procedure gutta percha adheres to and is removed by the heated spreader, and in consequence the coronal and middle parts of the root canal are

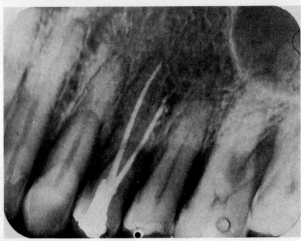

Fig. 153. |4. Filled by vertical condensation of gutta percha, with extrusion of filling material through accessory canals in distal aspect of buccal root (distally).

eventually incompletely filled. Segments of softened gutta percha are now introduced and condensed with pluggers to obliterate these parts of the canal.

The vertical condensation technique is especially useful where the creation of a ledge in the root canal wall during instrumentation prevents the insertion of a point to the apical limit. However, care has to be taken with this technique to avoid the extrusion of undue amounts of filling material into the periapical tissues.

d. Sectional method

The sectional method is another way of ensuring complete obliteration of a tapering or ovoid canal. First the apical section of the canal is filled. The remainder of the canal may be obliterated using either the same or another material.

One of three materials may be used to fill the apical section of the root canal, namely gutta percha, silver or amalgam. With both gutta percha and silver, the apical end of the canal is first coated with cement before introducing the root-filling point.

i. TECHNIQUE WITH GUTTA PERCHA (*Fig.* 154)

Gutta percha is generally used in combination with a cement for filling the apical section of the canal, although chloropercha can be employed.

A suitable point is selected and moulded to the apical end of the prepared canal in the manner described previously. The apical 4·0–5·0 mm of the point are cut off and attached by its coronal end to a warmed root canal plugger (*Fig.* 154). A suitable marker previously placed on the plugger, such as a disk of rubber dam, is adjusted so that its distance from the tip of the point corresponds to the working length. The gutta percha is then carefully coated with cement and carried to the apical limit on the plunger. Gentle pressure is exerted in an apical direction to ensure good adaptation. The plunger is detached from the gutta percha by swinging it from side to side, at the same time maintaining pressure apically.

The remainder of the canal is obliterated with some material which may, in the event of post crown construction later, be readily removed. For example, the canal

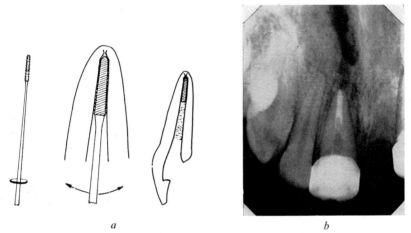

a   *b*

Fig. 154. *a*, Technique of filling with gutta percha by the sectional method. *Left*, Coated section of point attached to warmed root canal plunger, with marker in place; *Centre*, Detaching plunger from gutta percha after seating latter in position; *Right*, Completed root canal filling. *b*, Apical part of 1| root filled with gutta percha and cement by sectional method.

may be filled with a zinc oxide–eugenol cement by means of a spiral root filler and then gutta percha points inserted to ensure complete obliteration.

The main hazard of this method is that the section of gutta percha may become detached from the plunger before the apical limit is reached. The narrower the canal, the greater is the hazard. With most anterior and premolar teeth, the difficulty may be largely overcome by sinking the end of the plunger into the gutta percha for a distance of about 0·25 mm, and by ensuring that during insertion the long axis of the plunger corresponds to that of the root canal. The long axes of the plunger and the attached point must obviously coincide. Where the root canal is narrow mesiodistally, however, these measures may well be inadequate; in such a case it is better to use the lateral condensation method. The sectional technique is contraindicated in obviously curved canals.

ii. TECHNIQUE WITH SILVER (*Fig.* 155)

With silver a different technique is used (Nicholls, 1958). After the point has been fitted to the apical end of the canal, a deep groove is cut with a carborundum disk around the circumference of the silver about 4·0–5·0 mm from its tip, so that only a thin bar of metal is left connecting the two parts of the point. To facilitate removal of the coronal part of the point later, the silver projecting into the mouth beyond the occlusal measuring point is allowed to remain.

The part of the point apical to the groove is coated with cement and the point inserted to the determined length and seated firmly in position. The coronal end of the point is grasped firmly and, whilst maintaining gentle pressure in an apical direction, is moved to and fro both mesiodistally and buccolingually. Thus, the thin connecting bar of silver is weakened. The point is now rotated through 360° around its long axis two or three times. This completes the break in the metal and

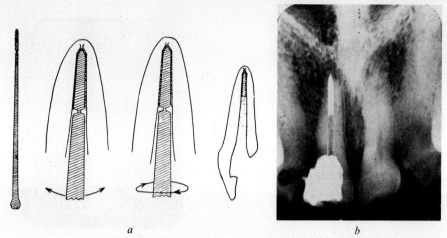

a   *b*

Fig. 155. *a*, Technique of filling with silver by the sectional method. *Left*, Point grooved and coated with cement apically; *Centre left*, weakening the connecting bar of silver after seating point in position; *Centre right*, Detaching coronal part of point; *Right*, Coronal part of silver point removed. *b*, Apical part of 1| root filled with silver and cement by sectional method. The coronal end of the silver has been covered with a layer of cement preparatory to post crown construction.

enables the coronal part of the point to be removed, so leaving the apical part cemented in position. As a check that the apical section of silver has not been dragged coronally, the coronal part of the point may be reinserted and its position relative to the occlusal measuring point verified. The coronal part of the canal may now be obliterated with gutta percha points and cement.

The sectional method of filling with silver also has hazards and drawbacks. It is important that the long axes of the two parts of the point coincide, and that the point is inserted in line with the long axis of the canal. In coating the point, cement should be confined to the apical section, since an excess around the coronal part impedes its removal. Since silver points smaller than size 40 or 50 cannot be grooved without buckling, the method is not applicable to narrow canals. In the event of treatment failing, removal of the apical part of the filling and retreatment by way of the root canal are not possible; in such a case, extraction or periapical surgery is necessary. This disadvantage is more apparent than real, however. A treatment which fails, assuming it to have been properly performed in the first instance, is usually corrected surgically.

Messing (1969) advocates another technique of sectional silver filling (*Fig.* 156). A section of silver with a screw thread at its coronal end is used. This screw thread engages in a hollow cylindrical handle. After coating the silver with cement and inserting it into position in the canal, the handle is unscrewed and removed. These apical silver fillings are available commercially in 3·0 mm and 5·00 mm lengths. The smallest size available is no. 45.

In root filling by the sectional method, some operators, in anticipation of post crown construction, fill only the apical part of the canal. This has two potential drawbacks. First, salivary contamination during post crown construction could

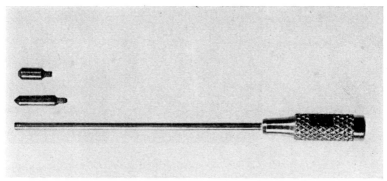

Fig. 156. Apical silver fillings (3·0 and 5·0 mm) and matching handle.

lead to a lesion of the supporting bone alongside the lateral aspect of the root should there be a lateral canal connecting the unfilled part of the main canal to the periodontal membrane. Although probably an uncommon complication, this is less likely when the entire canal is obliterated by a well-condensed filling. Secondly, it has been shown by Neagley (1969) that where post hole preparation impinges on an apical silver filling, leakage of the filling is likely to result, presumably due to disruption of the cement seal by the movement of rotary instruments against the silver or the heat they generate. Thus, saliva may penetrate alongside the silver, especially when pressure is exerted in an apical direction within the canal, as, for example, when an impression is taken of the preparation. In consequence, renewed periapical irritation is possible (*Fig.* 157). To prevent this, post hole preparation should stop short of the apical filling. Also, in case there should be a flaw in the seal of the apical filling, it is advisable to place a layer of cement over the coronal end of the silver point immediately after insertion of the root filling (*Fig.* 155*b*). The coronal end of the point used to fill the canal may be used to introduce and condense this plug of cement.

iii. TECHNIQUE WITH AMALGAM

Special carriers for the introduction of amalgam into the apical part of the root canal by way of the pulp chamber have been available for some years (Messing, 1958; Hill, 1967). An important limitation of these carriers was that their large diameter necessitated a considerable degree of enlargement of the root canal to permit introduction of the carrier to the apical region. Also, since they were fairly rigid, they could only be employed in virtually straight canals.

Recently, Dimashkieh (1975) has described a carrier consisting of an outer stainless-steel tube and an inner plunger, with a spring action to retract the plunger after ejection of the amalgam. The smallest size of carrier has an external diameter of 0·40 mm and so its use does not entail excessive enlargement of the root canal;

also, it is sufficiently flexible to be used in a slightly curved canal. After each increment of amalgam has been deposited apically, it is consolidated with a condenser slightly narrower than the matching carrier until the apical 4·0–5·0 mm of the canal have been filled.

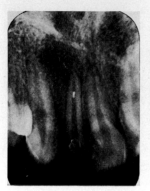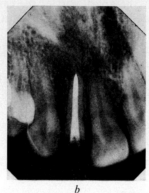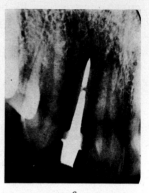

a   *b*   *c*

Fig. 157. 2]. *a*, Immediately before root canal treatment, showing periapical lesion; *b*, One year after root canal treatment and prior to post crown construction; there is virtually complete periapical repair: *c*, Two years after post crown construction; there has been a recurrence of periapical bone destruction, and it is evident that post hole preparation extended to the apical silver filling. There was no evidence of occlusal trauma.

In the foregoing descriptions of the sectional method of root filling, it has been stated that the apical filling is 4·0–5·0 mm long. In most teeth this leaves enough room for a post of adequate length should one be needed when the crown is restored. Where the root is relatively short, however, this may not be true. Since the post should be at least as long as the restored crown, the maximum length of the apical section of filling may be calculated by doubling the proposed length of the crown and subtracting this from the working length; this assumes that the latter is measured from an intact incisal or occlusal edge (*Fig.* 158).

TREATMENT OF THE PULP CHAMBER FOLLOWING ROOT FILLING

The materials used for root filling are opaque and reduce the translucency of the crown of the tooth if allowed to remain in the pulp chamber. Also, some root canal cements tend to discolour dentine. With an anterior tooth which is restored soon after root filling by a post crown, these considerations are obviously of no consequence. However, where part or all of the remaining natural crown is to be retained, the pulp chamber and the extreme coronal part of the canal should be cleared completely of root-filling material. This is carried out to a level 1·0–2·0 mm apical of the cervix of the tooth labially (*Fig.* 159). The pulp chamber is filled with a translucent material, such as one of the composites. Either the same or another material is used to restore the coronal opening into the pulp cavity.

As a prophylactic measure against subsequent loss of translucency of the crown following dehydration of the dentine, an attempt may be made immediately after root filling to fill the dentinal tubules coronally with a liquid having a refractive index similar to that of the tooth. Three different agents have been recommended for this purpose: an 80 per cent solution of chloral hydrate in distilled water, a 5 per cent solution of acrylic monomer in chloroform and silicone fluid of 3–30 centistokes viscosity. Although chloral hydrate solution has probably been advocated most frequently, Grossman (1974) prefers silicone fluid, since unlike the

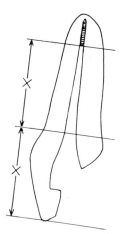

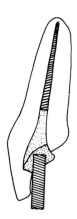

Fig. 158. If a post crown is likely to be necessary later and the root is to be filled by the sectional method, the maximum length of the apical section of filling equals the working length minus twice the proposed length of the crown (X). It is assumed the working length is measured from an intact incisal or occlusal edge.

Fig. 159. After filling a root canal, filling material should be removed to a level 1·0–2·0 mm apical of the cervix of the tooth labially. As a prophylactic measure against subsequent loss of translucency of the crown, a cottonwool pledget saturated with a suitable agent is sealed in the pulp chamber with gutta percha and pressure exerted on the latter with an orange-wood stick.

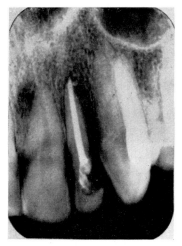

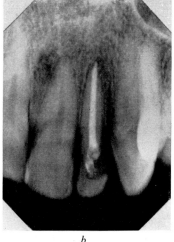

a   b

Fig. 160. |2. *a,* Immediately after root filling. A small excess of cement is apparent. *b,* Two years later the excess has virtually disappeared.

other two agents it does not evaporate and therefore remains permanently within the tooth.

Whichever is used, the openings of the dentinal tubules into the pulp chamber must be patent if any benefit is to be derived. To this end, fatty products resulting

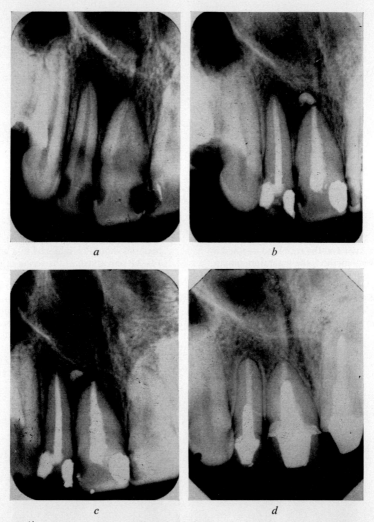

Fig. 161. 1|. *a*, Before treatment. There is obvious periapical destruction. *b*, Immediately after root filling. 1| has been grossly overfilled. *c*, Two months later the excess cement has moved and is apparently smaller. *d*, Six years later the excess cement has disappeared and periapical repair is virtually complete.

from pulpal decomposition must first be removed. Thus, where the pulp was necrotic, the walls of the pulp chamber are scrubbed first with a wool pledget moistened with chloroform, and then with a pledget moistened with alcohol. The pulp chamber is now dried and a third pledget saturated with one of the three agents described is inserted. The orifice of the pulp chamber is sealed with gutta percha, and heavy pressure—using, for example, a suitably trimmed orange-wood stick—is exerted for 30–60 seconds against the gutta percha to force the liquid into the dentinal tubules (*Fig.* 159). The pulp chamber is then dried and restored.

OVERFILLING

Occasionally, especially if instrumentation has extended beyond the apical foramen, root-filling material is extruded into the periapical region. Where the excess consists of a small amount of cement, or where a short length of point—say 1·0 mm

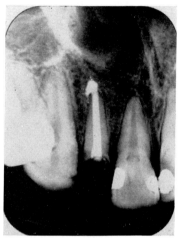

Fig. 162. 2|, which had an intact periapex, has been grossly overfilled by cement. The excess should be removed surgically as soon as possible.

or less—projects beyond the apical foramen, it is sufficient to apply a counter-irritant, such as tincture of iodine, to the buccal mucosa over the root apex, and, if not already done, to clear the tooth from occlusal contact with the opposing teeth. The patient is warned that there may be slight sensitivity for a few days. A small excess of cement is often eventually resorbed (*Fig.* 160).

With a relatively large excess of root-filling material, the position is less certain. Where a periapical lesion is present, a fairly large amount of excess cement is sometimes tolerated and does not interfere with periapical repair (*Fig.* 161). This is not so where the periapical bone is intact, however (*Fig.* 162); in such cases the excess material should be removed before symptoms of an acute apical periodontitis develop. When the excess consists of part of the gutta percha or silver point used to fill the tooth, the filling is removed and a new root filling inserted. If the point cannot be removed, or if the excess consists of cement, periapical surgery to remove the excess material is indicated. In the absence of a sinus from the periapical region, this should be performed immediately. If this is not possible, perforation of the buccal cortical plate, as described in Chapter 10, is indicated. By allowing the drainage of inflammatory exudate, this prevents the development of an acute apical periodontitis.

REFERENCES

Ainley J. E. (1970) Fluorometric assay of the apical seal of root canal fillings. *Oral Surg.* **29**, 753.

Barry G. N. and Fried I. L. (1975) Sealing quality of two polycarboxylate cements used as root canal sealers. *J. Endodontol.* **1**, 107.

Brady J. M. and del Rio C. E. (1975) Corrosion of endodontic silver cones in humans: a scanning electron microscope and X-ray microprobe study. *J. Endodontol.* **1**, 205.

Cooke H. G., Grower M. F. and del Rio C. E. (1976) Effects of instrumentation with a chelating agent on the periapical seal of obturated root canals. *J. Endodontol.* **2**, 312.

Dimashkieh M. R. (1975) A method of using silver amalgam in routine endodontics, and its use in open apices. *Br. Dent. J.* **138**, 298.

Dixon C. M. and Rickert U. G. (1938) Histologic verification of results of root-canal therapy in experimental animals. *J. Am. Dent. Assoc.* **25**, 1781.

Feldmann G. and Nyborg H. (1964) Tissue reactions to root filling materials. II, A comparison of implants of silver and root filling material AH26 in rabbits' jaws. *Odontol. Revy* **15**, 33.

Grossman L. I. (1958) An improved root canal cement. *J. Am. Dent. Assoc.* **56**, 381.

Grossman L. I. (1974) *Endodontic Practice*, 8th ed. London, Kimpton, pp. 299, 342.

Grossman L. I. (1976) Physical properties of root canal cements. *J. Endodontol.* **2**, 166.

Guttuso J. (1963) Histopathologic study of rat connective tissue responses to endodontic materials. *Oral Surg.* **16**, 713.

Higginbotham T. L. (1967) A comparative study of the physical properties of five commonly used root canal sealers. *Oral Surg.* **24**, 89.

Hill T. R. (1967) An amalgam carrier for use in endodontic treatment. *Dent. Practnr Dent. Rec.* **17**, 285.

Hunter H. A. (1957) The effect of gutta percha, silver points and Rickert's root sealer on bone healing. *J. Can. Dent. Assoc.* **23**, 385.

Langeland K. (1974) Root canal sealants and pastes. *Dent. Clin. North Am.* **18**, 309–27.

McComb D. and Smith D. C. (1976) Comparison of physical properties of polycarboxylate-based and conventional root canal sealers. *J. Endodontol.* **2**, 228.

McElroy D. L. (1955) Physical properties of root canal filling materials. *J. Am. Dent. Assoc.* **50**, 433.

McElroy D. L. and Wach E. C. (1958) Endodontic treatment with a zinc oxide–Canada balsam filling material. *J. Am. Dent. Assoc.* **56**, 801.

Marshall F. J. and Massler M. (1961) The sealing of pulpless teeth evaluated with radioisotopes. *J. Dent. Med.* **16**, 172.

Messing J. J. (1958) Obliteration of the apical third of the root canal with amalgam. *Br. Dent. J.* **104**, 125.

Messing J. J. (1969) Precision apical silver cones. *J. Br. Endodontic Soc.* **3**, 22.

Neagley R. L. (1969) The effect of dowel preparation on the apical seal of endodontically treated teeth. *Oral Surg.* **28**, 739.

Nicholls E. (1958) Sectional root filling with silver points. *Dent. Practnr Dent. Rec.* **8**, 241.

Nyborg H. and Tullin B. (1965) Healing processes after vital extirpation. *Odontol. Tidskr.* **73**, 430.

Sanders S. H. and Dooley R. J. (1974) A comparative evaluation of polycarboxylate cement as a root canal sealer utilizing roughened and non-roughened silver points. *Oral Surg.* **37**, 629.

Sargenti A. (1973) Is N2 an acceptable method of treatment? In: Grossman L. I. (ed.), *Transactions of the 5th International Conference on Endodontics*. Philadelphia, University of Pennsylvania, pp. 176–195.

Scheufele J. (1952) Untersuchungen und Erfahrungen mit dem Neuartigen Wurzelfullmittel Diaket. *Dtsch. Zahnarztl. Z.* **7**, 913.

Schilder H. (1967) Filling root canals in three dimensions. *Dent. Clin. North Am.* **11**, 723.

Schroeder A. (1954) Mitteilungen über die Abschlussdichtigkeit von Wurzelfüllmaterialen und Erster Hinweis auf ein Neuartiges Wurzelfüllmittel. *Schweiz. Monatschr. Zahnheilkd.* **64**, 921.

Seltzer S., Green D. B., Weiner N. and De Rensis F. (1972) A scanning electron microscope examination of silver cones removed from endodontically treated teeth. *Oral Surg.* **33**, 589.

Seltzer S., Maggio J., Wollard R. R., Brough S. O. and Barnett A. (1976) Tissue reactions to polycarboxylate cements. *J. Endodontol.* **2**, 208.

Sommer R. F., Ostrander F. D. and Crowley M. C. (1961) *Clinical Endodontics*, 2nd ed. London, Saunders, p. 235.

Spangberg L. (1969) Biological effects of root canal filling materials. 7, Reaction of bony tissue to implanted root canal filling material in guinea pigs. *Odontol. Tidskr.* **77**, 133.

Stewart G. G. (1958) A comparative study of three root canal sealing agents. *Oral Surg.* **11**, 1029, 1174.

Wach E. C., Hauptfuehrer J. D. and Kesel R. G. (1955) Endodontic significance of the penetration of S^{35}-labeled penicillin in extracted human teeth. *Oral Surg.* **8**, 639.

Weisman M. I. (1970) A study of the flow rate of ten root canal sealers. *Oral Surg.* **29**, 255.

FURTHER READING

Curson I. and Kirk E. E. J. (1968) An assessment of root canal-sealing cements. *Oral Surg.* **26**, 229.

Friend L. A. and Browne R. M. (1968) Tissue reactions to some root filling materials. *Br. Dent. J.* **125**, 291.

Grieve A. R. and Parkholm J. D. O. (1973) The sealing properties of root filling cements. Further studies. *Br. Dent. J.* **135**, 327.

Seltzer S. (1971) *Endodontology: Biologic Considerations in Endodontic Procedures.* New York, McGraw-Hill, pp. 259–75.

Chapter 9

Treatment plan and bacteriological control: postoperative repair and observation

TREATMENT PLAN AND BACTERIOLOGICAL CONTROL

1. Root canal preparation

It is less time-consuming if the root canal is prepared completely at one visit than if this procedure is spread over a number of visits. In the treatment of teeth with intact, or virtually intact, vital pulps, the absence of necrotic tissue within the root canal implies that contamination by micro-organisms is probably superficial and limited to that part of the pulp which has undergone necrosis in the region of the exposure. If the latter is cauterized by heat and the coronal part of the pulp removed first, therefore, the likelihood of infecting the apical region by completely preparing the root canal at one visit is small.

By contrast, where there is partial or complete necrosis of the radicular pulp, heavy contamination by micro-organisms is likely. To reduce the risk of exacerbation following upon the transmission of a large number of organisms in an apical direction, therefore, some operators consider it wiser to spend two or three visits in preparing such canals. However, this means that more attendances will almost certainly be necessary before the tooth is root-filled, since the antiseptic dressings used will not exert their maximum effect until the canal has been completely prepared. Also, although the likelihood of exacerbation may be greater when preparation is completed at one visit, its occurrence is not sufficiently frequent to constitute a major drawback. When it does occur, the cause may usually be traced to the careless use of instruments in the canal, often with the infliction of trauma on the periapical tissues. Complete preparation of the root canal at one visit, provided it is carefully performed, is therefore considered preferable.

2. Frequency of visits

Following root canal preparation of teeth with necrotic pulps, the risk of an acute exacerbation, with consequent inconvenience to both patient and operator, is largely eliminated if the second visit is within 24–36 hours of the first. Within this period of time really acute symptoms do not occur. Thus, if an acute apical periodontitis is developing, the operator is able to release and absorb the exudate before this has accumulated sufficiently to cause acute symptoms. The pulp cavity may then be redressed and resealed as part of the general plan of treatment. This arrangement need not be made where the pulp is vital, nor is it necessary where

174

there is a sinus from the periapical region, since this allows immediate drainage of exudate and therefore obviates acute exacerbation.

Otherwise, the frequency of visits is determined largely by the length of time for which the antiseptic dressing sealed within the pulp cavity remains effective. Once inserted, the antiseptic effect of the dressing gradually diminishes, owing to its dilution from the entry of tissue fluid through the apical foramen and possibly its diffusion into the periapical region. Thus, if the interval of time between appointments is unduly long, residual micro-organisms may multiply and the original

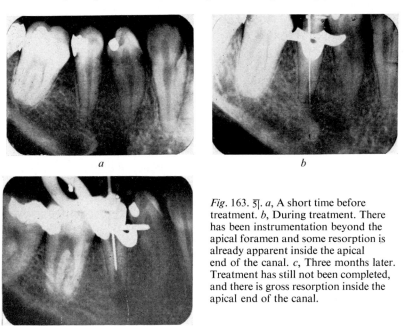

a

b

Fig. 163. ʒ. *a*, A short time before treatment. *b*, During treatment. There has been instrumentation beyond the apical foramen and some resorption is already apparent inside the apical end of the canal. *c*, Three months later. Treatment has still not been completed, and there is gross resorption inside the apical end of the canal.

c

benefit derived from placing the dressing will be lost. From this aspect the dressing should not be left unchanged for longer than 14 days (Chapter 7). Preferably it should be changed within 3–7 days.

Infrequent changing of antiseptic dressings also has the disadvantage that the seal to the pulp cavity is more likely to leak, due to washing away or breakdown of the cement. Furthermore, where the assessment of the working length was incorrect and instrumentation beyond the apical foramen has occurred, tissue from the periapical region sometimes grows into the canal through the widened foramen. This tissue interferes with root filling and, as *Fig.* 163 illustrates, is occasionally associated with resorption of the root.

3. Time of root filling

The root canal is filled when there are no clinical signs or symptoms of active disease.

The patient should no longer have pain or discomfort. The soft tissues overlying the root apex should not be swollen or inflamed. Any sinus originally present should have closed; this usually happens soon after the root canal is prepared. The tooth should not be tender to percussion. It should be no more mobile than the adjoining teeth, unless some condition not directly related to the periapical status, such as periodontal disease, exists.

Although exudation of tissue fluid into the canal may sometimes persist, it should be no more than slight. In this connection it should be remembered that antibiotic and other antiseptic pastes may be diluted by the entry of small amounts of periapical exudate between visits. Thus, when the pulp cavity is next opened, an antibiotic preparation often has a thin, creamy consistency; this is sometimes mistaken for pus.

If treatment is being controlled by bacteriological sampling of the root canal, there should be no evidence of the presence of micro-organisms.

Immediate root filling

Some operators, provided the pulp is vital and is without evidence of gross infection, insert a root filling immediately after preparation of the canal. This procedure, which is known as 'immediate root filling', has two main drawbacks. First, although it is improbable that an appreciable number of organisms remain after preparation, those which do may survive and cause periapical disease at a later date should there be a void in the apical part of the root filling allowing the entry of tissue fluid into the canal. The second drawback is that, following on the trauma of pulpectomy, haemorrhage may occur when the vasoconstrictor action of the anaesthetic solution eventually ceases. Since the root filling will prevent blood entering the root canal, haemorrhage into the periapical region may take place. Thus, a clinically apparent apical periodontitis may develop, with discomfort for the patient. It is therefore preferable to seal an antiseptic dressing in the canal and defer root filling to a second visit, especially as little additional time is involved by doing this.

4. Bacteriological control of treatment

For many years past, bacteriological testing—or, more accurately, microbiological testing—has been advocated as an aid in determining when the root canal may be filled. Currently the need for such testing is the subject of lively discussion. A brief account of this form of examination of the root canal will be given before discussing current thought on its value.

a. Methods

There are two methods of bacteriological testing, namely the stained smear and the bacteriological culture. In the smear method a sterile absorbent point is inserted to the apical part of the canal and manipulated to collect any micro-organisms present; unless wet with exudate, the canal is first moistened with sterile water or sterile normal saline. The point is now withdrawn and used to make a smear on a glass slide. This smear is dried and fixed, stained by Gram or a simple stain, and examined microscopically for micro-organisms.

The main disadvantage of the smear is that it is not sensitive enough for the detection of small numbers of organisms. Where bacteriological testing is employed, therefore, the culture method is normally used. In this method a sample is taken in the same way as in the smear method. The point is transferred from the canal to a tube or bottle of liquid culture medium, which is then incubated at 37 °C and periodically inspected for growth. In the meantime the canal is redressed and resealed and the patient dismissed.

b. Relation of bacteriological culturing to treatment

With an experienced operator, provided there are no clinical signs or symptoms of disease, root filling after removal of a necrotic pulp is generally performed immediately the specimen from the second or a succeeding visit has proved to be negative. Allowing for the delay necessary for incubating the specimen, this is normally at the third visit, assuming the canal was completely prepared at the first visit.

It has already been pointed out that the pulp cavity of a tooth from which an intact vital pulp has been removed should be no more than lightly contaminated. Thorough preparation reduces the contamination even further. Thus, one antiseptic dressing properly applied after preparation should eliminate any organisms remaining. In consequence, these teeth are generally filled at the second visit and bacteriological sampling is omitted. However, where a vital pulp shows extensive breakdown or suppuration, this approach cannot be safely adopted; such a case should be treated as if the pulp were necrotic, with root filling normally being performed at the third visit.

c. Technique of bacteriological sampling

The object of taking a culture sample is defeated if all reasonable steps to detect the presence of micro-organisms are not taken. Besides the qualities needed of the culture medium, which will be dealt with later, these steps include the manner in which the canal is sampled. Thus, the collection of organisms is facilitated if, in the absence of exudate, the canal is moistened and the absorbent point manipulated vigorously within the canal and left for at least 1 minute before removal. The point which is used should make close contact with the walls of the canal apically, since it is here that the presence of organisms is of most significance. There is a greater chance of collecting organisms if two or three points are used, separately or together, for sampling, especially if the apical foramen is wide or if the canal tapers appreciably. Sampling should not follow upon irrigation with antiseptic fluids, since these will reduce, albeit temporarily, the number of organisms present.

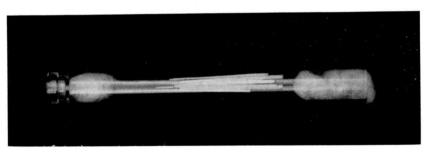

Fig. 164. Sterile absorbent paper points stored in a used local anaesthetic cartridge plugged with non-absorbent cottonwool.

Conversely, the time of both operator and patient will have been wasted if, due to extraneous contamination, a sample from a sterile canal shows growth, since this will result in root filling being deferred. For this reason a strict aseptic technique is essential. To maintain their sterility until they are used, the absorbent points used for sampling should be kept sealed in a separate container, such as an empty local anaesthetic cartridge plugged with non-absorbent cottonwool (*Fig*.164). If the tweezers which will grip the point have been used for some other purpose subsequent to their sterilization, they should be resterilized.

To reduce the risk of aerial contamination, each point should be transferred from its container to the root canal, and subsequently from the root canal to the culture medium, as quickly as possible. Since the side of the point will probably contact the rim of the opening into the pulp chamber, the lingual or occlusal surface of the tooth is scrubbed with a sterile wool pledget moistened with a suitable antiseptic, such as tincture of iodine, immediately prior to sampling. To avoid transfer to the culture medium, the antiseptic should not be allowed to enter the pulp chamber; also, the tooth surface should be dried of antiseptic with sterile wool pledgets.

d. Culture medium

It would be necessary to use a considerable number of culture media to support the growth of all the species of micro-organisms which might be present within a root canal. This is impracticable, and therefore a culture medium which will permit the growth of the greatest variety of organisms which may be present is used. A liquid culture medium, which allows immersion of the absorbent point used for

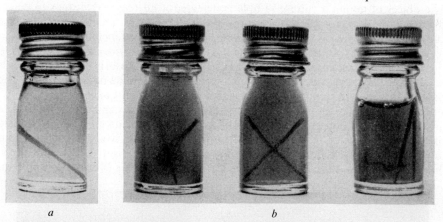

a   *b*

Fig. 165. *a*, A bottle of culture medium inoculated with an absorbent point. The medium is clear, denoting there is no growth. *b*, Bottles of medium inoculated with absorbent points and showing different forms of growth. *Left*, Turbidity throughout medium; *Centre*, Discrete colonies throughout medium; *Right*, Growth at bottom of medium, only evident after shaking the bottle.

sampling, is normally employed (*Fig*. 165). A screw-cap bottle of about 10 ml capacity may be used as the container.

The essential constituents of a typical medium are broth, glucose and agar. Glucose gives better growth of aciduric organisms, such as streptococci, whilst agar, by preventing convection currents within the liquid, permits a progressive decrease in oxygen tension from the top to the bottom of the medium. Thus, the growth of anaerobic as well as aerobic organisms is facilitated. The establishment of an anaerobic condition in the deeper parts of the medium may be further encouraged by the addition of sodium thioglycollate, which is a reducing agent. Dehydrated media in the form of granules or tablets are obtainable; they are reconstituted with water and the mixture is then sterilized in an autoclave to form the medium.

The culture medium is improved by the addition of serum, since this supports the growth of certain organisms which are demanding in their requirements and which otherwise would not be cultured. Unfortunately, since serum would be destroyed by autoclaving, it has to be added under aseptic conditions after the medium proper has been sterilized. It is often omitted, therefore. Similarly, penicillinase, which will inactivate any penicillin carried on the absorbent point from the canal to the medium, deteriorates at room temperature and is therefore commonly omitted.

e. Incubation and examination

The specimen is incubated at 37 °C for 7 days and periodically inspected.

Where there is no growth, the culture medium remains clear (*Fig.* 165*a*), whilst growth of organisms may result in a number of changes in appearance (*Fig.* 165*b*).

Evaluation of the bacteriological culture in treatment

Before discussing the value of the bacteriological culture, it should be pointed out that the eradication of micro-organisms is only one aspect of treatment. Irritation of the periapical tissues, and therefore periapical disease, may also be brought about by physical and chemical agents. Thus, the fact that cultures have been negative does not necessarily mean that treatment will be successful. Conversely, the fact that a root canal is filled whilst cultures still show growth by no means precludes a successful outcome to treatment. It is quite possible that residual organisms may be sealed from the periapical region by the root filling or, if pushed beyond the apical foramen at the time of filling, rapidly eliminated by the defences of the periapical region. The fact that these organisms would probably not be actively growing, due to the effect of the antiseptic dressings previously applied, would facilitate the latter process.

In recent years the need for bacteriological culturing and its validity in determining when to fill the root canal have been widely questioned. Two main objections to culturing have been raised, namely that both false positive and false negative results are possible, and that the presence of micro-organisms in an otherwise adequately treated root canal has no influence on the result of treatment.

False positive cultures may arise from a variety of sources and are for the most part avoidable. For example, salivary contamination from a leaking rubber dam or coronal restoration, the use of non-sterile instruments or paper points, or contamination of the paper point specimen from contact with the rubber dam, are all easily preventable.

Similarly, the frequency of false negative results can be reduced. Thus, the canal should be moistened prior to culturing, since the detection of organisms is more likely from a wet paper point than from a dry one (Marshall and Savoie, 1967). Some sources of false negative results are, however, unavoidable. For example, the paper point may fail to make contact with residual organisms; alternatively, the culture medium may fail to support the growth of these organisms. Because of limitations such as these, a negative bacteriological culture does not necessarily mean that the pulp cavity is free of micro-organisms. Thus, what is commonly called a 'sterile' root canal may well contain living organisms, although it is likely that these will be relatively small in number compared with those present before treatment was instituted.

Bacteriological culture tests do, therefore, have some limitations. However, this is true of other tests and methods of examination, such as pulp vitality tests and radiographic examination. By themselves, these limitations do not constitute sufficient reason for abandoning the test as a diagnostic tool to be used in conjunction with other tests.

The second objection to culturing, namely that the presence of organisms in a properly treated root canal has no influence on the result of treatment, is potentially of far greater significance. This objection is based mainly on the large-scale study of Seltzer et al. (1963), who obtained virtually the same rate of success 2 years after treatment whether the root canal yielded a positive or a negative culture specimen at the time of root filling. This finding received confirmation from the study of Seltzer et al., (1964), who concluded from experimental root canal treatment in dogs that the extent and severity of periapical inflammation were not related to the bacteriological state of the canal at the time of filling.

In contrast, other investigations have shown that a positive specimen from the root canal at the time of root filling is associated with a poorer prognosis than where a negative specimen is obtained. Thus, Engstrom et al. (1964) found that although there was no significant difference 1 year after root filling, 4–5 years after treatment pulpless teeth giving a positive specimen had a significantly higher failure rate than those yielding a negative specimen. Similar results were obtained in the treatment of teeth with vital pulps (Engstrom and Lundberg, 1965).

The influence upon prognosis of micro-organisms in the prepared root canal must therefore be regarded as an unresolved question. In discussing this, however, a distinction must be made between root canals which are filled despite the fact that they yield positive cultures, and those which are filled without any bacteriological examination whatsoever, since the two groups are not synonymous. Also, a distinction must be drawn between the results of workers who have considerable expertise in this field and of those who perform root canal treatment relatively infrequently. It was pointed out in Chapter 6 that the majority of infected root canals yield negative bacteriological specimens after thorough preparation. Thus, in the study of Stewart et al. (1969) well over 90 per cent of originally infected root canals gave negative specimens after being prepared and then sealed until the succeeding visit without the insertion of any antiseptic dressing. Applying these results to a hypothetical group of 110 infected teeth treated in the same way but without bacteriological control, the probable bacteriological status at the visit after root canal preparation would be:

Number of canals which would be negative, if examined: 99 (90%)
Number of canals which would be positive, if examined: 11 (10%)

Accepting for the moment the finding of Engstrom et al. (1964) that the failure rates following treatment of pulpless teeth are approximately 10 per cent for those positive and 25 per cent for those negative at the time of root filling, then root filling of the teeth should give the following results:

Of 99 probably negative canals: 10 would fail (10%)
Of 11 probably positive canals: 2 or 3 would fail (25%)

Thus, if no bacteriological control were to be used, the total number of failures would be 12 or 13. But if this same group of 110 teeth were to be treated with the aid of bacteriological control and root filling deferred until treatment with anti-septic dressings had resulted in each giving a negative bacteriological specimen, the number of failures would be 11 (10 per cent). In other words, bacteriological culturing to determine the time of root filling would reduce the total failure rate by 1 or 2 per cent.

Even though the bacteriological status of the canal at the time of root filling may influence the prognosis, therefore, it is hardly surprising that some workers maintain that the prognosis is as good without bacteriological control as with such control. However, the results of Stewart et al. (1969) which were cited earlier were those obtained by experts. For dentists who only occasionally perform this type of treatment, a considerably larger proportion of canals would be expected to contain residual necrotic material following preparation, and in consequence a larger proportion would yield positive specimens if cultured.

Thus, it may well be that the need for bacteriological control, and the potentially adverse effect of dispensing with it, is minimal for those who regularly root treat teeth and who, paradoxically, most often advocate such control, but rather greater for those who are less experienced and usually omit bacteriological control.

5. Synopsis of treatment

In the following stage-by-stage accounts of treatment it is assumed that a pre-operative radiograph has been taken, and that any acute condition involving the tooth has been eliminated (Chapter 10). All carious cavities suspected of com-municating with the pulp cavity will have been cleaned and dressed; similarly, all leaking fillings in the crown will have been replaced by dressings. Where the pulp is vital and is to be removed immediately, any exposure should have been cauterized by a hot instrument; where pulpectomy has been deferred from a previous visit, this step will have been omitted and the pulp will have been capped. Local anaes-thesia will have been used in all cases unless obvious periapical destruction is visible radiographically.

Cases may be divided into two groups, according to whether the pulp is vital and virtually intact, or shows obvious breakdown or suppuration, or is completely necrotic.

Group I: Intact, vital pulp
VISIT 1
(*a*) Apply rubber dam; (*b*) Scrub tooth surface with chemical antiseptic; (*c*) Cut access cavity to pulp chamber; (*d*) Remove coronal pulp, clean bulk of pulp chamber and cauterize by heat the surface of the radicular pulp; (*e*) Remove radicular pulp; (*f*) Insert reamer to a little short of probable level of apical limit and take radiograph; (*g*) Whilst film is being processed, complete cleaning of pulp chamber; (*h*) After processing film, assess working length; (*i*) Prepare canal to apical limit by reaming, filing and irrigation; (*j*) Fit gutta percha or silver point and take radiograph to check apical level; (*k*) Dress and seal pulp cavity.
VISIT 2
3–7 days later.
If there are clinical signs or symptoms of disease, treat as in Visit 2 of Group II cases (*below*).

If there are no clinical signs or symptoms of disease: (*a*) Apply rubber dam; (*b*) Scrub tooth surface with chemical antiseptic; (*c*) Remove seal to pulp chamber;

(*d*) Remove cottonwool and antiseptic dressing from Visit 1; (*e*) Remove remnants of antiseptic and any small amount of exudate with absorbent paper points; (*f*) Root fill; (*g*) Take radiograph to check on root filling; (*h*) Unless a post crown is to be made soon, treat walls of pulp chamber to maintain translucency of crown; (*i*) Either insert a permanent restoration in crown immediately, or insert a temporary restoration and arrange for its subsequent replacement.

Group II: Necrotic pulp, and vital pulp with obvious breakdown or suppuration
VISIT 1

(*a*) Apply rubber dam; (*b*) Scrub tooth surface with chemical antiseptic; (*c*) Cut access cavity to pulp chamber; (*d*) Remove bulk of necrotic tissue from pulp chamber and expose root canal; (*e*) Clean canal of pulpal fragments with a barbed broach; (*f*) Insert reamer to a little short of probable level of apical limit and take radiograph; (*g*) Whilst film is being processed, complete cleaning of pulp chamber; (*h*) After processing film, assess working length; (*i*) Prepare canal to apical limit by reaming, filing and irrigation; (*j*) Fit gutta percha or silver point and take radiograph to check apical level; (*k*) Dress and seal pulp cavity.

VISIT 2: 24–36 hours later
If a sinus is present, Visit 2 may be 3–7 days later.

(*a*) Apply rubber dam; (*b*) Scrub tooth surface with chemical antiseptic; (*c*) Remove seal to pulp chamber; (*d*) Remove cottonwool and antiseptic dressing from Visit 1; (*e*) Remove remnants of antiseptic with absorbent paper points; (*f*) If suitable facilities exist, take bacteriological sample; (*g*) Dress and seal pulp cavity.

VISIT 3: 3–7 days later
If there are no clinical signs or symptoms of disease then complete treatment by performing stages (*a*) to (*i*) of Group I, Visit 2.

If there are clinical signs or symptoms of disease then continue treatment by repeating stages (*a*) to (*g*) of Group II, Visit 2. Pay particular attention to stages (*a*), (*f*) and (*g*), and check that the root canal has been thoroughly prepared.

VISIT 4: 3–7 days later
If there are no clinical signs or symptoms of disease, complete treatment by performing stages (*a*) to (*i*) of Group I, Visit 2. If there are clinical signs or symptoms of disease, consider periapical surgery.

If root filling is performed but a negative culture has not been obtained, ensure that the tooth is kept under observation.

POSTOPERATIVE REPAIR AND OBSERVATION

1. Postoperative repair: prognosis

Following the removal of a vital pulp from a tooth, there is an acute inflammatory reaction which may be virtually confined to the remaining pulp apically or may involve the periodontal tissue around the apical foramen also. Hatton et al. (1928) and Seltzer (1971) point out that a phase of destruction accompanies the inflammatory response. Necrotic tissue is removed, and irregular areas of resorption occur in the dentine and cementum along the apical part of the root canal. Extension of the inflammation to the apical periodontal membrane may lead to resorption of alveolar bone and its replacement by granulation tissue. Provided the remaining pulp apically is not severely injured during root canal treatment and does not become infected, however, the inflammatory reaction resolves and repair occurs.

Fibrous tissue is elaborated in place of granulation tissue, and is in turn replaced by bone. There is a deposition of calcified tissue which fills in areas of root resorption and leads to a gradual narrowing of the canal apically. Fibrous or calcific

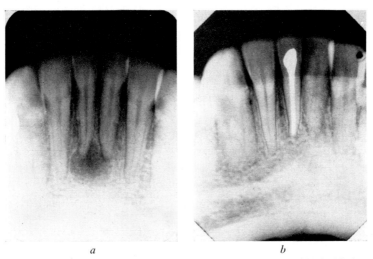

a   *b*

Fig. 166. T̄. *a,* Immediately before treatment. There is an obvious periapical lesion. *b,* Two years after treatment, periapical repair is complete.

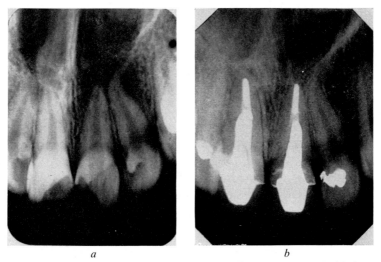

a   *b*

Fig. 167. ⌊1. *a,* Immediately before treatment. There is an obvious periapical lesion. *b,* Two years after treatment, periapical repair is complete.

tissue is formed over the apical end of the root filling, but it is rare for the latter to be sealed off completely with calcific tissue.

With a tooth having a necrotic pulp, the tissue in the vicinity of the apical foramen is already inflamed. Following successful root canal treatment, this inflammation gradually resolves. Resorbed areas of the apical surface of the root are repaired, and new bone is laid down to replace any which was destroyed. Granulation tissue in the unfilled apical part of the root canal is gradually replaced by fibrous tissue, and new periodontal fibres are formed around the apical part of

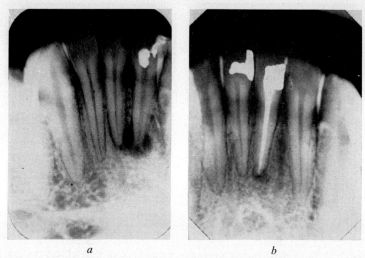

Fig. 168. ‖̄. *a*, Immediately before treatment. *b*, Ten years after treatment, repair is well advanced but is not complete.

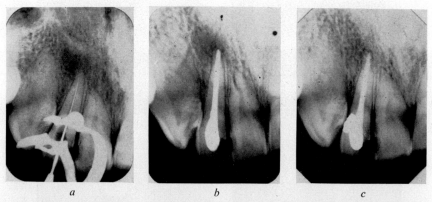

Fig. 169. 2‖. *a*, At the commencement of treatment. *b*, At the time of root filling 3 weeks later. The zone of periapical rarefaction is apparently larger, probably due to instrumentation beyond the apical foramen. *c*, Two and a half years later, repair is virtually complete.

the root to replace those which were destroyed. New cementum may be formed over the root-end (Weaver, 1947).

Most of the studies on the prognosis of non-surgical root canal treatment of permanent teeth report a success rate of 80–90 per cent, as assessed by clinical and radiographic criteria. The effect on prognosis of a periapical lesion is uncertain. Strindberg (1956), Seltzer et al. (1967), and Adenubi and Rule (1976) all report a higher failure rate for teeth with periapical lesions than for those with no such lesions. On the other hand, Grahnen and Hansson (1961), and evidently Harty et al. (1970), found no significant difference between the two groups.

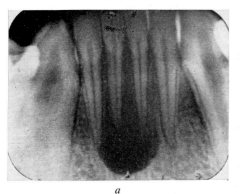

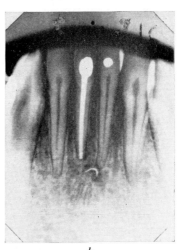

a

Fig. 170. ⊺⎸. *a*, Immediately before treatment. There is a large periapical lesion. *b*, Four years after treatment. The periapical lesion has healed with a radial pattern to the new trabeculae.

b

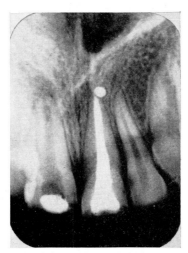

Fig. 171. The narrow zone of radiolucency around the excess root canal cement from ⎣1 is compatible with success.

Similarly, the influence of the pulpal status on the prognosis in those cases with no evidence of periapical destruction is uncertain; although it is generally held that success is more likely with a vital than with a necrotic pulp, in the study of Strindberg (1956) the converse was found to be true. Adenubi and Rule (1976) reported that the pulp status had no effect on the prognosis of such cases.

Seltzer et al. (1967) report that failures occurred more often with teeth which were crowned than with those which were not, especially posterior teeth with

7

periodontal disease. They suggest that occlusal trauma may have been responsible for the higher rate of failure.

2. Postoperative observation

Ideally, a root-filled tooth should be observed at regular intervals for as long as it remains within the patient's mouth. This is seldom possible, however, and it is therefore necessary to establish a period after which the result of treatment may be assessed with reasonable certainty. It should be emphasized that postoperative

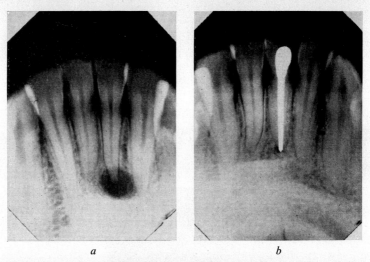

a   *b*

Fig. 172. ∏. *a*, Immediately before treatment. *b*, Two years after root filling. The small radiolucent zone around the excess point is compatible with success.

observation implies radiographic as well as clinical examination. As was pointed out in Chapter 1, clinical examination alone is of limited value in the diagnosis of chronic periapical disease, and should always be supplemented by radiographic examination.

Various authors suggest an observation period of 4–5 years before assessing the result of treatment (Strindberg, 1956; Grahnen and Hansson, 1961; Engstrom and Lundberg, 1965; Adenubi and Rule, 1976). However, a review of the literature (Nicholls, 1963) suggests that if treatment has been successful, most periapical lesions will show radiographic evidence of complete reconstruction within about 2 years (*Figs.* 166 and 167). Also, Seltzer et al. (1967) found that the majority of failures occurred within 2 years of treatment.

Once repair of a periapical lesion is complete, it is very probably permanent, provided the root filling is not disturbed and if periapical destruction following on periodontal disease or occlusal trauma is excluded. For these cases, therefore, clinical and radiographic inspection, say at 6-monthly intervals, for up to 2 years, or for a shorter period if there is evidence of complete reconstruction before this time, is usually satisfactory. Where it happens that observation beyond this time is possible, inspection should be performed annually.

Sometimes complete repair of a periapical lesion has not occurred after 2 years, although there is radiographic evidence of an obvious reduction in size. Occasionally, complete reconstruction is not evident even after several years (*Fig.* 168). Provided there is no clinical evidence of failure, observation of these cases should be continued. Where there is little or no reduction in size of a periapical lesion 2 years after root filling, failure may be assumed. Assessment after a 2-year period of observation is probably satisfactory also where the periapical region had a normal radiographic appearance immediately prior to treatment.

A temporary deterioration in the radiographic appearance of the periapical region occasionally occurs during or following root canal treatment, attributable to irritation of this region during treatment. Thus, there may be a slight increase in the size of a periapical rarefaction (*Fig.* 169), or a transient appearance of a new zone of rarefaction. Since these changes may take some time to disappear, a radiologic diagnosis of failure should not normally be made until at least 6 months after the completion of treatment. It is assumed, of course, that the radiographic change is slight, and that there is no clinical evidence of periapical disease.

Occasionally, the bone deposited during healing of a periapical lesion differs in radiographic density or trabecular pattern from that which existed prior to the advent of periapical disease or from that which exists around the adjoining teeth (*Fig.* 170). There is no evidence that such a variation is pathological. A narrow radiolucent zone of even width around an excess of root-filling material in the periapical region probably represents a capsule of connective tissue and is compatible with success (*Figs.* 171 and 172).

REFERENCES

Adenubi J. O. and Rule D. C. (1976) Success rate for root fillings in young patients. A retrospective analysis of treated cases. *Br. Dent. J.* **141**, 237.

Engstrom B., Hard Af Segerstad L., Ramstrom G. and Frostell G. (1964) Correlation of positive cultures with the prognosis for root canal treatment. *Odontol. Revy* **15**, 257.

Engstrom B. and Lundberg M. (1965) The correlation between positive culture and the prognosis of root canal therapy after pulpectomy. *Odontol. Revy* **16**, 193.

Grahnen H. and Hansson L. (1961) The prognosis of pulp and root canal therapy: a clinical and radiographic follow-up examination. *Odontol. Revy* **12**, 146.

Harty F. J., Parkins B. J. and Wengraf A. M. (1970) Success rate in root canal therapy: a retrospective study of conventional cases. *Br. Dent. J.* **128**, 65.

Hatton E. H., Skillen W. G. and Moen O. H. (1928) Histologic findings in teeth with treated and filled root canals. *J. Am. Dent. Assoc.* **15**, 56.

Marshall F. J. and Savoie F. L. (1967) Efficiency of endodontic culturing procedures using wet and dry paper points. *Oral Surg.* **23**, 806.

Nicholls E. (1963) Assessment of the periapical status of pulpless teeth. *Br. Dent. J.* **114**, 453.

Seltzer S. (1971) *Endodontology: Biologic Considerations in Endodontic Procedures.* New York, McGraw-Hill, pp. 235–47, 360–63.

Seltzer S., Bender I. B., Smith J., Freedman I. and Nazimov H. (1967) Endodontic failures—an analysis based on clinical, roentgenographic, and histologic findings, Part I. *Oral Surg.* **23**, 500.

Seltzer S., Bender I. B. and Turkenkopf S. (1963) Factors affecting successful repair after root canal therapy. *J. Am. Dent. Assoc.* **67**, 651.

Seltzer S., Turkenkopf A., Vito A., Green D. and Bender I. B. (1964) A histologic evaluation of periapical repair following positive and negative root canal cultures. *Oral Surg.* **17**, 507.

Stewart G. G., Kapsimalis P. and Rappaport H. (1969) EDTA and urea peroxide for root canal preparation. *J. Am. Dent. Assoc.* **78**, 335.

Strindberg L. Z. (1956) The dependence of the results of pulp therapy on certain factors. *Acta Odontol. Scand.* **14**, Suppl. 21, pp. 97, 100.

Weaver S. M. (1947) Root canal treatment with visual evidence of histologic repair. *J. Am. Dent. Assoc.* **35**, 483.

FURTHER READING

Morse D. R. (1971) The endodontic culture technique: an impractical and unnecessary procedure. *Dent. Clin. North Am.* **15**, 793–806.
Naidorf I. J. (1974) Clinical microbiology in endodontics. *Dent. Clin. North Am.* **18**, 329–44.
Seltzer S. (1971) *Endodontology: Biologic Considerations in Endodontic Procedures.* Chap. 8, Microbiologic aspects of endodontics. New York, McGraw-Hill, pp. 290–312.

Chapter 10

Treatment of acute pulpal and periapical conditions

Acute conditions of either the pulp or the periapical tissues often require separate treatment before preparation of the root canal may be performed, otherwise there is a risk of a spread of infection to the periapical region, or extension of an existing periapical infection. It has already been pointed out in Chapter 1 that, except following operative procedures, acute pulpitis does not constitute a histological entity, but is merely superimposed on regions of a pulp which is already chronically inflamed. The term 'pulpitis with acute symptoms' will therefore be used to describe these cases.

Acute inflammation of the periapical tissues may be largely confined to the apical periodontal membrane, constituting an acute apical periodontitis, or may have progressed further to form an acute periapical abscess. Although these two conditions are often the reason for instituting root canal treatment, on occasions they actually result from such treatment.

GENERAL PRINCIPLES OF TREATMENT

The aim in the treatment of each of the three conditions—pulpitis with acute symptoms, acute apical periodontitis and acute periapical abscess—is to convert an acute condition into a chronic one, and to relieve symptoms, particularly pain. The general principles of treatment comprise the drainage of inflammatory exudate, the provision of rest for the affected tissues and, where appropriate, the removal of the cause of the condition. In certain instances, supportive measures, such as the administration of antibiotics, are indicated. Analgesics, such as aspirin or codeine, are prescribed if considered necessary.

In all instances the affected tissues are rested by grinding to relieve the tooth of its occlusion with opposing teeth. Since the tooth under treatment is often sensitive to touch, the opposing teeth are usually reduced. Some operators advise this as a routine measure when a tooth is root-treated, whatever its pulpal or periapical condition.

Where treatment includes sealing of the pulp cavity, antiseptic dressings should be confined to the pulp chamber, so allowing further exudate to accumulate within the root canal.

Where it is necessary to leave the pulp cavity open to the mouth for the drainage of inflammatory exudate, a cottonwool pledget is placed within the pulp chamber to prevent blockage of the canal by food particles.

189

In all cases it is important to remember that the severity of the symptoms, although perhaps alarming, is largely unrelated to the prognosis.

PULPITIS WITH ACUTE SYMPTOMS

Where pulpal disease is due to caries, as is usually the case, the floor of the cavity should be cleaned completely, so that the resultant exposure allows the pulp to bleed freely and so wash away micro-organisms and reduce pulpal congestion. Subsequent treatment depends on whether there is visible evidence of suppuration.

1. Non-suppurative pulpitis

Where suppuration has not yet occurred, contamination of the pulp is probably superficial. There is therefore no objection to immediate pulpectomy. At the same time, there is no advantage in it, and where it is more convenient a sedative dressing should be inserted preparatory to pulpectomy, as described in the account of suppurative pulpitis.

Where immediate pulpectomy is decided upon, local anaesthesia, if not already obtained, will of course be necessary. After removing all caries, the exposed part of the pulp is cauterized by heat, the cavity dressed with a fast-setting zinc oxide–eugenol cement and the rubber dam applied. Where more than a few minutes have elapsed since injecting the local anaesthetic solution, a second injection is given before applying the rubber dam. Pulpectomy is now performed in an aseptic manner through an opening cut in the occlusal or lingual surface of the tooth. After the pulp has been removed, and if time permits, the radiographic examination necessary for assessing the working length of the tooth is made.

Haemorrhage will probably be fairly profuse following pulpectomy. It is allowed to continue for 1 or 2 minutes, after which the root canal is irrigated and all traces of blood removed from the pulp chamber. The pulp cavity is now dried and any residual haemorrhage arrested with absorbent points. An antiseptic dressing is placed in the pulp chamber and the latter sealed with cement. Arrangements are made to continue root canal treatment as soon as possible.

2. Suppurative pulpitis

Clinical evidence of suppuration denotes heavy contamination of the coronal pulp, and in consequence immediate pulpectomy carries the risk of thrusting organisms in an apical direction. Also, even though cauterization of the coronal surface of the radicular pulp may largely obviate this hazard, there still remains very often the problem of obtaining sufficiently profound anaesthesia to allow instrumentation within the pulp cavity, especially as intrapulpal injection is contraindicated by the infection present. For these reasons it is advisable to insert a sedative antiseptic dressing first, preparatory to removing the pulp shortly afterwards as a planned procedure.

Following the removal of caries and the escape of blood and pus from the site of exposure, the pulpal wound is washed with water or saline, or with an antiseptic fluid such as sodium hypochlorite, and is gently dried. The exposure is now covered with a wool pledget moistened with CMCP. Alternatively, a corticosteroid–antibiotic paste may be used. The cavity is dressed with a fast-setting zinc oxide–eugenol cement.

Where pulpal disease has resulted from some other cause, such as an exposure under a restoration, a similar procedure is followed. Pulpal disease due to the absence of a lining under a silicate or autopolymerizing acrylic restoration is usually without acute symptoms until the periapical tissues have been involved.

Following the treatment described, the patient should be seen again soon, preferably within 48 hours. By this time the condition will have improved sufficiently to allow pulpectomy.

ACUTE APICAL PERIODONTITIS

Acute apical periodontitis may exist in conjunction with a suppurative pulpitis, in which the pulp is partly necrotic, or with a totally necrotic pulp. Whatever the state of the pulp and the cause of the condition, the periodontal membrane is sensitive when the tooth is percussed. The tooth may be more mobile than the adjoining teeth.

1. Acute apical periodontitis in conjunction with suppurative pulpitis

By the time an acute apical periodontitis has developed following a suppurative pulpitis, a considerable part of the pulp is usually necrotic. Treatment is basically the same as with an uncomplicated case of suppurative pulpitis, except that wherever possible the pulp cavity is opened through the occlusal or lingual surface of the tooth, as for root canal treatment; the drainage of pus is thus facilitated. Treatment is performed in an aseptic manner, carious cavities being cleaned and dressed beforehand and the rubber dam applied. There should be the minimum of instrumentation in the pulp cavity compatible with obtaining the free escape of pus and blood. After gentle irrigation, the pulp chamber is dressed with an antiseptic and the occlusal or lingual opening sealed. The patient is seen again within 48 hours, when any residual vital pulp may be removed.

Occasionally the severity of the symptoms may tempt the operator to leave the pulp cavity open to the mouth for drainage. This is a mistake, since to do so increases the risk of acute exacerbation when the tooth is later sealed and root canal treatment continued, presumably due to increased contamination of the pulp cavity from exposure to saliva (Weine et al., 1975). Instead, the patient should be seen again within 24 hours to drain any further blood and pus, and the pulp chamber again dressed and sealed.

2. Acute apical periodontitis in conjunction with a necrotic pulp

a. Aetiology

An acute apical periodontitis associated with a necrotic pulp may arise from infection of the pulp cavity and be the reason for instituting root canal treatment in the first instance, or it may result from operative procedures within the pulp cavity.

Although injury to the periapex from the use of irritant antiseptics during treatment is not uncommon, the operative procedures which most often lead to acute apical periodontitis are those which force debris and micro-organisms beyond the apical foramen or inflict direct physical injury on the periapical tissues. Physical injury to these tissues occurs whenever instruments, antiseptic pastes, root-filling substances or other materials pass beyond the apical foramen.

Whatever the source of irritation, the reaction tends to be more severe when the periapical bone appears intact radiographically than when a periapical lesion is present, perhaps because of the greater opportunity for inflammatory exudate to accumulate in the latter type of case. Where micro-organisms constitute the source of irritation, an additional factor may be that the tissue defences are mobilized to a greater degree when a periapical lesion already exists. However, the presence of such a lesion does not mean that less caution need be exercised during treatment. Unless a sinus is already present or is created artificially, an acute exacerbation in such a case is by no means unusual following operative procedures beyond the apical foramen.

b. Treatment

Although the treatment which is given depends to some extent on the cause of the condition, it is usually possible to seal the pulp cavity at this visit. Treatment should therefore be performed in an aseptic manner.

Even though the pulp may be thought to be completely necrotic, local anaesthesia should be used if the root canal has not been treated previously, since vital tissue is sometimes present in the apical part of the canal. After opening the pulp chamber, the root canal is carefully cleared of as much necrotic pulp as is possible with barbed broaches and, if necessary, is gently reamed and irrigated to encourage drainage. The pulp cavity is left open for some minutes, exudate within the canal being periodically absorbed with paper points. During this time the radiographic examination necessary for assessing the working length is performed. An antiseptic dressing is then inserted in the pulp chamber, the occlusal or lingual opening sealed, and the patient seen again within 2 or 3 days, when thorough cleaning of the pulp cavity is generally possible. Should there be no drainage of exudate on initial opening of the pulp cavity, the patient should be seen again within 24 hours. If this is not possible, the pulp cavity should be left open to the mouth.

Where the condition occurs as an exacerbation during treatment, any dressing material, such as an absorbent point, is first removed, and the root canal carefully explored to ensure it is patent. Absorbent points are used to remove antiseptic drugs from the canal, which is then gently irrigated and dried. Absorbent points should be inserted slowly, otherwise pain, presumably as a result of forcing exudate in an apical direction, may be felt. The pulp cavity is now left open for some minutes and exudate periodically removed with absorbent points. Where previous treatment has been performed by another operator and the patient is being seen for the first time, the radiograph necessary for assessing the working length may now be taken.

Whilst the root canal is open the patient will usually experience a considerable reduction in pain, and the pulp cavity may then be dressed and sealed. There is generally no need to see the patient again before the next appointment for the continuation of root canal treatment is due. Sometimes, however, the treatment described provides no immediate relief. In such a case the patient should be seen again within 24 hours.

Occasionally, an uncomfortable periodontitis may result from slight overextension of a root filling into an originally intact periapical region. In these cases the application of a counter-irritant solution, such as tincture of iodine, to the buccal mucosa overlying the root apex is normally effective. However, if acute apical periodontitis has followed gross overfilling with a non-resorbable material, or if infection has been introduced or allowed to remain at the time of root filling, drainage is necessary. This is achieved by removing the root filling. Where this is not practicable, perforation of the buccal cortical plate over the root apex, preparatory to periapical surgery later, is indicated (p. 196). If this procedure is not feasible and it is thought that the periodontitis is due to infection, systemic antibiotic therapy is necessary if the tooth is to be retained.

ACUTE PERIAPICAL ABSCESS

Extension of an acute apical periodontitis into the adjoining bone results in an acute periapical abscess. This must be drained.

1. Drainage by opening of pulp cavity

Before the soft tissues in the vicinity of the root apex have become fluctuant, differentiation between an acute periapical abscess and an acute apical periodontitis associated with suppurative pulpitis may not be obvious. As was pointed out in Chapter 1, a radiograph of the periapical region may show no bone change. In these cases it is necessary to assess the state of the pulp and determine whether vital tissue is present before proceeding further.

When seen at this stage, a periapical abscess is drained by opening the pulp cavity and ensuring that the root canal is patent by the removal of pulpal remnants. Occasionally slight widening of the apical foramen with a no. 20 or 25 reamer may be necessary to promote drainage. The pulp cavity is left open to communicate with the mouth. Heat may be used to assist localization of the abscess, but should be applied within the mouth—for example, in the form of hot mouthwashes—and not to the surface of the face, since this would encourage extraoral drainage.

Although the dentine is insensitive to cutting, pain will be felt should pressure or vibration from the bur be transmitted to the apical periodontal membrane. Although only minimal pressure is needed when using air-turbine drills, stabilization of the tooth during opening of the pulp chamber is commonly necessary. Often, counter-pressure with a fingertip or a wool roll lightly applied to the buccal aspects of the teeth in the affected area is sufficient. In other cases, stabilization by means of impression compound moulded to the buccal surfaces of the crowns is necessary (*Fig.* 173). Very occasionally, pain is still felt despite these measures, and a general anaesthetic has to be given.

Because of the potential discomfort for the patient when opening the tooth, it is tempting to make only a small opening into the pulp chamber. This is a mistake. The opening which is cut must be wide enough to allow the removal of pulpal remnants if this is necessary for adequate drainage. Unless a general anaesthetic has been given, it will often be possible to perform the radiographic examination necessary for assessing the working length immediately drainage has been obtained.

Where an occlusal or a mesial or distal cavity is continuous with the cavity cut into the chamber, the wool pledget which is inserted to prevent food impaction may tend to be dislodged. If this is thought likely, the surface of the cavity is lightly varnished first so that the fibres of the pledget adhere to it. Alternatively, if the patient's condition permits, the adjoining carious lesion is cleaned and the entire cavity filled with a fast-setting zinc oxide–eugenol cement, in which is left a channel to accommodate a wool pledget.

It is better to leave the pulp cavity unsealed for a little too long rather than risk a recurrence of acute symptoms by sealing it too early. However, this does not mean that the pulp cavity should be left in free communication with the mouth for long periods of time, since this increases the likelihood of discoloration of the crown and may even lead to caries within the tooth. Normally, the acute symptoms

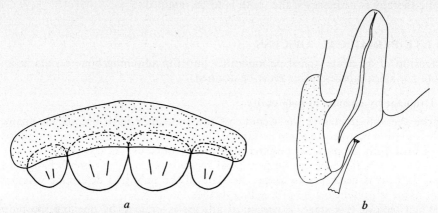

a   *b*

Fig. 173. Stabilization of a tooth with an acute periapical abscess during opening of pulp cavity, using impression compound. *a*, Occlusal view. *b*, View from mesial or distal aspect.

have largely disappeared within 2 or 3 days, and it is safe to prepare and seal the pulp cavity within a week.

2. Drainage by incision

Where the patient is first seen at a later stage in the development of the lesion and the intraoral soft tissues in the vicinity of the root apex are fluctuant, incision usually provides effective drainage. Opening of the pulp cavity is unnecessary provided root canal treatment is started within a few days, before the condition can recur following healing and closure of the wound. Occasionally, incision does not completely relieve the acute symptoms. In these cases, opening of the pulp cavity often leads to further drainage, suggesting that there was a localized collection of pus within the periapical bone with only a narrow communication through the cortical plate with the exterior (*Fig*. 174). Although intraoral swelling usually occurs in the buccal sulcus over the apex of the root, it occasionally forms palatally (*Fig*. 175), particularly with maxillary lateral incisor teeth and the palatal roots of maxillary molars.

The swelling is incised at its most dependent part. The incision should not extend into the gingival sulcus, since this would lead to an unsightly break in the gingival contour. Often the mucosal covering of the swelling is so thin that a light stroke with a scalpel is sufficient and no anaesthetic is needed. On other occasions a topical anaesthetic provides adequate anaesthesia. Sometimes the covering of the swelling is still quite thick, and either a nerve-block injection or a general anaesthetic is necessary. Premature closure of the incision, with possible recurrence of the acute condition, may be prevented by inserting a drain, such as an I-shaped piece of rubber dam, into the wound (*Fig.* 176), but this is rarely necessary if root canal treatment is begun within a few days.

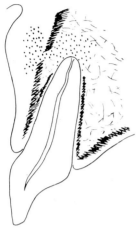

Fig. 174. Drainage of an acute periapical abscess by incision is occasionally insufficient, suggesting a localized collection of pus periapically with only a narrow opening in the cortical plate.

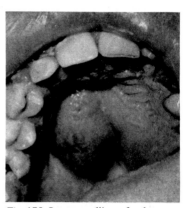

Fig. 175. Large swelling of palate from an acute periapical abscess.

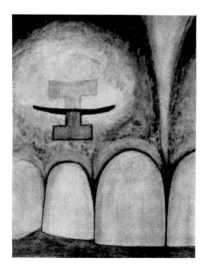

Fig. 176. The use of an I-shaped piece of rubber dam to prevent premature closure of the wound after incision of an acute periapical abscess.

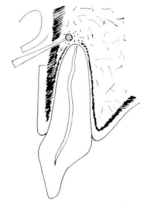

Fig. 177. Perforation of buccal cortical plate with a bur for drainage of an acute periapical abscess.

In very severe cases, both soft tissue incision and opening of the pulp cavity are performed to obtain the maximum possible drainage.

3. Drainage by perforation of cortical bone

Occasionally, neither incision nor opening of the pulp chamber is feasible as a method of draining an acute periapical abscess, the former being precluded because the cortical plate of bone is still intact, and the latter because the root canal is filled or is very narrow. In such a case it may be possible to obtain drainage by perforating the buccal cortical plate just beyond the root apex, using a round bur, about No. 6 (*Fig.* 177). This operation is sometimes called 'transmucous bone trephining', or 'artificial sinus technique'. Although not essential, it is better to reflect a small flap in the region of the apex first.

4. Antibiotic therapy

For patients whose general health is normal, systemic antibiotic therapy is not necessary provided that effective drainage is established. Where the general symptoms are very pronounced, however, or where the swelling is spreading rapidly, the systemic administration of an antibiotic, typically penicillin, is indicated. In these cases the patient's temperature and pulse should be taken, and other supportive measures, such as rest in bed, instituted.

Systemic antibiotic therapy is justified in certain other instances. An obvious example concerns patients whose medical histories suggest possible endocardial disease, for instance those who have had rheumatic fever. Again, with a molar tooth where the tissues are not yet fluctuant and the root canals are very narrow, perforating the cortical plate with a bur may not be feasible. Under these circumstances the systemic administration of an antibiotic may provide the only means of reducing the acute condition sufficiently to permit root canal treatment.

5. Subsequent treatment

Where drainage has been obtained by incision and the soft tissues have healed, the irritation caused by subsequent cleaning and preparation of the pulp cavity may lead to renewed abscess formation. To prevent this, root canal preparation is best carried out before complete closure of the incision.

Where the pulp cavity has been left open for drainage, subsequent closure is sometimes followed by an acute exacerbation. This may be avoided by ensuring that sealing of the pulp cavity does not follow immediately upon preparation of the root canal, and is performed only in the presence of a reasonably clean canal. The root canal is first prepared, but the pulp cavity is left open to the mouth for drainage. A few days later the pulp cavity is irrigated to remove debris, an antiseptic dressing inserted in the pulp chamber, and the tooth sealed. No reaming or filing is performed at this second visit. At a subsequent visit the canal is prepared one or two sizes larger to eliminate dentine contaminated from contact with saliva.

REFERENCE

Weine F. S., Healey H. J. and Theiss E. P. (1975) Endodontic emergency dilemma: leave tooth open or keep it closed? *Oral Surg.* **40**, 531.

FURTHER READING

Seltzer S. (1971) *Endodontology: Biologic Considerations in Endodontic Procedures.* New York, McGraw-Hill, pp. 164–70.

Chapter 11

Periapical surgery

In a small minority of cases it is necessary to supplement root canal treatment by periapical surgery in order to ensure a favourable prognosis.

There are three forms of periapical surgery, namely apicectomy, apical curettage and apicectomy with reverse filling of the root canal. In describing these procedures, it is assumed that there is adequate access to the operative field and that sufficient of the root will remain following surgery to support the tooth firmly in its socket. The amount of root necessary for this depends on various factors, amongst the more obvious of which are the length of the crown, the extent of any periodontal destruction present, and the nature of the occlusion and of the opposing teeth. With a single-rooted tooth it is desirable that at least one-half, and preferably more, of the original length of the root remains attached to the alveolus.

It is also assumed that there are no systemic or local contraindications to surgery. Any systemic disease liable to interfere with repair should have been controlled. There should be no evidence of acute inflammation in or close to the region to be operated upon.

Treatment should be performed as aseptically as is possible within the mouth. Thus before use all instruments are sterilized. A clean field is obtained before operation; the teeth and mucous membrane in the area are cleaned of cellular debris and mucinous material.

Periapical surgery is normally performed under local anaesthesia. With a highly apprehensive patient, preoperative sedation is indicated. Oral diazepam, 5 mg three times daily, starting the evening before treatment, is usually effective.

The following account of periapical surgery, although concerned mainly with anterior and premolar teeth with 'closed' root apices, is in its broader aspects largely applicable also to molar teeth and to teeth with open apices. Further details of the surgical treatment of these last two groups of cases are given in Chapters 12 and 13 respectively.

GENERAL CONSIDERATIONS

Before dealing with the different forms of periapical surgery, certain considerations common to each will be discussed.

1. Indications

The possible indications for periapical surgery have already been covered in Chapter 3, but will be considered again briefly.

197

a. Inaccessibility of apical region of canal

Periapical surgery is indicated most commonly where adequate preparation and filling of the root canal to within a short distance of the apical foramen are not possible by way of the pulp chamber. The prime object of surgery in such cases is to remove, or to facilitate effective treatment of, the apical part of the canal. As a general rule, surgery is indicated in the treatment of a tooth with a necrotic pulp where a level within 2·5–3·0 mm of the root apex cannot be reached. With a vital pulp a greater discrepancy is probably permissible, and non-surgical treatment may sometimes be successful even though access cannot be gained to the apical 4·0– 5·0 mm of the root canal. Such cases may be observed and periapical surgery performed only when shown to be necessary.

b. Perforation of apical part of root

If a perforation of the apical part of the root cannot be adequately cleaned and filled by way of the pulp chamber, it may be possible to eradicate it by removing this part of the root surgically.

c. Periapical disease associated with a foreign body periapically

Sometimes periapical disease is associated with the presence in the periapical tissues of a foreign body. If this cannot be removed by way of the pulp chamber, periapical surgery may be indicated.

d. Failure of previous root canal treatment

Where root canal treatment has been adequately performed but has failed, there is usually little point in repeating it. Instead, periapical surgery may be performed, the object being to eradicate some unfavourable factor, such as an additional root canal or a void in the root filling, which has escaped detection.

e. Persistence of periapical irritation during treatment

Sometimes, despite thorough cleaning and medication, periapical irritation persists. With these cases periapical surgery may be performed. Again, the object is to eliminate any unfavourable factor which may have escaped detection. Occasionally, especially in the maxillary premolar region, persistent discomfort is associated with an apical fenestration, with the root apex in direct contact buccally with the overlying soft tissues, without any intervening bone.

f. Adjacent abnormalities

It is sometimes expedient to include periapical surgery in the treatment of a tooth when an immediately adjacent abnormality, such as a supernumerary tooth, has to be eliminated surgically.

Periapical surgery is not indicated merely because a periapical lesion appears radiographically to be large or to have a circumscribed outline, or because a tooth with periapical disease shows resorption of the root apex. Where postoperative observation of a tooth with a large lesion will not be possible, however, it is safer to include periapical surgery in the treatment and remove the lesion.

Teeth with incompletely formed root apices and necrotic pulps can generally be treated successfully without surgical intervention (Chapter 13). Surgical treatment is not indicated for teeth with transverse root fractures and necrotic pulps coronally unless there is evidence of bone destruction around the apical fragment, indicating pulpal necrosis apically, or unless removal of the apical fragment is needed to allow the insertion of an endodontic stabilizer (Chapter 14).

2. Teeth amenable to periapical surgery

Periapical surgery is used most commonly in the treatment of anterior teeth, since access to these is good. Sometimes, where access is reasonable, the operation is performed on premolar and molar teeth. In these cases the radiographs of the region should be carefully studied to determine the proximity of the maxillary antrum, or of the inferior dental canal or mental foramen. Where there is a definite risk of trauma to the inferior dental or mental nerve, the case for retaining the tooth would have to be very strong indeed before embarking on periapical surgery, and, needless to say, the significance of injury to these structures would have to be fully explained to the patient. Similarly, where the creation of an extensive opening into the antrum is likely, the operation is contraindicated. This does not apply if only a small perforation is likely, however, such a lesion apparently healing quite readily provided the wound is clean.

3. Treatment plan

Normally, treatment is divided into two separate stages, the tooth being root-filled first and periapical surgery performed afterwards. One of three different methods may be followed. First, the pulp cavity may be cleaned and dressed with an anti-septic, and root filling and surgery carried out at a subsequent visit. Secondly, surgery may be performed after root filling the tooth at a previous visit; Smith (1952) has shown that, provided the intervening interval does not exceed 24 hours, there is little or no danger of exacerbation. Thirdly, the root canal may be prepared and filled immediately prior to, and at the same visit as, surgery.

With the last method, there is obviously no opportunity to seal an antiseptic medicament in the pulp cavity, although electrolytic medication may be used, or a chemical antiseptic may be applied for a short period, before filling. Also, the fact that the canal has only just been cleaned makes contamination of the surgical field periapically more likely, although this risk may be largely obviated by careful instrumentation of the canal in the presence of an antiseptic fluid, such as sodium hypochlorite. A further disadvantage is that the visit at which surgery is performed is lengthier than when part or all of the root canal treatment necessary is carried out at a preceding visit; this is an important factor when, as with a child, co-operation is likely to be limited, or where two or more teeth are to be treated concurrently. Because of these considerations, one of the first two methods is more commonly used.

An alternative form of treatment is to fill the root during the course of periapical surgery, or immediately before the wound is closed and the operation completed. This method has significant disadvantages. Isolating the root-end to prevent seep-age of blood into the canal during root filling may prove troublesome. Prolonging the operation places a greater strain on the patient and makes loss of anaesthesia before completion of the operation more likely than when the tooth is root-filled beforehand. Also, the fact that it is necessary to change from surgical instruments to root canal instruments, and then back to surgical instruments, is less conducive to efficient operating. Sometimes, however, this method has to be employed. For example, when there is a profuse exudate into the canal which cannot be con-trolled, a better apical seal is obtained by inserting the filling after the periapical lesion has been removed rather than before. Again, if an instrument has been broken in the apical part of the canal and is too long to remove in one piece with the root apex, preparation and filling of the apical part of the canal are only possible after the root apex has been removed and the instrument pulled out by way of the bony wound or pushed in the opposite direction into the pulp chamber and so out of the tooth (*Fig.* 178).

Whenever possible with this last plan of treatment, complete preparation of the root canal is carried out prior to surgery, otherwise the bony wound may be contaminated unnecessarily by dentine fragments and micro-organisms from the root

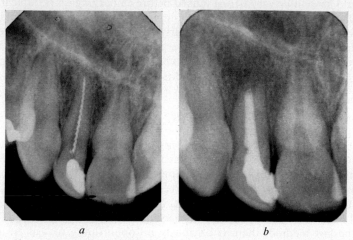

a   b

Fig. 178. 2]. *a*, Broken file which prevents root canal filling before apicectomy.
b, Appearance immediately postoperatively.

canal. Apicectomy with reverse filling of the root canal forms an exception to this general rule, since preparation of the apical part of the canal usually has to be done in its entirety after surgery. Also, with a broken instrument which cannot be removed with the root apex, although as much preparation as possible is performed beforehand, the completion of preparation is only possible after the instrument has been removed.

4. Root canal treatment

The importance of thorough root canal treatment cannot be overemphasized. The standard of root canal treatment is no less important merely because periapical surgery is to be performed. Inadequate preparation or filling of the root canal is likely to impede periapical repair and may well jeopardize the success of treatment, however well the surgical phase is performed (*Fig.* 179). The entire procedure should be regarded as one in which the inclusion of surgery is necessary for a successful outcome to root canal treatment. The latter should be performed as thoroughly and with the same regard to asepsis as when surgery is not included in treatment.

Where the tooth is already root-filled but treatment has failed, the object of surgery is to determine and eliminate the cause of failure. To equate periapical surgery in such a case with the removal of diseased periapical tissue and no more is to remove the manifestation of failure but to ignore its cause. Sometimes this cause may not be directly associated with the existing root filling; for example, a radicular cyst may have formed, or a radiolucent foreign body may be present periapically. Typically, however, the cause is associated with the existing root filling in that the latter does not seal the root canal effectively.

Where the tooth is root-filled preparatory to surgery, it is sometimes advocated that filling material deliberately be extruded beyond the apical foramen into the periapical tissues in order to facilitate location of the root-end during surgery.

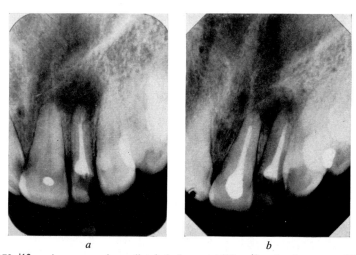

a   *b*

Fig. 179. |12. *a*, Appearance immediately before root filling |1 and apicectomy of |12. *b*, Three and a half years later there is very little improvement in the periapical state, due to inadequate root fillings in |12.

Although this procedure is not really necessary if a careful surgical technique is followed, there is no objection to it provided surgery is carried out before there is time for acute periapical inflammation to develop. Indeed, in some cases deliberate overfilling may be necessary in order to achieve a satisfactory apical seal. However, overfilling should not be preceded by deliberate widening of the apical foramen during root canal preparation, since this eliminates the 'stop' at the apical end of the prepared canal and encourages haemorrhage into the latter during filling. Thus, the apical seal to the root canal, upon which the result of treatment largely depends, is likely to be spoiled. Also, dentine fragments and micro-organisms are likely to be carried by reamers and files into the periapical tissues, so contaminating the surgical field unnecessarily.

It has already been pointed out that the application of some form of antiseptic agent to the root canal is still possible even though the pulp cavity is to be cleaned at the same visit as surgery. Although many operators omit this stage and rely entirely on thorough preparation and filling of the canal, an attempt to eliminate any organisms remaining would seem desirable. Electrolytic medication, using a current of 5 mA for 6 minutes, is sometimes recommended for this purpose. A more convenient method is to apply CMCP to the canal on a closely fitting absorbent point whilst preparations are made to root fill the tooth. The canal is dried immediately prior to insertion of the root filling.

5. General surgical technique

a. Armamentarium
The armamentarium necessary for periapical surgery is shown in *Fig.* 180.

b. Anaesthesia
Even though part or all of the region may have already been anaesthetized to allow root canal treatment, if more than a few minutes have elapsed, fresh injections are given as a safeguard against the loss of anaesthesia during treatment.

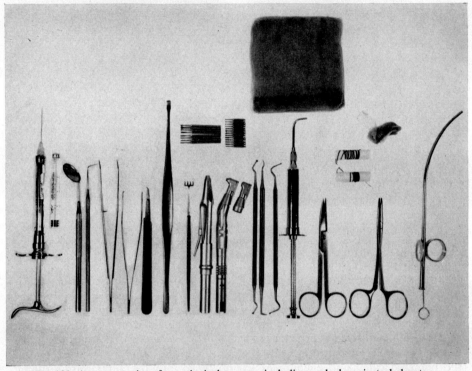

Fig. 180. Armamentarium for periapical surgery, including scalpel, periosteal elevator, retractor, excavators and Mitchell's trimmer for curetting diseased periapical tissue, Hunt syringe, scissors, needle holders and Magill's suction tube. Instruments needed for treatment of the root canal are not included.

Although some workers advocate an infraorbital injection for a maxillary anterior tooth, subperiosteal injections buccally are invariably effective. These have the added advantage of producing vasoconstriction locally, so reducing haemorrhage during surgery. They are spaced about 6·0 mm apart and should span the entire length of the flap which is planned. They are given slowly to avoid distending the tissues unnecessarily and so reducing access later. Particular care should be taken to obtain complete anaesthesia palatally. For anterior teeth an injection into the incisive foramen is preferable, whilst for premolar teeth injections are made locally.

Incomplete anaesthesia of the maxillary incisor region during periapical surgery is sometimes attributed to sensory innervation of this region through the floor of the nose. Because of this, some operators advocate, as an additional measure, packing the floor of each nostril with ribbon gauze moistened with 10 per cent cocaine solution. This procedure is unnecessary provided that the local anaesthetic injections are correctly sited and made.

In the mandible an inferior dental nerve-block injection, to include the lingual nerve, is given. It is advisable to supplement this by subperiosteal injections, administered in the same way as in the maxilla; particular care should be taken with mandibular anterior teeth to avoid unnecessary distension of the tissues, since access to the periapical regions of these teeth can be difficult. When the operative field is close to the midline, a lingual injection is given on the opposite side to allow for cross-innervation.

c. Preparation of patient

A sterile towel is placed over the apron covering the patient's chest; materials such as swabs may then be rested on the towel immediately before being used. It is good practice to apply a towel from the front to the back of the head to cover the patient's hair, so keeping the latter well clear of the operator's hands. With a patient who is likely to become apprehensive at the sight of instruments, this towel may also be used to cover the eyes.

The patient is instructed to close on a gauze square which has been folded on itself two or three times and placed between the upper and lower teeth. This enables both lips and cheeks to be retracted farther than if the mouth were open, so giving more access. The gauze serves to absorb saliva, and is changed as necessary during treatment.

The teeth and mucous membrane in the region of the operative field, including the mucosal surface of the lip or cheek, are dried with a wool roll or gauze. If the operator wishes, a suitable antiseptic solution, such as a 0·5 per cent alcoholic solution of chlorhexidine, may be applied to the mucosa using a wool roll. However, it is doubtful that this achieves more than a temporary reduction in the number of organisms in the region.

d. Flap

An incision is now made buccally over the alveolar process and a flap reflected. The incision is made right down to bone so that the mucoperiosteum may be lifted as one layer. The flap is reflected with a periosteal elevator until it is well clear of the levels of the root apices, as judged from the preoperative radiographs, and, if available, from the recorded length of the tooth under treatment. With long-standing lesions which have perforated the buccal cortical plate, fibrous adhesions may make reflection difficult. These adhesions are severed with a scalpel rather than torn with the elevator.

The line of incision and the resultant flap should provide adequate access to the periapex and apical region of the root under treatment, and bleeding points along the incision should not be in close proximity to the region under treatment. Where one tooth is to be treated, a flap three times longer in span than the mesiodistal width of the crown, with vertical relieving incisions extending to the buccal sulcus, is usually adequate (*Figs.* 181 and 182). The line of incision should be such that the subsequent line of closure rests directly on bone and is not over the dead space of the bony wound.

One of two basic flap designs may be used. An undulating incision parallel to and about 3·0–4·0 mm from the gingival crests may be made in the attached gingiva (*Fig.* 181) or the flap may be lifted from the gingival sulci around the teeth (*Fig.* 182). With the latter design, an inverse bevel incision may be used should there be concomitant periodontal disease. There are two possible disadvantages of an incision involving the gingival sulci. Firstly, it is occasionally followed by some

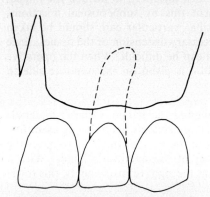

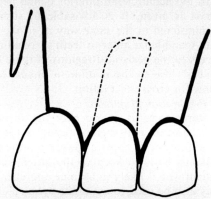

Fig. 181. Incision for periapical surgery is about three times longer in span than the mesiodistal width of the crown (|2). The horizontal incision is about 3·0 mm from, and roughly parallel to, the gingival crests.

Fig. 182. A flap design which allows not only periapical surgery but also periodontal surgery. The span of the flap is similar to that in *Fig.* 181.

gingival recession, which may result in the margin of an artificial crown being exposed to view. Secondly, if there is a dehiscence with direct contact buccally between the coronal part of one of the roots and the overlying soft tissues, the tissues may fail to reattach to the root following replacement of the flap, with resultant pocket formation. These disadvantages do not apply to the first type of flap (*Fig.* 181), and provided the periodontal condition is satisfactory this is the type normally used.

e. Removal of bone and location of root apex

Buccal bone is removed until the root apex and any associated periapical lesion are clearly in view. Either chisels or burs, or both, may be used for this purpose. If burs—which are more popular—are used, cutting is much easier and faster if an assistant with a syringe keeps up a steady flow of sterile normal saline over the area. A generous supply of various sizes of fissure and round burs, both straight and right-angle, should be available.

Particular care should be taken over this part of the operation, since much time, and tissue, may be wasted looking in the wrong position for the apex of a root. When a periapical lesion is present and part of the buccal cortical plate has been lost, enlargement of the bony opening towards the approximate position of the root apex makes location of the latter quite easy. With an intact buccal plate, however, location of the apex is not so straightforward, especially in the absence of periapical destruction. In this latter type of case the length of the tooth, if recorded, is a useful guide in deciding where to penetrate bone. When a periapical lesion is present, bone is penetrated over it, about 2·0–3·0 mm beyond the apex and roughly in line with the apical part of the root canal (*Fig.* 183). When the periapical region is intact, bone is generally penetrated directly over the root, 2·0–3·0 mm short of the apex (*Fig.* 184).

Other factors besides the length of the tooth must be considered when assessing the position of the root apex. For example, mesial or distal inclination of the tooth or curvature of the root may result in the apex being some millimetres from its

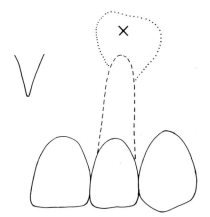

Fig. 183. Where there is a periapical lesion but the buccal cortical plate is intact, bone is penetrated at X, about 3·0 mm beyond the apex in line with the apical part of the root.

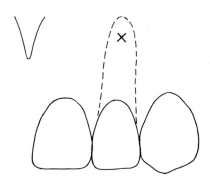

Fig. 184. Where there is no periapical destruction, bone is penetrated at X, directly over the root, 2·0–3·0 mm short of the apex.

anticipated position. For an accurate assessment of the probable mesiodistal position of the root apex it is important to view the field from a position at right-angles to the general line of the arch in the vicinity of the tooth, and not to allow the patient's head to tilt to the left or right (*Fig.* 185). With incisor teeth the field will be viewed from directly in front of the patient.

The buccolingual inclination of the crown and the configuration of the buccal plate give a reasonable idea of the thickness of bone over the root apex; the inclination of instruments previously inserted into the root canal provides another good guide. With the exception of mandibular incisors, whose apices may be situated lingually, the root apices of anterior teeth are generally close to the labial cortical plate. The apices of single-rooted premolars and of the buccal roots of two-rooted maxillary first premolars also are normally close to the buccal plate. The buccal cortical plate is thicker in the mandible than in the maxilla.

Unless the root apex is to be removed, care should be taken not to mutilate it when using burs to cut bone. In the absence of periapical destruction, differentiating between the labial or buccal surface of the root and the adjoining bone may not be easy. However, if the periodontal membrane is located by tracing with a probe its exposed line of attachment to the root, the latter may be recognized (*Fig.* 186).

f. Removal of diseased periapical tissue and foreign bodies

One of the prime requisites for success in root canal treatment—irrespective of whether it is supplemented by surgery—is that the pulp cavity be effectively sealed from the periapical tissues. In consequence, it is important that whenever possible the apical end of the root filling is inspected during periapical surgery. This is true

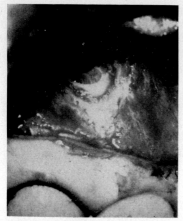

Fig. 185. In assessing where to penetrate bone, the patient's head should be upright. In this photograph, tilting results in the root-end appearing to lie midway between 1| and |1.

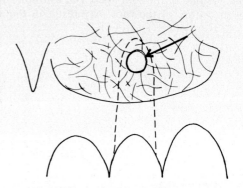

Fig. 186. Location of the periodontal membrane (arrowed) with a probe is useful when differentiating between bone and root.

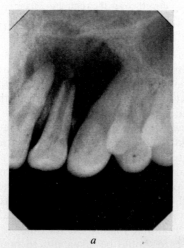

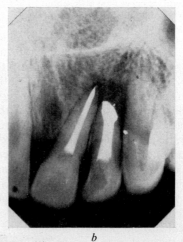

a   b

Fig. 187. |12. *a*, Preoperative condition. *b*, Considerable new bone formation is evident 18 months postoperatively, even though only enough of the lesion to gain access to the root apices was removed.

even if previous X-ray films indicate the root filling to be satisfactory, since voids in the buccal or lingual part of the filling are not usually apparent on a radiograph.

To permit inspection of the apical end of the root filling, part at least of any periapical lesion present has to be eliminated. In view of the undoubted potential for repair of such a lesion once all sources of irritation have been eradicated, it might be argued that no further part of it need be removed, and this may indeed sometimes be true (*Fig.* 187). However, such an approach does not allow for the possibility that cystic change has occurred. Also, diseased periapical tissue constitutes the most troublesome source of haemorrhage, and therefore the main hindrance to vision. In consequence, a periapical lesion is normally eradicated to all intents and purposes in its entirety, so that the sides and base of the wound are formed entirely by bone. Depending on the nature of the operation, the removal of diseased periapical tissue may be completed before or after treatment of the root apex. To facilitate description, however, this aspect of treatment will be dealt with in its entirety before treatment of the root apex is discussed.

In some instances, particularly in the anterior region of the mandible where the root apices are close together, the complete removal of a lesion would result in severing the neurovascular bundles leading to the pulps of adjacent, uninvolved teeth. In treating such cases, elimination of the lesion, whilst being as complete as possible, may stop a little short of the adjacent root apices; this assumes that no evidence of cyst formation is seen during treatment. Where there is extensive bone destruction, however, this procedure would result in the retention of a considerable amount of the lesion. In these cases a partial regeneration of bone, with a consequent reduction in size of the lesion, may sometimes be achieved by 'decompressing' the lesion (*Fig.* 188). This is done by perforating the overlying buccal cortical plate and then inserting a rubber dam drain in the manner described in Chapter 10 to prevent closure of the wound. The patient is seen periodically and the drain changed as necessary until there is radiographic evidence of sufficient bone regeneration to permit removal of the remainder of the lesion without damage to the adjacent teeth. Instead of rubber dam, Freedland (1970) suggests the use of a narrow polyethylene or polyvinyl tube.

In removing a periapical lesion, care must also be taken not to open the nasal cavity or the maxillary antrum, or a neurovascular canal; the roots of adjacent teeth must not be damaged. The preoperative radiographs should be consulted as necessary during the operation. Perforation of the palatal plate of bone by instruments with destruction of the overlying periosteum leads to what is commonly called an 'operative defect' (*Fig.* 189). Here, fibrous tissue rather than new bone is formed, even though bone regeneration in the vicinity of the root-end proceeds normally. It is especially likely to occur with maxillary lateral incisors (Persson, 1966; Rud et al., 1972c).

Diseased periapical tissue is removed with curettes or excavators. Small tags of tissue which tend to resist these instruments may be brushed away with round burs. The pointed end of a Mitchell's trimmer is often useful for relatively inaccessible areas. Any foreign body known to be present is removed. The removal of an excess of root-filling material presents little difficulty, since it is usually plainly visible. A broken instrument may be more difficult to locate, however, and fragments of tissue removed from the wound should be carefully examined for its presence before they are discarded.

It is particularly during the removal of diseased periapical tissue that haemorrhage may prove troublesome, and it is at this stage especially that an aspirator to remove blood from the field of operation is useful. If an aspirator is not available, it may be necessary to discontinue the operation periodically while the field is dried with wool rolls or gauze squares.

As more softened tissue is removed, the orifice of the bony wound may have to be enlarged to provide adequate access to the remainder of the lesion. Once removal of the latter is complete and access to the root apex is satisfactory, the margins of the opening into the bony wound are rounded. Thus, should subsequent treatment

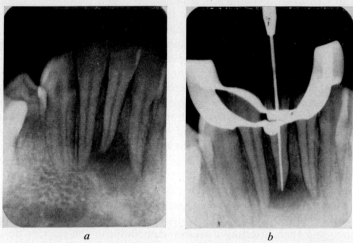

a   *b*

Fig. 188. ⊤|. *a*, Periapical lesion immediately before 'decompression'. *b*, The lesion is considerably smaller 3 months after decompressing it through the buccal cortical plate.

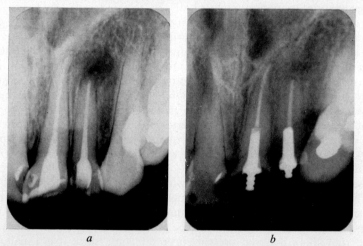

a   *b*

Fig. 189. |2. *a*, Immediately after apicectomy. *b*, One year later, repair by new bone is evident, but there is a radiolucent area 2·0–3·0 mm beyond the root-end, representing an 'operative defect' where the palatal periosteum was destroyed.

of the root apex prove time-consuming, any slight loss of anaesthesia towards the end of the operation should not prove inconvenient, since work on the sensitive part of the wound will already have been completed. With complete removal of the lesion the major source of haemorrhage is eliminated, and bleeding is significantly less.

g. Treatment of root apex

The treatment carried out on the root apex varies according to the operation being performed. Irrespective of the form treatment takes, however, it is important that the final apical surface of the root is inspected both visually and with a probe to ensure that there are no obvious voids around the periphery of the filling and that the adjoining dentine is hard. An exception to this rule is the case in which the root canal has deliberately been filled to excess in anticipation of periapical surgery. Here, inspection should be unnecessary.

h. Completion of operation

When treatment of the root apex has been completed, the wound is cleaned by irrigation with sterile normal saline, or, if this is not available, with local anaesthetic solution from a cartridge. It is then inspected to ensure that all debris has been removed, allowed to become covered with blood and finally closed with sutures. Although packing of the bony cavity with an absorbable material is sometimes advocated, the relatively small size of the wound generally makes this unnecessary. Insufflation with antibiotic powders is also unnecessary.

The number of sutures required depends largely on the length of the incision. If only one tooth has been treated, two or three are normally sufficient. Wounds in the anterior part of the lower jaw are more liable to tear open than those in the corresponding region of the upper jaw, probably because of the mobility of the lower lip. Thus for similar operations, more sutures tend to be used in the mandible than in the maxilla. Where the flap has been raised from the gingival sulci, a periodontal pack may be applied.

Periapical surgery is commonly followed by moderate postoperative swelling, and various enzyme and antihistamine preparations have been advocated from time to time to control this. The efficacy of such preparations is uncertain and their use is not normally indicated. Systemic antibiotic therapy is needed only where the wound is particularly extensive or shows evidence of heavy contamination at the time of surgery, or where there is a definite systemic indication. However, if an anti-inflammatory drug is used, or if the patient is already on systemic corticosteroid treatment, systemic antibiotic therapy is indicated.

A radiograph is taken either immediately postoperatively or a few days later when the sutures are removed, so as to provide a basis for comparison with later radiographs in assessing postoperative healing.

i. Variations in surgical technique

There are many variations in general surgical technique other than the few already mentioned. For example, some operators do not suture the wound, whilst others insert a rubber drain into it. A trephine may be used to remove the periapical lesion and the overlying bone. Removal of a periapical lesion, and even of the root apex itself, by way of the root canal has been described.

Variations such as these, however, are practised by relatively few operators, and have therefore not been included in the preceding account.

6. Postoperative instructions to patient

Before the patient is dismissed, definite verbal instructions are given for the postoperative care of the wound. If preoperative sedation was used, it is advisable to give the patient a written copy of the instructions.

The patient is warned that swelling of the face in the region of the wound is likely. This may be controlled by applications of cold—in the form of a clean cloth soaked in cold water, or two or three ice cubes wrapped in a handkerchief—to the outside of the lip or cheek. If time permits, these applications are made for about 10 minutes each hour for 1–2 days. With this treatment there is little obvious swelling after 2–3 days.

Apart from a few hours immediately postoperatively, actual pain is uncommon following periapical surgery, but discomfort, in the form of slight soreness, is often experienced. It may be satisfactorily controlled with a mild analgesic. Because of the inflammatory response to the trauma of the procedure, the tooth may become slightly mobile and tender to touch.

The patient is instructed to avoid any strenuous activity until the next day, since this tends to make the wound bleed. A reminder is given about the care needed for the first few days when brushing the teeth in the vicinity of the wound. The patient is also warned not to retract the lip or cheek to inspect the region. The use of mouthwashes may be started 24 hours postoperatively; a hydrogen peroxide mouthwash is useful after operations on posterior teeth, since postoperative swelling makes these more difficult to brush.

The sutures are normally removed 4–5 days after the operation. Although some operators leave them longer, the patient may find their presence irritating after a few days.

7. Complications of periapical surgery

Apart from swelling and discomfort, and ecchymosis, which occasionally occurs, complications of periapical surgery are rare. They may be listed as follows:

a. Anaesthesia

Occasionally after operations on maxillary incisor teeth, the patient states that the region about the tooth feels numb; this usually disappears within a few weeks. Anaesthesia of the lower lip due to damage to the mental nerve during an operation on a mandibular premolar tooth may persist for a much longer period, however.

b. Devitalization of pulp of adjacent tooth

Devitalization of the pulp of a tooth adjacent to the one under treatment, due to damage to the neurovascular bundle leading to the tooth, is most likely in the mandible anteriorly. If the complication is noticed during the course of surgery and if time permits, the tooth is root filled during the operation. Otherwise the tooth is root filled directly there has been sufficient soft-tissue healing to permit treatment.

c. Damage to root of adjacent tooth

The radiograph taken immediately postoperatively may show that the root of an adjacent tooth has been damaged by burs (*Fig. 190*). In such a case the damaged tooth is observed radiographically in the same way as the treated tooth.

d. Acute infection and breakdown of wound

The author has not seen a case of acute infection and breakdown of a periapical wound except following inadequate surgical treatment without proper regard to asepsis. The initial treatment of such a case is to eliminate the acute symptoms which exist, if necessary with the aid of systemic antibiotic therapy. Before periapical surgery is repeated in the area, it must be verified that there are no local or systemic contraindications to treatment.

e. Perforations of nasal cavity or maxillary antrum
Provided an adequate surgical technique has been followed and the wound is clean, a small opening into the nasal cavity or maxillary antrum seems to be followed by uneventful healing. The bony cavity is allowed to fill with blood before the wound is closed, and the patient is warned against blowing the nose for a few days.

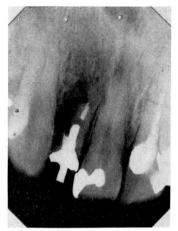

Fig. 190. 1|. A cut can be seen in the distal surface of the root level with the root-end of 2|, on which apicectomy had evidently been performed.

Systemic antibiotic therapy is indicated if there is any doubt about the cleanliness of the wound.

8. Postoperative repair and observation

Coolidge and Kesel (1956) discuss the literature on healing following surgery of the periapical region, and point out the resemblance to that which occurs after vital pulpectomy and root filling. The latter has already been covered in Chapter 9.

An inflammatory reaction occurs in the periapical region, with some resorption of the adjoining bone. There may be resorption of the cut apical surface of the root. With resolution of the inflammatory process, repair takes place. New bone is laid down and a band of fibrous tissue forms over the cut surface of the root. In some cases of apicectomy the dentine exposed by the operation, but not the root filling itself, becomes covered by a deposit of acellular cementum, in the outer part of which are embedded the ends of new periodontal fibres (Andreasen and Rud, 1972a). Sometimes small areas of ankylosis may occur between bone and root, whilst the new bone which is formed may differ in radio-opacity and structure from the adjoining bone (Rud et al., 1972a).

Cases treated by periapical surgery are observed in the same way as those in which root canal treatment has not been supplemented by surgery. Clinical and radiographic examinations are carried out at 6-monthly intervals until the radiographic appearance suggests complete healing. Should inspection beyond this period be possible, it is performed annually.

The literature on the average period necessary for repair is sparse. In the study of Smith (1952), complete regeneration of bone was normally evident radiographically 1 year after treatment. Boyne et al. (1961) found that where the diameter of labial plate destroyed was less than 8·0 mm, regeneration of cortical bone was complete within 5 months. Rud et al. (1972a) concluded that where the result was radiologically uncertain 4 years following treatment, failure was probable. Once healing was complete, later deterioration did not occur (Rud et al., 1972b).

APICECTOMY

Apicectomy is probably the most commonly practised form of periapical surgery. One of the earliest references to the operation is that of Farrar (1884).

The operation of apicectomy includes not only the elimination of diseased periapical tissue but also the removal of the root apex of the causative tooth. The operation is sometimes called 'root resection' or 'root amputation', but these terms are less desirable and are now used infrequently.

1. Rationale of root apex removal

Three main advantages derive from removing the root apex. First, by sectioning the root at an appropriate level and angle, an effective apical seal to the root canal may be ensured. Secondly, access is improved to diseased periapical tissue lingually to the root. Thirdly, unfilled apical branches of the main root canal, which may have been invaded by micro-organisms, are eliminated. At one time this last factor was thought to constitute the major advantage of, and thus the justification for, apicectomy. Whilst these branches are no doubt of some significance, their importance relative to that of the apical seal to the canal has in the past probably been overestimated. As will become apparent in discussing apical curettage, it is also improbable that elimination of the apical cementum confers any advantages.

Apicectomy also exposes to the periapical tissues many dentinal tubules which may be contaminated at their pulpal ends by micro-organisms. Although in the past this has sometimes constituted a criticism of this operation, it is extremely unlikely that it is of real significance. Indeed, Andreasen and Rud (1972b) have demonstrated that new cementum may be deposited over the cut ends of such tubules.

2. Prognosis

The available reports indicate the prognosis to be very favourable following root filling and apicectomy. Blum (1930, 1932), Phillips and Maxmen (1941) and Smith (1952) quote success rates of 96 per cent and 97 per cent, 99 per cent and 100 per cent respectively, although the publication of Phillips and Maxmen, whilst based on more than 600 apicectomies, gives few data. Grossman et al. (1964) found that almost 75 per cent of cases showed complete periapical repair and over 21 per cent partial repair when examined 1–5 years after treatment. Harty et al. (1970) report a success rate of over 90 per cent; there was a significantly higher failure rate with teeth associated with periapical radiolucency than with those with no radiolucent area. The most unfavourable reports are probably those of Persson (1966), Mattila and Altonen (1968) and Nordenram and Svardstrom (1970), who obtained success rates of 55 per cent, 54·5 per cent and 64 per cent respectively, whilst Harnisch (1963) reports that almost 30 per cent of cases showed residual periapical rarefaction.

3. Technique

Following location of the root-end, bone is removed so that the buccal surface of the root apex is exposed in its entirety for a distance of about 3·0–4·0 mm. A fissure bur is used to separate the root apex from the supporting bone mesially and distally (*Fig.* 191). If diseased periapical tissue is present, most of it is eliminated after the root apex has been removed, since greater access is then available.

As little of the root is removed as is necessary to obtain satisfactory access to diseased periapical tissue, if present, and to ensure that the apical end of the canal

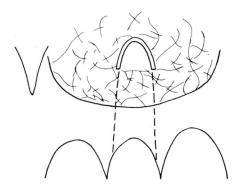

Fig. 191. Separation of the root apex from the bone mesially and distally.

is effectively sealed. Since bone but not root will regenerate, it is better to enlarge the bony opening than to cut away an excessive amount of the root. It is difficult to give an estimate of the maximum length of root which may reasonably be removed, especially as its real significance is in determining how much root remains. Much depends on the periodontal status of the remaining part of the root and the amount of stress taken by the tooth. As a rough guide, the root length should wherever possible be reduced by no more than 3·0–4·0 mm (*Fig.* 192), and preferably by less. However, the removal of a greater length than this is occasionally unavoidable, as, for example, when the root has to be sectioned coronal to a perforation on its palatal surface.

A fast-running bur is used to remove the root apex. Although convex, flat and concave shapes to the apical surface of the remaining root have all been advocated at one time or another, there seems no proof that any one of these is associated with a superior prognosis. No doubt because it represents the most convenient approach, most operators cut the root with fissure burs, so that the apical surface of the root-end is flat. This may be done either by working from side-to-side in a coronal direction from the root apex or by actually sectioning the root at the requisite level. If the latter method, which is the more popular, is followed, due allowance must be made for the width of the fissure bur in deciding on the level of section. Cutting of the root, like the removal of bone, is much easier and faster if done in the presence of a suitable coolant, such as sterile normal saline.

The root is cut in such a plane that the apical surface of the root-end faces buccally, so facilitating inspection of the end of the root filling (*Fig.* 193). The mesiodistal direction in which the root is cut is that which gives best access to diseased periapical tissue; this commonly, but not invariably (*Fig.* 192), results in a horizontal cut. Although it has occasionally been advocated that the root be trimmed flush with the final base of the bony cavity, this is not only unnecessary but actually undesirable if it entails excessive loss of root structure. However, where there is an apical fenestration, with direct contact between the root and the

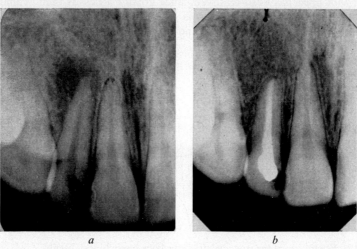

a   *b*

Fig. 192. 2|. *a*, Preoperative appearance. *b*, Appearance 7 years after apicectomy; 3·0–4·0 mm of the root were removed. The root filling, although occupying the entire root canal, appears to be short of the root-end, which faces distally.

overlying soft tissues buccally, the root should be planed back until its surface is within the outline of the buccal cortical plate. Also, in treating a two-rooted premolar, the buccal root has to be shortened rather more than usual in order to obtain access to the palatal root (*Fig.* 194).

If the root filling is inserted beforehand it is important that it is completely set when the root apex is removed. In using burs to remove the apex of a root filled with gutta percha, tearing of the filling may tend to spoil the apical seal. Although the gutta percha may be readapted with warmed plastic instruments, it is difficult to achieve as good an adaptation as existed originally; also, shrinkage of the gutta percha may occur. By contrast, silver cuts without tearing to give a relatively smooth surface to the sectioned filling. Not surprisingly, therefore, there is less disruption of the apical seal with a silver filling than with gutta percha (Cunningham, 1975). However, prolonged exposure of silver to tissue fluid can lead to corrosion with the formation of highly irritant compounds (Chapter 8). For this reason gutta percha is probably preferable to silver; should clinical examination of the cut apical surface of the filling reveal defects, the insertion of a reverse root filling is indicated.

Instead of gutta percha or silver, the apical end of the root canal may be filled with amalgam (Chapter 8). Although this avoids the problems of tearing or irritation from corrosion of the filling, Harty et al. (1970) found no significant difference in failure rate between teeth filled with amalgam and those filled with gutta percha or silver and a cement.

Following removal of the root apex, some operators attempt to seal the exposed dentinal tubules opening on to the apical surface of the root by applying silver nitrate solution for a few seconds and then reducing it with eugenol. There seems no proof that this has any beneficial effect. If the procedure is adopted, the solutions must be confined to the apical surface of the root. Each is applied on a small wool pledget or a wood point.

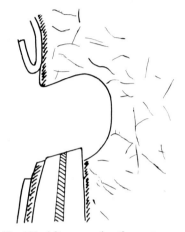

Fig. 193. After removing the root apex, the root-end should face buccally.

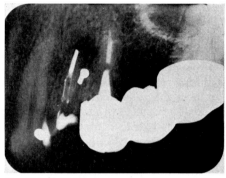

Fig. 194. |4. Following periapical surgery. The buccal root (distally), into which a reverse amalgam filling has been inserted, has been shortened more than usual in order to gain access to the palatal root (mesially).

Radiographs taken after apicectomy usually show the apical end of the root projecting beyond the end of the root filling, even though the latter is known to obliterate the canal completely (*see Figs.* 178 and 192). This is true even if the buccolingual plane of the cut apical surface is horizontal, and is due to projection of the X-ray beam in a downward or upward direction relative to the cut surface. Where the root has been cut so that the apical surface faces buccally, as described previously, the discrepancy on the radiograph between the end of the filling and that of the root is even greater.

4. Variations of apicectomy technique

Certain terms are sometimes used to describe special forms of apicectomy. The drawbacks of these forms of apicectomy compared with that in which root canal treatment is carried out first and surgery is performed at a second visit, which is known simply as apicectomy, have already been discussed.

a. Immediate apicectomy
The expression 'immediate apicectomy' means that the operation is performed immediately after, and at the same visit as, preparation and filling of the root canal.

b. Post-apicectomy filling
The term 'post-apicectomy filling' denotes that the root canal is prepared and filled during surgical treatment, after removal of the root apex. A variation of this

form of apicectomy is to defer removal of the apex until after the root filling has been inserted.

c. Apicectomy with immediate post crown cementation

If the tooth is to be restored by a post crown, it is possible to make this before surgical treatment. After preparation of the root canal, the tooth is prepared and impressions taken. At the next visit, apicectomy is performed; before the wound is closed, the crown is tried in and the metal core trimmed so that the apical end of the post is flush with the cut apical surface of the root. The prepared root canal is then coated with phosphate cement and the core seated in position. When set, excess cement is removed from the wound and the operation completed. The overlying jacket crown is then cemented in position.

This method of treatment has no generally recognized title. The advantages claimed for it are, first, that by utilizing the entire length of the root, displacement of the restoration from a tooth with a short root is less likely, and second, that the end of the post may be closely adapted by burnishing to the apical surface of the root during setting of the cement. There is no doubt that the first advantage, in so far as it may obviate the need for auxiliary retention, is a real one. However, the second advantage is hardly likely to apply if a cast post—and therefore presumably a hard gold—is used.

Apart from the need to keep the root canal dry during cementation of the core, the technique has two main drawbacks. First, since the post extends to the apical end of the root, contamination of the periapical tissues by saliva is inevitable if subsequently the post should become loose. Secondly, the seal provided apically by the phosphate cement used to cement the core is inferior to that given by other materials. If the technique is used, therefore, it is better to root fill the extreme apical end of the canal separately. This may be done by trimming the end of the post so that it is a millimetre or so short of the apical surface of the root and then root filling the space beyond either through the root canal immediately before cementing the core or by way of the bony wound after cementation.

APICAL CURETTAGE

In apical curettage, the removal of diseased periapical tissue is followed by curettage and smoothing of the cementum of the root apex, with rounding of the end of the root. The root apex is not excised.

Apical curettage has been practised for many years. In a lengthy description published in 1925, Roy stated he had had 25 years' experience of the operation, whilst Farrar, in 1884, referred to scraping roots softened at their apices. The operation is sometimes known as 'periapical curettage'.

1. Rationale; apical currettage versus apicectomy

It is usually claimed or implied by the advocates of apical curettage that an important reason for the failure of some root canal treatments is that whereas the main root canal and its branches are accessible to antiseptic drugs, the lacunae and canaliculi of the apical cementum are beyond their reach. Thus, since the lacunae and canaliculi are also beyond the reach of the tissue defences, infection stemming from them can only be eliminated by their removal. The fact that this can be accomplished by merely curetting the cementum covering the root apex, rather than by actual excision of the latter, enables the root length to remain virtually unreduced (*Fig.* 195).

The conservation of root structure is an undoubted advantage of apical curettage. However, the rationale for curetting the apical cementum, as opposed to leaving it untouched, seems to be based on little evidence of a convincing nature. Although micro-organisms may invade the lacunae and canaliculi in experimental animals, both Barker and Lockett (1971) and Morse (1973) point to the lack of evidence of this occurring in human teeth. In 66 cases of suspected failure of periapical surgery,

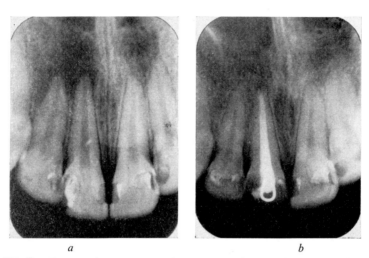

a   *b*

Fig. 195. 1|. *a*, Preoperative appearance. *b*, Two years after apical curettage. The root length is virtually the same. There is advanced but incomplete periapical bone regeneration.

Andreasen and Rud (1972b) found micro-organisms in the apical cementum in only two instances. Moreover, apical curettage has definite disadvantages, namely that access to diseased periapical tissue lingually to the root may be difficult, and that much periapical bone may have to be removed to enable inspection of the apical end of the root filling. If the apical seal is known to be adequate and there is sufficient access to diseased periapical tissue, then apical curettage rather than apicectomy may be performed. Usually, however, the operator is not completely sure that the apical seal is adequate, especially where surgical treatment is being performed on a case in which non-surgical treatment has failed. In consequence, apical curettage is performed far less commonly than apicectomy. Possible indications are the presence of a foreign body in the periapical region and the existence of a lesion situated mainly beyond the root apex (*Fig.* 195).

2. Prognosis

The only comparative report on the prognoses of apicectomy and apical curettage seems to be that of Rud et al. (1972c). These workers found no significant difference in the prognoses of the two procedures, with a success rate of 76 per cent.

3. Technique

Since the root apex must not be cut unnecessarily, it is preferable to penetrate bone beyond rather than directly over the root. Diseased periapical tissue is removed. In case the periapical lesion has undergone cystic change, the apical cementum is curetted to remove adherent epithelium. Excavators or burs are used for this purpose; long-shank contra-angle excavators may be needed where the lesion has involved the lingual surface of the root. Burs are used to round and trim the end of the root until it is flush with the root filling. Although root filling may be carried out after the root has been trimmed, it is generally performed prior to surgery. The filling should be set by the time the root comes to be trimmed.

APICECTOMY WITH REVERSE FILLING OF ROOT CANAL

It has already been pointed out that periapical surgery is most commonly indicated where the apical part of a root canal cannot be adequately prepared and filled by way of the pulp chamber and where removal of this region of the canal is considered necessary for a favourable prognosis. Usually the length of root involved is relatively small and it is possible by apicectomy to eliminate it completely and so ensure an adequate apical seal. Sometimes, however, it is too great to eliminate by apicectomy alone, and preparation and filling of the apical end of the untreated part of the canal are carried out by way of the bony wound following apicectomy.

This operation is known as apicectomy with 'reverse', or 'retrograde', filling of the root canal. The publications of Garvin (1919, 1942) indicate it has been in use for many years.

1. Indications

The factors which may prevent adequate treatment of the apical part of the canal by way of the pulp chamber, and which may therefore constitute indications for apicectomy with reverse filling, have been considered in Chapter 3. Some of these factors are illustrated in *Fig.* 198.

Apicectomy with reverse filling is also indicated when inspection of the surface of the cut root face during routine apicectomy reveals the root filling to be defective or to be surrounded by softened dentine (*Fig.* 198 *f* and *g*), assuming that the removal of more root structure to eradicate the fault is contraindicated.

2. Prognosis

Harty et al. (1970) report a failure rate of 11 per cent following apicectomy and reverse root filling with silver amalgam. Buchs and Reul (1962) give an extensive review of the European studies which have been performed, and these evidently quoted success rates varying from 18 to 92 per cent. Of their own cases, Buchs and Reul found that only 34 per cent were successful. However, in each of these studies the material used to fill the root-end was copper amalgam, which is known to cause severe irritation. Comparing teeth treated by root filling with gutta percha and apicectomy with those treated by apicectomy and reverse filling with amalgam, Rud et al. (1972b) quote success rates of 83 and 72 per cent respectively; the difference was statistically significant.

Kopp and Kresberg (1973), using gold foil to fill the root-end, obtained a success rate of 90 per cent.

3. Technique

The major part of the root canal, provided it is accessible, is prepared and filled by way of the pulp chamber before the operation.

Preparation of the untreated apical part of the canal remaining after apicectomy usually consists of enlarging it with burs to form a well-defined cavity in the root-end.

a. Surgical treatment

The salient features of the surgical phase of the procedure, including the ways in which it differs from other apicectomy operations, are as follows. The mesiodistal span of the incision is made rather longer than in other forms of apicectomy, since

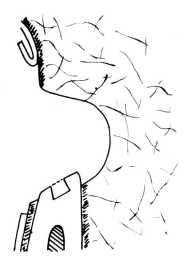

Fig. 196. In apicectomy with reverse filling, the root-end is cut to give a more pronounced buccal slope than with apicectomy alone. Also, the orifice of the bony wound is wider. The buccal and lingual walls of the root-end cavity incline lingually towards its floor.

besides providing more access for treatment of the root-end, this keeps any bleeding points along the line of incision farther from the mesial and distal margins of the bony cavity, and farther therefore from the root-end. If the root is already short—due, for example, to previous apicectomy—and it is important to conserve as much of its length as possible, bone is penetrated beyond the root apex rather than buccally to the root.

Wherever possible the supero-inferior size of the buccal orifice of the bony wound is made greater than that of the lingual base; this is accomplished mainly at the expense of the border of the wound which is farther from the root apex. Moreover, the root-end is cut to give a more pronounced buccal slope than is used in apicectomy alone (*Fig.* 196). Each of these measures improves visibility and increases access to the cut root surface, so facilitating treatment of the apical end of the root canal.

In case there should be some loss of anaesthesia before the completion of treatment, it is especially important to complete the removal of diseased periapical tissue and to round the margins of the opening in the alveolus before going on to treat the apical end of the canal. An added advantage of this approach is that with the removal of diseased tissue the main source of haemorrhage is eliminated, and so further treatment is facilitated.

b. Preparation of root-end cavity

The apical orifice of the root canal—the position of which may be confirmed by exploration with a probe—should now be visible and sufficiently accessible to allow the apical part of the canal to be prepared to a depth of about 1·0–2·0 mm. The initial cutting, which is done with round burs slightly larger than the apical orifice of the root canal, is confined to the immediate periphery of the canal and is continued until this periphery is completely eliminated. The cavity is then widened mesiodistally and buccolingually with larger round burs until it is large enough to permit adequate filling; wherever possible the base of the cavity is undercut, using

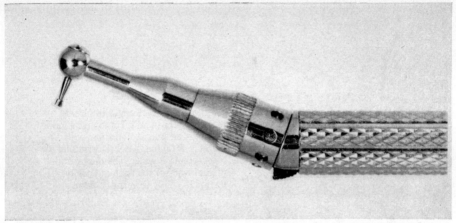

Fig. 197. The Kavo Contra-angle Handpiece, No. 126a Microhead.

small round or inverted cone burs. The mesiodistal and buccolingual dimensions of the final cavity depend on the original cross-sectional shape of the canal and on the amount of root structure available, but normally the outline is roughly circular and about 1·0–2·0 mm in diameter. Because of the buccal approach used during preparation of the cavity, its buccal and lingual walls usually incline lingually towards its floor (*Fig.* 196). This buccal approach should be borne in mind during cavity preparation and care taken not to perforate the lingual aspect of the root or to so weaken the lingual wall of the cavity that it is likely to fracture during condensation of the root-end filling.

If calcification of the pulp cavity has occurred and the apical orifice of the canal cannot be detected, the cavity in the root-end is prepared so as to include the site which the canal would normally have occupied.

The apical surface of the root should be carefully examined to ensure that the orifice of a second root canal has not been overlooked, especially in maxillary premolar and mandibular incisor teeth. Where an additional canal is present, either a separate cavity (*Fig.* 198*k*) or one large cavity (*Fig.* 198*i*) may be prepared, depending on the amount of dentine between the two orifices.

Usually a right-angle handpiece with a miniature head, used with burs of standard length, is satisfactory for preparation of the root-end cavity. Where access is very limited, the Kavo Contra-angle Handpiece, No. 126a, is occasionally useful (*Fig.* 197); with the bur inserted, this measures just over 10·0 mm from the cutting end of the bur to the far side of the head.

The position of the operator when cutting the cavity, and also when filling it, is important. Maximum access and vision are usually obtained if the operator is behind and to the side of the patient. It is also useful if the reverse side of a mouth mirror can be used to hold the flap in a retracted position. This is best done by the operator rather than by the assistant, since then the edge of the mirror may be lodged and held at such an angle against the line of attachment of the flap to the underlying bone as to reflect the maximum amount of light on to the root face.

After cutting of the cavity has been completed, the root-end is isolated by packing the floor of the surrounding bony cavity with ribbon gauze. Debris remaining in the root-end cavity is now removed by irrigation with sterile saline or local anaesthetic solution. The gauze pack is then removed and a fresh one inserted, and the root-end cavity dried with absorbent paper points bent at an appropriate angle.

By this time haemorrage into the bony wound is usually so slight that it offers no hindrance to filling of the root-end cavity. In those cases where it does prove troublesome, three main methods are available for its control. Provided there is no systemic contraindication to its use, a 0·4 per cent adrenaline solution may be used to moisten the pack. Although some workers object to the use of such a concentrated adrenaline solution, the author has seen no adverse effect from its application; needless to say, the solution is used sparingly. Alternatively, instead of using gauze, the root-end may be isolated by packing the bony wound with oxidized cellulose. Lastly, the entire bony wound may be filled with bone wax, which is then carved away to expose the root-end. Although often effective, each of the last two methods sometimes allows seepage of blood over the root-end.

c. Filling of root-end cavity

The insertion of a reverse filling provides one of the few opportunities the operator ever has to treat the apical end of a root canal by direct vision and to ensure beyond doubt that it is properly cleaned, shaped and filled. The completed root-end cavity should be clean, free of debris and dry, with a well-defined, regular outline. It should be filled with the same care that is used in filling the crown of a tooth.

i. MATERIALS

Many materials have been advocated for reverse root filling, including copper amalgam, silver amalgam, gold foil and cements.

The relatively poor results obtained with copper amalgam have already been mentioned; they are no doubt due at least in part to the rather severe irritation this material is known to cause (Dixon and Rickert, 1933; Mitchell, 1959). The use of cohesive gold foil pellets, as recommended by Kopp and Kresberg (1973), would probably appeal only to those who already use this material for coronal restorations. Reverse root fillings of polycarboxylate cement have been demonstrated to give a relatively poor seal (Barry and Fried, 1975; Barry et al., 1975), whilst the report of Persson et al. (1974) indicates that teeth filled with a zinc oxide–polyvinyl cement (Cavit) have a significantly poorer prognosis than those filled with amalgam.

Fast-setting zinc oxide–eugenol cements have also been recommended for reverse root filling, mainly because of their ease of manipulation (Nicholls, 1962). However, Hunter (1957) found that one such cement, namely Rickert's cement, was resorbed following implantation into experimental animals, whilst Nielsen (1963) claims that such cements are not resistant to tissue fluids. Unpublished data of the author confirm that resorption or dissolution of these cements does in fact occur

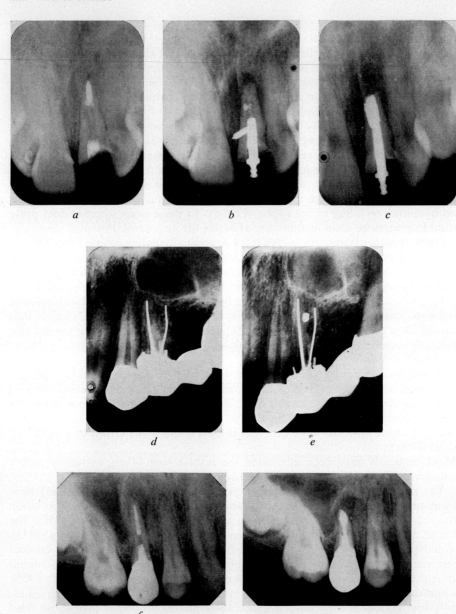

Fig. 198. Some indications for apicectomy with reverse amalgam filling of the root canal. *a*, *b* and *c*, ⌊1: Perforation of the apical part of the root during post crown preparation led to an ingrowth of tissue and displacement of the apical section of silver point. Both the apical part of the root and the perforation were filled with amalgam. *d* and *e*, ⌊4: An extra root, suspected because of pronounced radio-opacity 'distally' to the palatal filling, was thought to account for periapical tenderness. Exploratory surgery revealed a second buccal root. *f* and *g*, 5⌋: Periapical disease developed following root filling. Apicectomy revealed the root filling to be inadequate. *h* and *i*, ⌐12: The ⌐1 probably contains

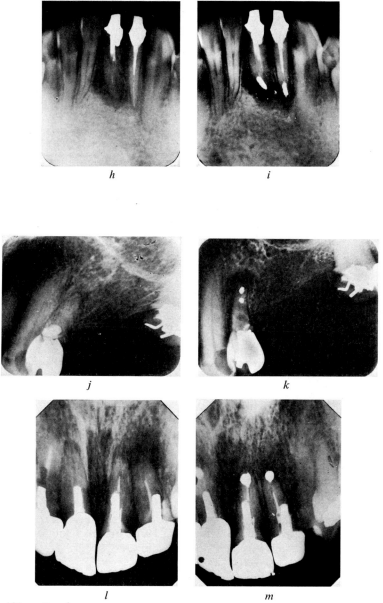

Fig. 198 *continued*

a broken instrument, and perhaps $\overline{2}$ also. At the level at which the roots were sectioned, separate buccal and lingual canals existed in both teeth. Since these were close together, a single cavity including both canal orifices was prepared in each root and filled. *j* and *k*, $\underline{|4}$: Apicectomy was performed because of calcification of pulp cavity. At the level at which the root was sectioned, separate buccal and palatal canals existed. Since these were some distance apart, separate cavities were prepared and filled. *l* and *m*, $\underline{|12}$: Post crowns prevented access to the apical regions of these teeth.

in a minority of teeth some years after insertion (*Fig*. 199), and occasionally leads
to recurrence of periapical disease.

Silver amalgam, although relatively difficult to handle in the confined space
available, is the material of choice for reverse root filling. Friend and Browne
(1968) found that although silver amalgam caused a severe initial reaction, it was
well tolerated 3 months following experimental implantation, whilst Feldmann and
Nyborg (1962) concluded that the irritation from this material was less than that
from gutta percha.

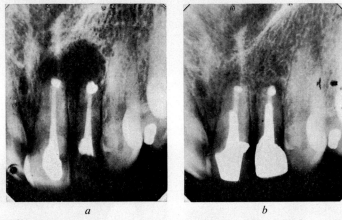

a   *b*

Fig. 199. |12. *a*, Immediately after apicectomy and reverse filling with fast-setting zinc
oxide–eugenol cement; *b*, Five years later, there has been resorption or dissolution of
the cement fillings, although periapical repair is well advanced.

The use of a zinc-free amalgam alloy is sometimes advocated, mainly to avoid
the excessive delayed expansion which occurs when a zinc-containing amalgam is
contaminated by blood during insertion. Although a zinc-free alloy is occasionally
useful where there is poor access and therefore a greater opportunity for contamination, in general it is preferable to devote additional time to the control of haemorrhage rather than rely on such an alloy to offset the effects of contamination.

It is feasible that contact between a zinc-containing amalgam and an existing
gold post in the root may lead to electrolytic action with the formation of zinc
carbonate, and there is some evidence that the latter may have an irritant or anti-
genic effect on connective tissue (Martin et al., 1976). Where a gold post is present,
therefore, there is a case for using a zinc-free alloy.

ii. FILLING WITH SILVER AMALGAM

Large particles of amalgam are difficult to control. They tend to fall from the end
of the root onto the surrounding gauze, and thence, when the gauze is removed,
into the bony wound, where they may be overlooked.

When using silver amalgam, therefore, only a small quantity is placed in the
cavity at a time. The material may be transferred to the root-end cavity with one
of the special carriers described in Chapter 8, or with a miniature amalgam carrier
of the type depicted in *Fig*. 200. Alternatively, College tweezers may be used, or the
amalgam may be fixed by gentle pressure to the end of a serrated plugger or silver-
plated plastic instrument. Small hand condensers are used to pack the amalgam

until the cavity is slightly overfilled. The filling is then trimmed flush with the apical surface of the root, the excess material being worked buccally and carefully removed with excavators. Any large fragments of amalgam which have fallen lingually to the root-end are removed.

d. Completion of operation

In removing the pack or bone wax following completion of the filling, care should be taken to avoid dropping small fragments of material into the wound. Before the latter is closed with sutures it is irrigated and then inspected for excess amalgam

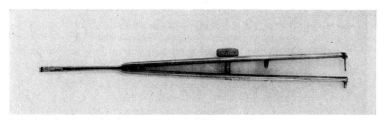

Fig. 200. Amalgam carrier for reverse root filling.

and any residual wax. If small particles of amalgam remain, they are removed by gentle prising with an excavator or probe away from the bony surface rather than by curetting, which tends to burnish the material into the alveolar bone.

4. Variations of technique

When a tooth with an open apex is treated by apicectomy with reverse filling, a rather lengthier technique than that previously described is followed. A full account is given in Chapter 13.

Sommer (1946) describes a different technique of reverse filling of the root canal following apicectomy, which he calls 'indirect resection'. In this technique, burs are not used to prepare a root-end cavity. Instead, the apical part of the canal is prepared with files bent at right-angles about 6·0 mm from their tips, and is filled with a section of silver point smeared with cement. The point is inserted with its butt end facing the bony wound. It is driven into position by tapping on a flat plastic instrument placed against its butt end. After the cement has set, the point is trimmed flush with the apical surface of the root.

REFERENCES

Andreasen J. O. and Rud J. (1972a) Modes of healing histologically after endodontic surgery in 70 cases. *Int. J. Oral Surg.* **1**, 148.

Andreasen J. O. and Rud J. (1972b) A histobacteriologic study of dental and periapical structures after endodontic surgery. *Int. J. Oral Surg.* **1**, 272.

Barker B. C. W. and Lockett B. C. (1971) Utilization of the mandibular premolars of the dog for endodontic research. *Aust. Dent. J.* **16**, 280.

Barry G. N. and Fried I. L. (1975) Sealing quality of two polycarboxylate cements used as root canal sealers. *J. Endodontol.* **1**, 107.

Barry G. N., Heyman R. A. and Elias A. (1975) Comparison of apical sealing methods: a preliminary report. *Oral Surg.* **39**, 806.

Blum T. (1930) Root amputation: a study of one hundred and fifty-nine cases. *J. Am. Dent. Assoc.* **17**, 249.

Blum T. (1932) Additional notes on root amputation, including a study of thirty-eight new cases. *J. Am. Dent. Assoc.* **19**, 69.

Boyne P. J., Lyon H. W. and Miller C. W. (1961) The effects of osseous implant materials on regeneration of alveolar cortex. Oral Surg. 14, 369.

Büchs H. and Reul L. (1962) Zur Frage der Knochenregeneration nach Wurzelspitzenresektion mit Retrograder Abfüllung. Dtsch. Zahnarztl. Z. 17, 1635.

Coolidge E. D. and Kesel R. G. (1956) A Textbook of Endodontology, 2nd ed. London, Kimpton, pp. 292–97, 331–39.

Cunningham J. (1975) The seal of root fillings at apicectomy: a scanning electron microscope study. Br. Dent. J. 139, 430.

Dixon C. M. and Rickert U. G. (1933) Tissue tolerance to foreign materials. J. Am. Dent. Assoc. 20, 1458.

Farrar J. N. (1884) Radical and heroic treatment of alveolar abscess by amputation of roots of teeth. Dent. Cosmos. 26, 79, 135.

Feldmann G. and Nyborg H. (1962) Tissue reactions to root filling materials. I, Comparison between gutta percha and silver amalgam implanted in rabbit. Odontol. Revy. 13, 1.

Freedland J. B. (1970) Conservative reduction of large periapical lesions. Oral Surg. 29, 455.

Friend L. A. and Browne R. M. (1968) Tissue reactions to some root filling materials. Br. Dent. J. 125, 291.

Garvin M. H. (1919) Foci of infection in relation to non-vital teeth. J. Natl. Dent. Assoc. 6, 195.

Garvin M. H. (1942) Root resection. J. Can. Dent. Assoc. 8, 126.

Grossman L. I., Shepard L. I. and Pearson L. A. (1964) Roentgenologic and clinical evaluation of endodontically treated teeth. Oral Surg. 17, 368.

Harnisch H. (1963) Heterogenous bone plugs in root resection. Int. Dent. J., Lond. 13, 620.

Harty F. J., Parkins B. J. and Wengraf A. M. (1970) The success rate of apicectomy: a retrospective study of 1016 cases. Br. Dent. J. 129, 407.

Hunter H. A. (1957) The effect of gutta percha, silver points and Rickert's root sealer on bone healing. J. Can. Dent. Assoc. 23, 385.

Kopp W. K. and Kresberg H. (1973) Apicoectomy with retrograde gold foil: a new technique. N. Y. State Dent. J. 39, 8.

Martin L. R., Tidwell E., Tenca J. I., Pelleu G. B. and Longton R. W. (1976) Histologic response of rat connective tissue to zinc-containing amalgam. J. Endodontol. 2, 25.

Mattila K. and Altonen M. (1968) A clinical and roentgenological study of apicoectomized teeth. Odontol. Tidskr. 76, 389.

Mitchell D. F. (1959) The irritational qualities of dental materials. J. Am. Dent. Assoc. 59, 954.

Morse D. R. (1973) Does culturing contribute to endodontic success? In: Grossman L. I. (ed.), Transactions of the 5th International Conference on Endodontics. Philadelphia, University of Pennsylvania, pp. 91–100.

Nicholls E. (1962) Retrograde filling of the root canal. Oral Surg. 15, 463.

Nielsen T. H. (1963) The ability of 39 liquid chelating agents to form cements with metal oxides, respecting their usability as root-filling materials: a preliminary communication. Acta Odontol. Scand. 21, 159.

Nordenram A. and Svärdström G. (1970) Results of apicectomy. Swed. Dent. J. 63, 593.

Persson A. G. (1966) Bedömning av resultatet efter rotamputation. Sven. Tandläk. Tidskr. 59, 219.

Persson G., Lennartson B. and Lundstrom I. (1974) Results of retrograde root-filling with special reference to amalgam and Cavit as root-filling materials. Sven. Tandläk. Tidskr. 67, 123.

Phillips W. A. and Maxmen H. A. (1941) A practical root resection technique for young permanent anterior teeth. Dent. Dig. 47, 60.

Roy M. (1925) Le curettage apical. Odontologie 43, 5

Rud J., Andreasen J. O. and Jensen J. E. M. (1972a) Radiographic criteria for the assessment of healing after endodontic surgery. Int. J. Oral Surg. 1, 195.

Rud J., Andreasen J. O. and Jensen J. E. M. (1972b) A follow-up study of 1000 cases treated by endodontic surgery. Int. J. Oral Surg. 1, 215.

Rud J., Andreasen J. O. and Jensen J. E. M. (1972c) A multivariate analysis of the influence of various factors upon healing after endodontic surgery. Int. J. Oral Surg. 1, 258.

Smith H. W. (1952) Alveolar bone regeneration. Oral Surg. 5, 225.

Sommer R. F. (1946) Essentials for successful root resection. Am. J. Orthodont. 32, 76.

FURTHER READING

Luebke R. G. (1974) Surgical endodontics. Dent. Clin. North Am. 18, 379–91.

Chapter 12

Root canal treatment of molar teeth

The principles of root canal treatment of anterior teeth apply to molar teeth also. Provided these principles are observed, the treatment of molar teeth, although more time-consuming, has a good prognosis. However, because of their position in the arch and the anatomical characteristics of their pulp cavities, the treatment of molars does present special problems.

1. SELECTION OF TEETH FOR TREATMENT

Various factors merit special attention when assessing the suitability of a molar tooth for root canal treatment, namely the access available, the number of root canals and the anatomy of each, and the possibility of an incomplete longitudinal fracture of the tooth. Although clinical and radiographic examination of the tooth will yield considerable information, very often these factors can only be fully investigated when the pulp cavity is actually opened and explored. For this reason the patient's first visit for treatment should be regarded as a preliminary one at which the tooth is investigated further and a more definite assessment made of the prognosis, although other measures, such as the cementation of a copper band, may also be performed.

a. Access

One of the most obvious but commonly overlooked considerations in determining the feasibility of treatment is the extent to which the patient can open the mouth. There must be enough room for the introduction of instruments into each canal, and the amount of opening required must be maintained for the major part of each session of treatment. The actual degree of opening needed will depend partly on the working lengths of the various canals, and partly on the mesiodistal angle of the coronal part of each canal.

The working lengths of the various canals are determined by the root lengths and the state of the clinical crown. Relatively long instruments will be needed for a tooth with intact buccal and lingual cusps and long roots, and a considerable degree of opening will therefore be required. Far less opening will be needed for a tooth with a broken-down crown, since not only will there be more room between its occlusal surface and that of the opposing tooth, but also the working lengths of the canals will be less, so enabling shorter instruments to be used.

Mesial inclination of a canal in a gingivo-apical direction will hinder the insertion and use of instruments, since the opening of the canal into the pulp chamber will face distally. In consequence the handle of the instrument will be located further distally, where the room between the arches is less. Conversely, distal inclination of a root canal facilitates instrumentation, since the instrument handle is positioned further mesially (*Fig.* 201). It is partly for this reason that the treatment of the mesial and mesiobuccal canals of mandibular and maxillary molars respectively tends to present difficulty. On occasions, satisfactory access can only be obtained by the deliberate reduction of a mesial cusp, so providing more visibility and enabling shorter instruments to be used. Where the subsequent coronal restoration will in any case involve cuspal reduction, it is obviously advantageous to attend to this before beginning root canal treatment.

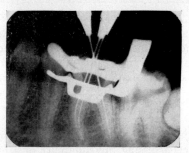

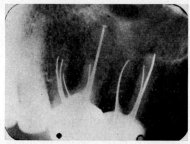

Fig. 201. ⌐6. The insertion of instruments into mesial canals may be difficult if their orifices face distally.

Fig. 202. |6. The mesiobuccal root had 3 canals; none was penetrable in the apical part of the root.

A mesial tilt to a tooth or the absence of an opposing tooth will, of course, facilitate access and reduce the opening required.

b. Number of root canals

In recent years root canal anatomy has been the subject of considerable investigation, and it is now realized that many molar teeth possess 4 root canals, or even more (*Fig.* 202). Although a few molars do have less than 3 canals, the latter number should in general be regarded as a minimum rather than a norm.

Most mandibular molars have 2 mesial canals, and these have separate apical foramina in from 40 per cent (Burch and Hulen, 1972) to 77 per cent (Ainamo and Löe, 1968) of teeth. Almost 30 per cent of mandibular first molars were found by Skidmore and Bjorndal (1971) to have 4 root canals, due to the presence of a second distal canal; in almost 40 per cent of teeth with this anatomy the 2 distal canals had separate apical foramina.

Seidberg et al. (1973) found that over 60 per cent of maxillary first molars had a second mesiobuccal canal; in 40 per cent of such teeth the extra canal had a separate apical foramen. In confirming the former finding for both first and second molars, Pomeranz and Fishelberg (1974) report that only 30 per cent of mesiobuccal roots with more than 1 canal had a single apical foramen; occasionally a second distobuccal canal was found. In another study (Weine et al., 1969) 37·5 per cent of maxillary first molars were found to have 2 mesiobuccal canals with a common apical foramen, whilst 14 per cent had 2 canals with separate foramina.

Thus, care should be taken not to overlook a second mesiobuccal canal in the maxilla, or a second distal canal in the mandible. A minimum of two preoperative radiographs should be taken, using different horizontal angulations. Undue width or radio-opacity to a root, or a canal which does not follow a central course within the root, may indicate the presence of an additional canal. After the coronal pulp has been removed from the tooth and the major root canal orifices located, the floor of the pulp chamber should be examined visually and with a probe for the presence of extra openings. The orifice of a second mesiobuccal canal, when present, is normally lingual but close to that of the main canal.

c. Anatomy of individual root canals

The radiographic inclination, width, curvature and density of each canal are carefully studied, particular attention being paid to mesial canals in mandibular

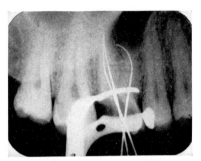

Fig. 203. 6|. A 90° curvature of the apical part of the mesiobuccal root canal was negotiable because it was gradual.

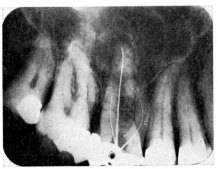

Fig. 204. 6|. Curvature of the mesio-buccal canal throughout its length necessitates bending of the coronal part of an instrument, which is wider and less flexible.

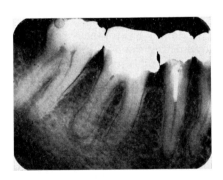

Fig. 205. 6|. Irregular root canal calcification, probably due to previous pulpotomy or pulp mummification.

teeth, and to mesiobuccal canals in maxillary teeth. Narrowness *per se* does not usually prevent access to the apical region, but if a canal is also curved, access may prove much more difficult. A gradual curvature is obviously easier to negotiate than a sudden one. A curvature of the canal near its apical end, provided it is not sudden, can usually be negotiated because of the flexibility of reamers and files at their tips (*Fig.* 203). Curvature of the canal further coronally presents more difficulty, because this necessitates bending of the coronal part of each successive instrument, which is wider and therefore less flexible (*Fig.* 204); there is therefore a greater risk of instrument breakage, and a greater likelihood of surgical treatment being needed. Occasionally, irregular calcification within the root canal space is apparent, particularly where there is evidence of previous pulpotomy or pulp mummification (*Fig.* 205); access to the apical region may not be possible in such cases.

d. Incomplete longitudinal fracture

Sometimes an incomplete longitudinal fracture or crack occurs in a posterior tooth, giving rise to symptoms for which there is no immediately apparent cause. The teeth in the painful region may have deep restorations, but sometimes are caries-free and unrestored, or have restorations of unexceptional depth. Sometimes, but not invariably, there is a history of bruxism or clenching. Pain is felt only during mastication, especially of hot or cold foods, but often only in certain positions of the mandible. Unless there is actual pulpal involvement, vitality tests give normal results and radiographic examination reveals no abnormality. Typically it is not possible to reproduce the intensity of the pain by the application of heat and cold to the tooth, and there is little or no sensitivity to percussion.

Usually the causative tooth, or at least the region of the tooth, may be located by having the patient bite on a wool roll or wooden tongue spatula held over different teeth in turn. The involved cusp or cusps may then be identified by placing a mounted rubber polishing wheel or similar object over each cusp in turn and instructing the patient to close and exert biting pressure; pain may be felt during closure or on the release of biting pressure. Although the removal of an existing restoration involving the occlusal surface or the cutting of a cavity to eliminate the occlusal fissures may fail to demonstrate any abnormality, application of a dye such as methylene blue or tincture of iodine to the base of the cavity will result in staining of the fracture line. The latter is often at the junction of the pulpal and buccal or lingual wall, and runs predominantly in a mesiodistal direction. Sometimes part of the tooth will actually break off during preparation of the cavity or when sideways pressure is exerted with a probe at the base of the buccal or lingual wall, but usually there is no discernible movement of the fractured part.

Cameron (1964), who uses the term 'cracked tooth syndrome' in referring to these cases, found that they only occurred after the age of 35 years, and that the mandibular second molars were the most commonly involved teeth. Occasionally an anterior tooth with no history of trauma is associated with an incomplete vertical fracture (Linaberg and Marshall, 1973), but in the author's experience this occurs only when the tooth has been root-filled.

The treatment of these teeth depends on the position of the fracture line. Where part of the tooth actually breaks away without exposing the pulp, there is immediate cessation of symptoms and an appropriate restoration may be placed. If the fracture line is at the base of a buccal or lingual cusp which does not move or break away, and if there are no symptoms suggesting pulpal involvement, crowning is indicated to prevent actual separation of the fractured part.

When the fracture line is situated over the roof of the pulp chamber, extending from the mesial to the distal aspect of the tooth, the prognosis is far less favourable. If independent movement of the buccal or lingual aspect of the tooth is discernible (*Fig.* 206), or if a fracture line is evident in the base of the pulp chamber after removal of the coronal pulp, extraction is indicated. Otherwise, an attempt may be made to conserve the tooth, but the patient should be warned that the long-term prognosis is uncertain, especially as removal of the roof of the pulp chamber leads to further weakening of the tooth. In all instances the tooth should first be splinted with a tightly fitting band. If an extensive cavity is present, it is restored with amalgam, with the insertion of pins both buccally and lingually to the fracture line to prevent separation of the two sides of the tooth. Access for root canal treatment is obtained through the amalgam, following which a full crown is constructed.

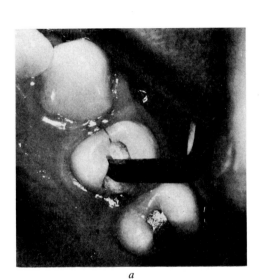 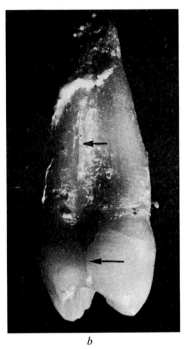

a   *b*

Fig. 206. |4. *a*, Untreatable longitudinal fracture extending through mesial marginal ridge. Independent movement of the two parts of the tooth could be demonstrated by gentle leverage with a plastic instrument; *b*, After extraction; the fracture (*arrowed*) extends apically along the root.

Sometimes an incomplete longitudinal fracture occurs in a tooth with a necrotic pulp, with no symptoms attributable to the fracture itself. Because of the absence of unusual symptoms, these cases are easily overlooked until there is separation of part of the tooth, which may actually occur during the course of root canal treatment. The base of any existing cavity and that of the access cavity should routinely be inspected before actually opening the pulp chamber, therefore. The same criteria as with a vital pulp govern whether root canal treatment is continued.

2. TREATMENT OF ACUTE CONDITIONS

Opening of the pulp chamber may not provide satisfactory drainage of an acute periapical abscess because of the narrow calibre of some molar root canals. Unless abscess formation is sufficiently advanced to allow incision, systemic antibiotic therapy may be the only means of reducing the acute condition sufficiently to permit root canal treatment. Perforation of the buccal plate apically with a bur is generally not feasible as a means of obtaining drainage, owing to the difficulty of access and the risk of impinging upon major anatomical structures such as the maxillary antrum.

3. PREPARATORY PROCEDURES

Where the tooth is being treated through an extensive restoration, such as a crown, the restoration should be examined for leakage and marginal caries which might communicate with the pulp cavity. If the tooth serves as a bridge abutment it should be checked that the bridge is not loose on the tooth, since this will lead to salivary contamination of the pulp cavity.

The application of a rubber dam is essential for the root canal treatment of molar teeth. Despite the limited access, only the tooth under treatment need usually be isolated. If extra working room is needed an adjacent tooth, preferably posterior to that being treated, is also isolated; a clamp is applied to the more posterior tooth. Often the presence of a large mesial or distal cavity in the tooth makes the cementation of a band necessary, partly to facilitate isolation and to retain a temporary restoration, but especially to prevent cuspal fracture.

Sometimes the tooth will have been restored with a temporary crown or used to support a temporary bridge. Such temporary restorations are best removed when opening the pulp cavity, since better access and vision are thereby achieved. Whether the restoration is allowed to remain in place during subsequent treatment, or is removed and later replaced at each visit, depends on the circumstances of the individual case. If retention is good, the restoration may be left in place during treatment; after access to the pulp cavity has been completed, a suitable opening is made in the occlusal surface of the restoration, which is then recemented prior to assessment of the working length of each canal. Where retention is limited or access poor, the restoration is allowed to remain intact, but is removed at each visit. This precludes contamination of the pulp cavity due to loosening of the restoration between visits, and, by reducing the working lengths of the various canals, allows shorter instruments to be used.

4. ACCESS TO PULP CAVITY

Mesiodistally in both maxillary and mandibular molar teeth the pulp chamber occupies roughly the middle one-third of the crown. The opening made occlusally is also roughly in the middle one-third of the crown mesiodistally, therefore. The precise shape and extent of the opening depend partly on the positions of the orifices of the various canals. Thus, the mesiodistal width of the opening in a maxillary first molar will generally be greater buccally than palatally, since at least 2 canals will be situated buccally (*Fig.* 207a). Similarly, the buccolingual width of the opening in a mandibular first molar is usually greater mesially than distally (*Fig.* 207b).

It should be emphasized that openings of these shapes, although common, are by no means invariable. The final opening should be such as to allow all parts of the pulp chamber floor to be inspected. Also, the angle of the coronal part of the canal may necessitate a larger opening. Thus, curvature of the canal may result in the shanks of reamers and files contacting a side wall of the cavity (*Fig.* 208). Such contact leads to unnecessary deflection of the relatively wide and inflexible coronal part of the instrument, and so needlessly increases the risk of instrument breakage.

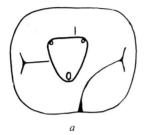 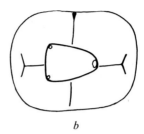

a   *b*

Fig. 207. *a*, Outline of opening into pulp cavity of maxillary molar; *b*, Outline of opening into pulp cavity of mandibular molar.

A further requirement of the final opening, therefore, is that its side walls should not make contact with instruments inserted to the apical limit of each root canal.

After applying an antiseptic solution to the tooth surface, an occlusal cavity of roughly the required shape is prepared; the floor of the cavity is examined to ensure that no fracture line is present. The pulp chamber is now opened with a large round bur. With maxillary molars the head of the bur is placed mesially to the oblique ridge, close to the centre of the mesial fissure. With mandibular molars the head of the bur is placed midway along the mesiodistal fissure of the tooth. The suggestion of Gottlieb (1938) that the bur be directed towards the widest canal when penetrating the roof of the pulp chamber is particularly useful in reducing the risk of unwittingly crossing a shallow pulp chamber and perforating its floor (*Fig.* 209). In the maxilla the bur is directed slightly palatally, and in the mandible distally.

Removal of the roof of the pulp chamber is completed with round burs cutting from within the pulp chamber outwards towards the occlusal surface of the tooth. Excavators are used to remove the coronal pulp, after which the pulp chamber is cleaned of debris and its floor inspected. In locating the orifices of the various root canals, it should be noted that in maxillary molars the coronal opening of the distobuccal canal is mesial to, rather than in line with, the tip of the distobuccal cusp, and that in mandibular molars the orifice of the mesiolingual canal is buccal to the tip of the corresponding cusp. The various root canal orifices tend to be located peripherally to a central dome formed by the floor of the pulp chamber, the dull grey colour of which is quite characteristic. Particular care should be taken not to damage this floor, since its configuration assists in locating the root canal orifices.

The next stage in treatment at the first visit is to remove gross necrotic material or vital pulp from the wide palatal or distal canal, following which an instrument is inserted to the probable apical limit of each canal and the cavity walls cut back wherever they make contact with the projecting instruments. Radiographs are now taken to determine the working lengths of the various canals, and to confirm that the apical parts of these will be accessible; this aspect of treatment will be discussed presently. The pulp cavity is then dressed with an antiseptic preparation and sealed.

Thus, the first visit, which usually lasts about 45 minutes, is concerned only with certain preparatory stages of treatment essential for adequate preparation of the root canals at a later stage, and with the assessment of prognosis. For a tooth with a vital pulp, treatment consists essentially of pulpotomy, at least so far as the

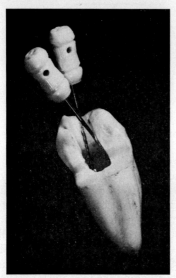

Fig. 208. Access to the mesiobuccal canal (*right*) is unsatisfactory, since the shank of the instrument is deflected by the side-wall of the cavity; access to the mesiolingual canal (*left*) is satisfactory.

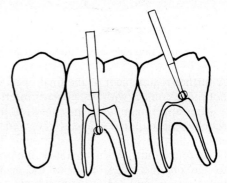

Fig. 209. The risk of unwittingly penetrating a shallow pulp chamber and perforating its floor (6) is reduced by directing the bur towards the wide distal canal (7).

finer canals are concerned. Root canal preparation is not usually performed at the first visit since it would result in an unduly long appointment; instead it is deferred to a second visit 24 hours to 7 days later. However, for convenience of description an account of root canal preparation will be given before discussing antiseptic medication and sealing of the pulp cavity.

5. ASSESSMENT OF WORKING LENGTHS

A fairly accurate idea of the working length of each canal may be obtained by direct measurement from carefully taken preoperative radiographs. With mandibular molars, such measurements should provide a reasonably accurate guide to the working length of each canal, since relatively undistorted radiographs of these teeth are easily obtained. A reamer or file of appropriate size, and with some form of measuring device, such as a silicone rubber marker, set at the appropriate length, is inserted into each canal to a level 1–2 mm short of the estimated apical limit (*Fig*. 210). The level of the rubber marker should coincide with some convenient occlusal measuring point, usually the tip of the nearest cusp.

Sometimes one radiograph is sufficient to give a clear and reasonably undistorted view of the apical region of each canal. On other occasions, for example where it is difficult to separate the images of different roots or where one or more of the roots contains two canals, two or more radiographs are necessary. Thus, a minimum of two radiographs would be needed for a mandibular molar with two mesial and two distal canals, one taken for the two lingual and one for the two

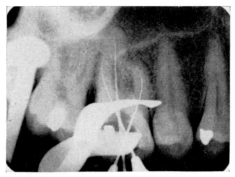

Fig. 210. 6|. In assessing the working length of each canal, a reamer or file is inserted to a level 1–2 mm short of the estimated apical limit.

buccal canals, with the films suitably marked for ease of identification. The rubber dam frame or strap is removed during radiographic examination to facilitate accurate positioning of the films.

The working length of each canal is assessed in the same manner as with anterior teeth. The apical limit to preparation and filling should be 1·0–1·5 mm short of the root apex.

6. ROOT CANAL PREPARATION

The depth of penetration of all instruments used in preparing molar root canals should be controlled with the aid of suitable measuring devices, such as rubber markers. It is especially important in finer canals not to thrust instruments into the periapical region, since the narrow calibre of these canals impedes drainage of the resultant periapical exudate.

Either hand instruments or special engine-driven instruments, or both, may be used for root canal preparation. The insertion of both types of instrument is facilitated by widening the coronal opening of each canal to the shape of a funnel with a root canal orifice enlarger (*Fig.* 211).

a. Preparation with hand instruments

The wider palatal and distal canals of molar teeth have a distinct taper and are prepared in the same way as those of anterior teeth. Instruments 25 mm long are suitable for most teeth, and these canals may generally be enlarged to a size no. 40 or 50 instrument.

Instruments 21 or 25 mm long are used for the narrower mesial and buccal canals. The distobuccal canals of maxillary molars are often relatively straight and in consequence may often be enlarged to a size no. 40 instrument. With this exception, however, these canals normally show some degree of curvature and in consequence cannot usually be enlarged apically beyond a size no. 30 or 35 instrument without the risk of instrument breakage or root perforation.

It is most important during preparation of a curved canal not to create a ledge in the wall of the canal, since this makes subsequent negotiation of the canal apical to the ledge difficult. The canals are therefore kept moist during preparation, using, for example, one of the EDTA preparations described in Chapter 6. Each

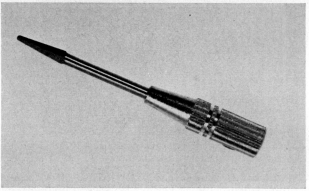

Fig. 211. Root canal orifice enlarger.

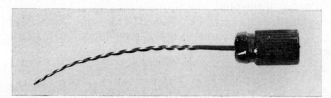

Fig. 212. Instrument bent to a gentle curve before use.

instrument is bent to a gentle curve before use (*Fig*. 212). Instruments should be used in strict numerical sequence. Periodic irrigation is indicated to prevent dentine shavings being packed apically by subsequent instrumentation. Whilst some workers rely largely upon reamers to prepare the apical part of the root canal, others prefer to use K-type files with a reaming action; there is some evidence that the latter method of enlargement is more likely to produce a preparation which is circular in cross-section (Jungmann et al., 1975).

If difficulty is experienced in introducing the next larger size of instrument to the apical limit, an intermediate size may be made at the chairside, as suggested by Weine et al. (1970). Thus, shortening the apical end of a no. 25 file by 1·0–1·5 mm produces a size roughly midway between nos. 25 and 30; the apical end of an instrument modified in this way will need to be smoothed and reshaped.

Preparation of a curved canal is further complicated by the fact that the enforced curvature of instruments apically and the tendency of each instrument to straighten to its original form may result in uneven enlargement of the canal. The study of Weine et al. (1975) suggests that whether reamers or files, or both, are used for root canal preparation, the 'outer' concave wall of the curved apical part of the canal is enlarged to a greater degree than the 'inner' convex wall (*Fig. 213a, b*). Instead of the prepared root canal tapering progressively to the apical limit, therefore, it may instead flare apically, with the narrowest part of the preparation roughly at the midpoint of the curvature. This in effect leads to a shortening of the root canal, so that if progressively larger instruments are inserted to the same working length, perforation of the curved root surface, or actual 'transportation' of the apical foramen across this surface, may eventually occur (*Fig. 213c, d*).

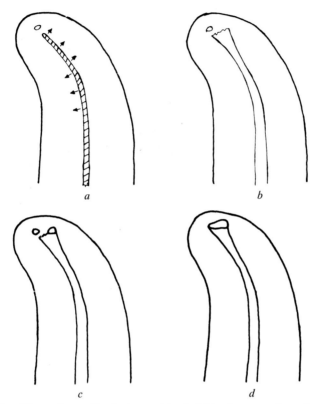

Fig. 213. *a*, The tendency of an instrument to straighten in a curved canal may lead to more dentine being removed from the regions arrowed than elsewhere; *b*, Resultant flaring of apical region of canal; *c*, Flaring of apical region of canal may be followed by perforation if progressively larger instruments are used to the same length; *d*, Alternatively, the apical foramen may be 'transported' across the root surface.

The more curved the apical part of the canal the greater will be the tendency for the prepared canal to be flared apically and to deviate from a circular outline in cross-section. In consequence, the less accurately will a matching silver point fit the prepared canal apically, and the greater will be the likelihood of leakage of the cement seal and corrosion of the silver from exposure to tissue fluid. Somewhat paradoxically, therefore, the type of case in which the relative rigidity of silver facilitates the passage of the root-filling point to the apical end of the canal is often that in which the use of silver is most dubious, and in which gutta percha is more suitable, despite the tendency of the latter to buckle upon insertion into a curved canal.

To minimize this tendency for flaring of the apical part of a curved canal, as well as to ensure that the wider coronal and middle parts of the canal are properly cleaned and to facilitate the passage apically of a gutta percha point when this material is used, a serial or step method of preparation, previously advocated by

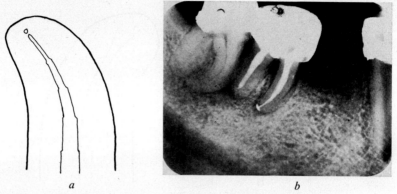

a   *b*

Fig. 214. *a*, Diagrammatic representation of serial preparation of the root canal; *b*, 7|, Filling of mesial root following serial preparation; some filling material has been extruded periapically, and also through a lateral canal on the mesial aspect of the coronal part of the mesial root.

Clem (1969), has been developed by Schilder (1974). In this method the apical part of the canal is first enlarged to about a size no. 25 or 30 instrument. Successively larger instruments up to about size no. 60 or 70 are then used, but each instrument is inserted only as far as that level at which resistance is encountered; periodically the largest size of instrument to reach the apical limit is used to check the patency of the apical part of the canal. Thus, there is a progressive reduction in the depth of penetration of instruments (*Fig.* 214). As a result of widening of the canal coronally, further enlargement of the apical part of the canal may subsequently be possible.

This technique is very useful where there is a significant curvature of the root canal, and facilitates both the passage apically of a gutta percha point and condensation of the root filling. Also, there is some evidence that it results in a cleaner root canal apically (Coffae and Brilliant, 1975) and in more aspects of the root canal being reached by instruments (Walton, 1976).

b. Preparation with engine-driven instruments

Special types of reciprocating contra-angle handpieces may be used in root canal preparation. The Giromatic, which has a rotary action, is used in conjunction with special barbed broaches or Hedstroem files, which are made to turn to and fro through 90° (*Fig.* 215). The broaches are available in 21 and 29 mm lengths, and in sizes 15–80 inclusive. The files are made in lengths of 21, 25 and 29 mm, in sizes

8–90 inclusive. The same instruments may also be used with the Kavo Endo Handpiece, which has a similar action to the Giromatic.

The Cardex Racer handpiece (*Fig.* 216) is used in conjunction with conventional short-handle files, which are made to move vertically up and down through a distance of about 2·5 mm. The depth of penetration of each file is controlled by a shoe which rests against the occlusal surface; the level of the shoe is adjusted according to the working length.

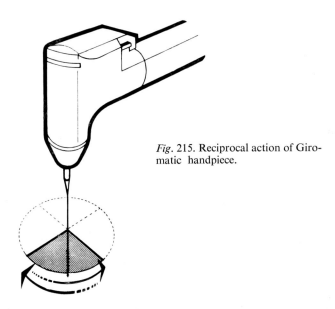

Fig. 215. Reciprocal action of Giromatic handpiece.

A number of *in vitro* investigations have been carried out into the effectiveness of these instruments. Molven (1970) compared the amount of canal enlargement obtained using different instruments for the same period of time. Files used by hand gave greater enlargement than those used in the Racer instrument; Giromatic broaches were the least effective for canal enlargement. O'Connell and Brayton (1975) assessed the quality of root canal preparation produced by hand instrumentation, by the Giromatic handpiece using both broaches and files, and by a handpiece employing a similar principle to the Racer instrument. Hand instrumentation was found to produce better preparations with less extrusion of debris through the apical foramen than engine-driven instruments. Similarly, in a comparison of preparation with Giromatic instruments and various hand instruments, Mizrahi et al. (1975) found that Giromatic broaches were the least effective in cleaning the root canal. Klayman and Brilliant (1975) found that serial preparation gave significantly better results than Giromatic instruments in cleaning the apical parts of root canals, whilst the study of Weine et al. (1976) indicates that both Giromatic and Racer-type handpieces lead to more apical flaring of canals with sharp apical curvatures than do hand instruments. Fromme and Guttzeit (1972), however, found that Giromatic broaches produced a very smooth surface to the dentinal wall of the root canal.

There is little evidence, at least from *in vitro* studies, that root canal preparation is any faster with engine-driven than with hand instruments. Although it is sometimes claimed that a fine Giromatic broach will negotiate a canal which has defied the passage of a hand instrument, this has not been the author's experience, nor that of Molven (1968) or Klayman and Brilliant (1975). Comparison of the finest broach (no. 15) with a no. 15 reamer reveals the former to be wider, due to the projecting barbs, whilst a no. 8 Giromatic file is about the same width as a no. 15

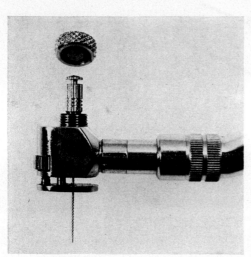

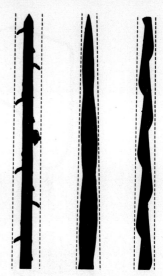

Fig. 216. Exploded view of head of Cardex Racer handpiece, with locking cap (*above*), and adjustable shoe on undersurface of head.

Fig. 217. Comparative widths of no. 15 Giromatic broach (*left*); no. 15 reamer (*centre*); and no. 8 Giromatic file (*right*; × 26). The Giromatic file has a flattened end.

reamer (*Fig.* 217). Although less access may be needed once the broach or file is in place within the root canal, due to the size of the handpiece head the actual introduction of an engine-driven instrument requires more room than does a hand instrument grasped in suitable instrument-holding forceps.

The use of engine-driven files moving rapidly in a vertical direction, as in the Racer instrument, would seem undesirable in view of the risk of thrusting dentine fragments and necrotic pulp in an apical direction; there is also evidence that they tend to produce ledges hindering further instrumentation of the canal (Weine et al., 1976). It is doubtful whether root canals can be as effectively enlarged and shaped with Giromatic broaches as with hand instruments, whilst Giromatic files can produce ledges in the wall of a curved canal, no doubt due to their flattened ends (*Fig.* 217). Nonetheless, Giromatic-type instruments can be useful in root canal preparation. Once a pathway to the apical region has been discovered in a canal with a ledge along its course, elimination of the ledge is often easier and quicker with a Giromatic broach than with a hand file. Giromatic broaches do not break unless abused and are useful in agitating irrigating solutions in the root canal, so helping to dislodge debris. In view of the previously quoted finding of Fromme and

Guttzeit (1972), there may be some advantage in using these broaches at the completion of hand instrumentation with the object of smoothing the root canal wall. Although there is a danger of creating a ledge when using Giromatic files in the curved part of a root canal, these instruments may be useful for widening the straight coronal part of the canal.

7. ANTISEPTIC MEDICATION

Either chemical antiseptics or antibiotics are used for antiseptic medication of molar teeth. Electromedication can be applied to these teeth, but is rarely used, if only because for the patient it prolongs what are already lengthy attendances.

Some degree of periapical irritation with the formation of exudate is common following root canal preparation. The antiseptic dressing used immediately following such preparation should be confined to the pulp chamber, so allowing exudate to drain into the root canals. Needless to say, dressings should not be inserted into root canals until the latter have been cleaned of pulpal tissue and will accommodate them.

Chemical antiseptics are normally applied on a wool pledget placed over the base of the pulp chamber, and the diffusibility of the preparation plus capillary action relied upon to carry the drug in an apical direction. If it is decided to use an absorbent point to apply the drug to a fine root canal, the point is introduced in a dry rather than a moist state to prevent it buckling upon insertion. The butt end of the point is folded over and a moistened wool pledget is placed in the pulp chamber to wet the point and to act as a 'reservoir' of the drug.

Care should be taken when introducing antibiotic pastes into fine canals not to extrude paste into the periapical region. To prevent sudden jamming in the canal with consequent breakage, spiral root fillers are best used by hand rather than in a handpiece. A reamer used with the same counter-clockwise action as in coating a canal with root-filling cement may also be employed. Surplus paste on the floor of the pulp chamber is removed.

The wool pledget used to apply the chemical antiseptic or to cover the antibiotic paste should be pressed firmly against the base of the pulp chamber so as to leave sufficient room for a thick cement seal to the pulp cavity. The pledget should cover the entire base of the pulp chamber to prevent occlusion of a root canal orifice by cement. To avoid the risk of breakage of the cement seal before the next appointment, it is important to check that it does not make occlusal contact with the opposing teeth.

8. ROOT FILLING

The tooth is judged to be ready for root filling by the same criteria as are used for anterior teeth. The filling of each canal is best performed as a separate procedure, and the least accessible canal—normally the mesiobuccal in both maxillary and mandibular teeth—is filled first. Before each canal is filled it is dried with an absorbent point and small wool pledgets are inserted in the orifices of the remaining unfilled canals to prevent their blockage by surplus cement.

The advantages and disadvantages of gutta percha and silver as root-filling materials and the techniques of root filling were discussed in Chapter 8. Gutta percha is the material of choice for molar teeth, especially for curved canals where instrumentation may have led to flaring of the apical part of the preparation. Where it is decided to root fill with silver, its use should be limited to relatively straight canals where flaring is unlikely to have occurred (*see Fig.* 202).

The root-filling points are fitted and checked radiographically at the visit preceding that at which the tooth is root-filled. Before removal from the tooth they are cut level with a suitable reference point occlusally, so providing a check on their complete insertion at the time of root-filling. The radiograph may reveal a gutta

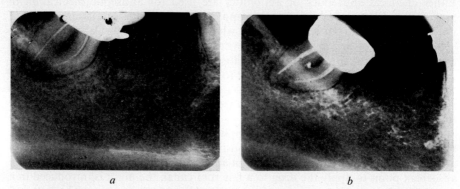

a	*b*

Fig. 218. 7̄|. *a,* Trial insertion of gutta percha points; *b,* After root filling. The lubricant action of the root canal cement has enabled the gutta percha point in the mesial canal to be inserted further apically. Some filling material has been extruded through a lateral canal on the distal aspect of the mesial root.

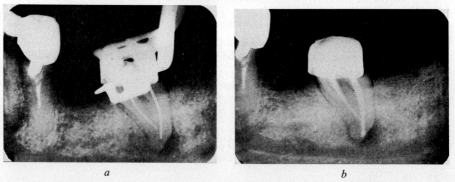

a	*b*

Fig. 219. |7̄. *a,* Trial insertion of gutta percha points. The point in the distal canal is about 2 mm short of the apical limit; *b,* After root filling by vertical condensation.

percha point to be slightly short of the known apical limit. This is of no consequence since the lubricant action of the root canal cement and the pressure used in inserting the point will seat it in its correct position (*Fig.* 218). If the vertical condensation technique of filling is to be used, each point should bind and stop about 2·0 mm short of the apical limit (*Fig.* 219).

A fitted silver point should encounter resistance on insertion only in the apical 3–4 mm of the canal, which it should fit tightly; it should obviously extend to the apical limit. Sometimes the selected point stops a little short of the apical limit, whilst the next smaller size, although it can be inserted to the correct level, does not fit tightly. This can be rectified by gripping and rotating the apical 3–4 mm of the larger point within a folded sandpaper disk (Schilder, 1967), so thinning it. After cementation of a silver point there are usually obvious regions in the middle and coronal parts of the canal where the point does not fit closely; to ensure that these are obliterated, sections of gutta percha point are heated and softened and then condensed vertically alongside the silver.

After the completion of root filling with gutta percha, excess material at the orifices of the canals is removed with a hot plastic instrument and a layer of zinc oxide–eugenol cement packed against the base of the pulp chamber to occlude the orifices of any accessory canals communicating with the supporting periodontium. Where silver has been used, the projecting points are reduced in length with a pair of fine scissors; cement is then packed against the base of the pulp chamber, and the points either bent over and embedded in the cement or cut flush with the surface of the cement when the latter has set.

9. POSTOPERATIVE OBSERVATION AND PROGNOSIS

Molar teeth are observed postoperatively in the same way as other teeth. With correct case selection, the prognosis of non-surgical treatment of molar teeth is good (*Fig.* 220). Indeed, the studies of Strindberg (1956) and Grahnen and Hansson

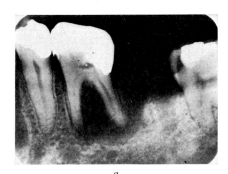 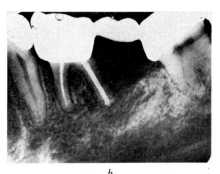

a   *b*

Fig. 220. ⌐6. Before treatment. A large periapical lesion is present; *b*, Eighteen months after root filling. Periapical repair is complete. The referring dentist had constructed a bridge in the intervening period.

(1961) indicate that the success rate with these teeth is, contrary to popular belief, higher than with other teeth.

10. SURGICAL TREATMENT OF MOLAR TEETH

The surgical treatment of molar teeth may take one of three forms, namely periapical surgery, radisectomy or hemisection.

a. Periapical surgery

The selection of teeth for periapical surgery, including the influence of the proximity of the maxillary antrum and the inferior dental canal on selection, was discussed in Chapter 11. A particularly relevant consideration in the surgical treatment of molar teeth is access, which needs to be good. An important factor influencing the amount of access is the degree to which the cheek can be retracted when the teeth are in occlusion. Because of the restricted access, treatment is more time-consuming than with anterior teeth. Unless root fillings are already present, therefore, the canals should be filled prior to surgery.

It is generally more satisfactory to reflect a flap from the gingival crevices of the teeth, especially in the mandible. If during treatment it is found that access for periapical surgery is inadequate, this type of flap will facilitate radisectomy or hemisection as an alternative form of treatment. Because of the restricted amount

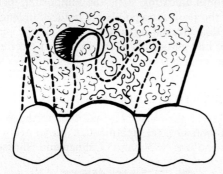

Fig. 221. In periapical surgery on molar teeth, access is improved by cutting back at an angle the mesial border of the bony wound. The flap is normally reflected from the gingival crevices.

of room, and in some instances the proximity of the antrum or inferior dental canal, access to the root apex has to be gained by removing the bone directly overlying the apical part of the root rather than beyond, whatever the periapical status. The amount of access to the root-end can be increased to some extent by cutting back at an angle the mesial border of the bony wound (*Fig.* 221), so permitting, at least in part, an approach from the front of the mouth and at the same time improving visibility. The extent to which this can be done is of course controlled by the proximity of adjacent structures, including other roots.

The buccal roots of maxillary molars are in close proximity to the overlying cortical plate, which is relatively thin. Adequate access to these roots is therefore generally possible, even at the rear of the mouth (*Fig.* 222). The cut root face apically should be examined for the presence of a separate second canal, especially with a mesiobuccal root. Where an additional canal is found it may be too close to the periphery of the root to allow the preparation of a suitable root-end cavity; under these circumstances the root is progressively shortened until the canal is more centrally placed (*Fig.* 223). Access to the palatal root of a maxillary molar is gained from the palatal aspect but is usually inadequate for satisfactory examination and treatment of the root-end; in consequence these roots are not usually amenable to periapical surgery.

The buccal cortical plate is much thicker in the mandible than in the maxilla, and several millimetres of bone may have to be penetrated before the root apex is exposed. Access to the root-end and illumination of the bony wound are consequently less satisfactory, and sometimes a considerable reduction in root length is necessary to gain reasonable working room (*Fig.* 224). Access to a mandibular molar therefore needs to be good if the tooth is to be treated by periapical surgery.

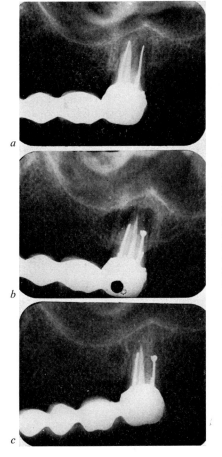

Fig. 222. |7. a, Prior to periapical surgery. A dentine pin had been inserted into each buccal canal to support an amalgam core. Both buccal canals had been overfilled. The distobuccal root is associated with a periapical lesion. b, Immediately following apicectomy of each buccal root, with reverse amalgam filling of the distobuccal root. c, Nineteen months postoperatively, there is advanced periapical repair mesiobuccally, and complete repair distobuccally.

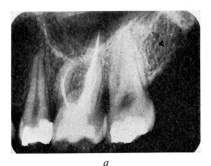
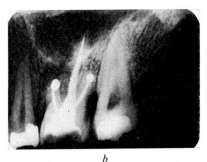

a   b

Fig. 223. |6. a, Prior to periapical surgery. The tooth was associated with persistent tenderness in the buccal sulcus; b, Immediately following apicectomy and reverse amalgam filling of each buccal root. The mesiobuccal root had to be shortened more than the distobuccal root to facilitate inclusion of a second canal in the root-end cavity.

Because of the depth of the root apex in bone, unless there is extensive periapical destruction, any significant error in the position or angle at which bone is penetrated may lead to difficulty in locating the apex. It is especially important, therefore, that the preoperative radiographs are closely studied beforehand for root inclination and curvature, and that due allowance is made for any tilting of the tooth. It is obviously useful if the working length of the root under treatment is known. The bony wound should be periodically inspected to ensure that the correct course is being followed by cutting instruments. Although either right-angle or straight instruments

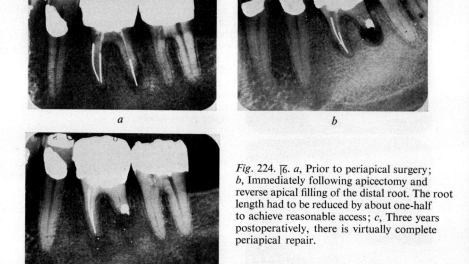

a

b

c

Fig. 224. ⌐6. *a,* Prior to periapical surgery; *b,* Immediately following apicectomy and reverse apical filling of the distal root. The root length had to be reduced by about one-half to achieve reasonable access; *c,* Three years postoperatively, there is virtually complete periapical repair.

may be used for bone removal, removal of the root apex is more readily accomplished with right-angle instruments; the use of standard length burs in conjunction with a miniature head provides better visibility during the latter procedure. Care should be taken during apex removal not to leave a sliver of dentine projecting on the lingual aspect of the root. Where the insertion of a reverse filling is necessary, it should include all untreated or inadequately treated canals at the level at which the root is sectioned (*Fig.* 225).

Altonen and Matila (1976) quote a success rate of 81 per cent following treatment of molar roots by periapical surgery, and state that reverse root filling was associated with a lower rate of success.

b. Radisectomy and hemisection

Removal of an entire root from a multi-rooted tooth is sometimes necessary. In radisectomy, all or most of the overlying part of the crown is left, whereas in hemisection it is removed. Although sometimes regarded as recent innovations, the publications of Farrar (1884) and Black (1887) show that both procedures have been practised for many years. The study of Bergenholtz (1972) indicates that with proper case selection these forms of treatment have a good prognosis.

The indications for the two procedures are somewhat similar and may be endodontic, periodontal or restorative in nature. For example, a root canal may be obstructed by calcification or previous root canal treatment and may not be amenable to periapical surgery, or there may be severe periodontal bone loss limited to one root of the tooth, or it may be necessary to convert a trifurcation into a bifurcation to facilitate plaque control. Alternatively, there may be advanced

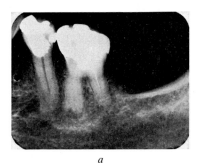 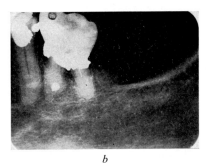

a   *b*

Fig. 225. ⌐6. *a*, Prior to periapical surgery. The tooth had evidently been root-filled many years previously, but the mesial root was associated with a periapical lesion; *b*, Eight years after apicectomy and reverse filling of the mesial root to include the openings of both mesiolingual and mesiobuccal canals. Periapical repair is complete.

unrestorable caries or a vertical fracture involving the roots. Where the base of the pulp chamber has been exposed by caries or trauma, hemisection is indicated. In the maxilla the use of both radisectomy and hemisection is normally confined to the removal of one or both buccal roots.

In both procedures, there should obviously be sufficient periodontal attachment remaining after treatment to support the tooth; the periodontal and periapical condition of each remaining root should therefore be carefully assessed. To ensure that it is possible to treat adequately each of the roots which is to remain, root canal filling is normally performed prior to surgery. An exception to this rule occurs when treatment is being performed for periodontal reasons and a period of postoperative observation is needed to assess the response to treatment. Here, rather than root treat the tooth needlessly, pulpotomy is performed as an interim measure; alternatively, if radisectomy is carried out, the radicular pulp is capped at its site of exposure during root removal. If the tooth has already been root-filled, the existing fillings should be satisfactory, or capable of being made so.

Apart from these requirements, there should be no evidence that the root to be removed is fused apically with another root. Also, the furcation should not be situated so far apically that an excessive amount of supporting bone would have to be removed to expose the site of root division. It is because of this last factor that radisectomy and hemisection are seldom performed on two-rooted maxillary premolars. Since some degree of trauma and resultant inflammatory resorption of bone are unavoidable, particularly in the mandible, both procedures are contraindicated where the roots of the tooth are close together with minimal interradicular bone.

1. *Radisectomy* (*Fig.* 226)

This procedure is also known as 'radectomy' or 'root amputation'.

Although conserving the mesiodistal dimension of the tooth, and thereby the contact areas with adjacent teeth, radisectomy has obvious drawbacks compared with hemisection. Since the crown overlying the extracted root is not removed, this part of the tooth becomes unsupported and the remaining roots are subjected to non-axial stresses during mastication. Where the crown is relatively intact, these undesirable effects may be partially offset by reduction of the occlusal table bucco-lingually over the extracted root. Similarly, the development of a food-trap between

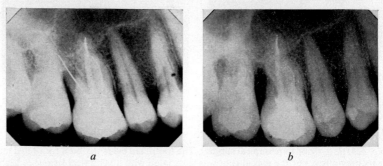

a   *b*

Fig. 226. 6|. *a*, Gross periodontal bone loss around distobuccal root; *b*, Immediately after radisectomy of distobuccal root.

the unsupported part of the tooth and the gingival tissues may be largely prevented by cutting back the undersurface of the crown at the time of radisectomy so that it is well clear of the gingival tissues, as suggested by Amen (1966). In the mandible, however, the presence of ridges running mesiodistally on the undersurface of the tooth between the two roots makes plaque control difficult in the region of the furcation following its exposure to the mouth. Burch and Hulen (1974) found that these bifurcation ridges were present in 76 per cent of mandibular molars.

Because of these drawbacks, hemisection is generally preferable to radisectomy. However, where the tooth is splinted to other teeth by some form of fixed appliance, it is expedient to perform radisectomy. Occasionally, radisectomy is performed on an anterior or premolar tooth, the natural crown being left in situ within an overlying appliance (*Fig.* 227).

In radisectomy the coronal part of the root to be removed is filled by way of the pulp chamber with a material, such as amalgam, which will be insoluble on sub-sequent exposure to saliva. This may be accomplished by reaming the coronal 2–3 mm of the canal with instruments up to no. 100 and using root canal pluggers to condense amalgam into this part of the canal and the adjoining pulp chamber. If the tooth is already root-filled, a reverse 'root' filling of amalgam is inserted after root removal. Recontouring of the crown to reduce the occlusal table is performed before root removal, so avoiding the unnecessary introduction of debris into the wound.

A flap is reflected from the gingival crevices. Unless already destroyed by periodontal disease, bone is removed to expose most of the root length. Fissure burs are used to section the root in the vicinity of the cemento-enamel junction, care being taken to avoid damaging an adjacent root. A fairly wide gap is made between the undersurface of the crown and the root to facilitate removal of the latter. Very often the coronal part of a molar root is appreciably wider bucco-lingually than mesiodistally and a check should be made that it has been separated completely from the overlying crown. This is normally obvious from visual examination, but should be checked by gentle leverage against the root, when no movement of the crown should be apparent. Provided exposure of the root is adequate, it should now be possible to prise it from its socket with elevators. If difficulty is encountered, further bone should be removed to expose the entire root

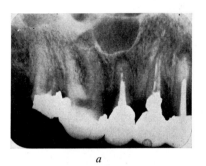 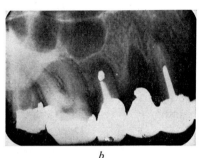

a   b

Fig. 227. 4|. *a*, The 4|, which was splinted to 5| and 3|, was associated with advanced periodontal disease and caries of the root; 5| and 3| were associated with periapical lesions; *b*, The 4| was treated by radisectomy, leaving the natural crown within the over-lying appliance. The 5| was treated by apicectomy and reverse apical filling, which are also indicated for 3|.

length. Complete exposure of the buccal aspect of the root is normally necessary in the mandible, where judicious removal of some interradicular bone may also be needed because of the concave cross-sectional shape of the adjoining root surface.

Following root removal, granulation tissue in the region of the furcation is curetted and the bony margins of the socket contoured to blend with the cortical plate over the adjoining roots. The cut undersurface of the tooth is smoothed and sharp margins at its junction with the sides of the crown rounded with stones; it is also examined to ensure that the amalgam seal is satisfactory and that there is no evidence of the opening of a second canal. The wound is now closed with sutures.

2. Hemisection

In hemisection the crown is sectioned in a vertical plane so as to separate the root to be removed. This enables the root, together with the overlying part of the crown, to be extracted in an occlusal direction, instead of having to be prised out sideways, as in radisectomy. Hemisection is generally an easier procedure than radisectomy in the treatment of mandibular molars, where the latter procedure can be difficult. Although the term 'hemisection' is, strictly speaking, applicable only to the treat-ment of a two-rooted tooth, it is also used to describe similar procedures on three-rooted teeth.

As in radisectomy, the canal of each root to be retained is best filled prior to surgery. The tooth is sectioned with long tapered air-turbine diamonds, cutting from the gingival region towards the occlusal surface. In the mandible this cut

9

extends buccolingually over the bifurcation. In the maxilla, where the operation is normally used only for the removal of buccal roots, the cut is made from the buccal aspect to the centre of the occlusal surface, and thence to the mesio- or disto-palatal surface of the crown. Reflection of a flap facilitates accurate positioning of the cut, but unless indicated for periodontal surgery, is often unnecessary in the mandible, where radiographs provide an accurate guide to the position of the bifurcation.

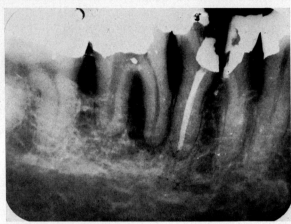

Fig. 228. 6̄|. During hemisection a radiographic check was made prior to extraction of the mesial root, to ensure that the tooth had been sectioned through the centre of the furcation.

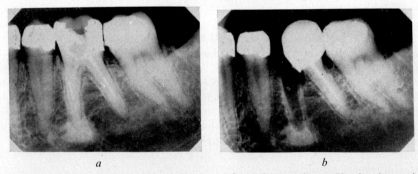

a	*b*

Fig. 229. |6̄. *a*, Fragments of broken instruments in the mesial root. Hemisection, rather than radisectomy, was decided upon because the sclerosed bone apically might have made radisectomy difficult. *b*, Immediately after removal of mesial root by hemisection and application of a temporary crown.

The crown should be accurately sectioned over the centre of the furcation and not towards the root to be removed, otherwise a sliver of tooth substance will be left projecting in the region of the future socket; if necessary a radiograph is taken to check this (*Fig.* 228). Care should be taken when cutting through the base of the pulp chamber not to cause needless damage to the underlying bone.

Complete separation is checked by passing a probe from the undersurface of the crown in an occlusal direction and by demonstrating independent movement of the two parts of the tooth. Before extracting the root, the remaining natural crown is reshaped as necessary to receive a temporary crown pending a permanent restoration (*Fig.* 229). Following extraction the temporary crown is cemented and, where appropriate, the wound closed with sutures.

Occasionally hemisection is performed but, instead of extracting one of the roots, each is retained and restored. This form of treatment is normally confined to a

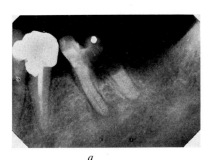
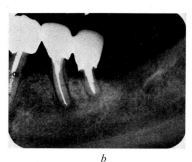

a   *b*

Fig. 230. ⌐7. *a*, The floor of the pulp chamber has been perforated by caries; the roots are widely separated; *b*, Following root canal treatment and hemisection, with the retention of both roots. Provisional restorations have been placed.

mandibular molar with periodontal bone loss limited to the bifurcation region, or where the floor of the pulp chamber has been perforated by caries or trauma. The procedure is contraindicated unless the roots of the tooth are sufficiently splayed to allow cleaning of the 'interdental' region by the patient following restoration (*Fig.* 230).

REFERENCES

Ainamo J. and Löe H. (1968) A stereomicroscopic investigation of the anatomy of the root apices of 910 maxillary and mandibular teeth. *Odontol. Tidskr.* **76**, 417.

Altonen M. and Matila K. (1976) Follow-up study of apicoectomised molars. *Int. J. Oral Surg.* **5**, 33.

Amen C. R. (1966) Hemisection and root amputation. *Periodontics* **4**, 197.

Bergenholtz A. (1972) Radectomy of multirooted teeth. *J. Am. Dent. Assoc.* **85**, 870.

Black G. V. (1887) In: Litch W. F. (ed.), *The American System of Dentistry*, Vol. 1, Part 4. Edinburgh, Pentland, pp. 990–2.

Burch J. G. and Hulen S. (1972) The relationship of the apical foramen to the anatomic apex of the tooth root. *Oral Surg.* **34**, 262.

Burch J. G. and Hulen S. (1974) A study of the presence of accessory foramina, and the topography of molar furcations. *Oral Surg.* **38**, 451.

Cameron C. E. (1964) Cracked-tooth syndrome. *J. Am. Dent. Assoc.* **68**, 405.

Clem W. H. (1969) Endodontics: the adolescent patient. *Dent. Clin. North Am.* **13**, 483–93.

Coffae K. P. and Brilliant J. D. (1975) The effect of serial preparation versus nonserial preparation on tissue removal in the root canals of extracted mandibular human molars. *J. Endodontol.* **1**, 211.

Farrar J. N. (1884) Radical and heroic treatment of alveolar abscess by amputation of roots of teeth. *Dent. Cosmos* **26**, 79, 135.

Fromme H. G. and Guttzeit R. (1972) Experimental investigation of mechanical and chemical root canal enlargement and the adhesion of root filling materials. *Quintessence Int.* **3**, 27.

Gottlieb B. (1938) *Dentistry in Individual Phases.* Tel-Aviv, Haaretz. Quoted by Grossman L. I. (1955) *Root Canal Therapy*, 4th ed. London, Kimpton, p. 209.

Grahnen H. and Hansson L. (1961) The prognosis of pulp and root canal therapy. A clinical and radiographic follow-up examination. *Odontol. Revy* **12**, 146.

Jungmann C. L., Uchin R. A. and Bucher J. F. (1975) Effect of instrumentation on the shape of the root canal. *J. Endodontol.* **1**, 66.

Klayman S. M. and Brilliant J. D. (1975) A comparison of the efficacy of serial preparation versus Giromatic preparation. *J. Endodontol.* **1**, 334.

Linaburg R. G. and Marshall F. J. (1973) The diagnosis and treatment of vertical root fractures: report of a case. *J. Am. Dent. Assoc.* **86**, 679.

Mizrahi S. J., Tucker J. W. and Seltzer S. (1975) A scanning electron microscopic study of the efficacy of various endodontic instruments. *J. Endodontol.* **1**, 324.

Molven O. (1968) Engine and hand-operated root canal exploration. *Odontol. Tidskr.* **76**, 61.

Molven O. (1970) A comparison of the dentin-removing ability of five root canal instruments. *Scand. J. Dent. Res.* **78**, 500.

O'Connell D. T. and Brayton S. M. (1975) Evaluation of root canal preparation with two automated endodontic handpieces. *Oral Surg.* **39**, 298.

Pomeranz H. H. and Fishelberg G. (1974) The secondary mesiobuccal canal of maxillary molars. *J. Am. Dent. Assoc.* **88**, 119.

Schilder H. (1967) Filling root canals in three dimensions. *Dent. Clin. North Am.* **11**, 723–44.

Schilder H. (1974) Cleaning and shaping the root canal. *Dent. Clin. North Am.* **18**, 269–96.

Seidberg B. H., Altman M., Guttuso J. and Suson M. (1973) Frequency of two mesiobuccal root canals in maxillary permanent first molars. *J. Am. Dent. Assoc.* **87**, 852.

Skidmore A. E. and Bjorndal A. M. (1971) Root canal morphology of the human mandibular first molar. *Oral Surg.* **32**, 778.

Strindberg L. Z. (1956) The dependence of the results of pulp therapy on certain factors. *Acta Odontol. Scand.* **14**, Suppl. 21, p. 100.

Walton R. E. (1976) Histologic evaluation of different methods of enlarging the pulp canal space. *J. Endodontol.* **2**, 304.

Weine F. S., Healey H. J., Gerstein H. and Evanson L. (1969) Canal configuration in the mesio-buccal root of the maxillary first molar and its endodontic significance. *Oral Surg.* **28**, 419.

Weine F. S., Healey H. J., Gerstein H. and Evanson L. (1970) Pre-curved files and incremental instrumentation for root canal enlargement. *J. Can. Dent. Assoc.* **36**, 155.

Weine F. S., Kelly R. F. and Bray K. E. (1976) Effect of preparation with endodontic handpieces on original canal shape. *J. Endodontol.* **2**, 298.

Weine F. S., Kelly R. F. and Lio P. J. (1975) The effect of preparation procedures on original canal shape and on apical foramen shape. *J. Endodontol.* **1**, 255.

FURTHER READING

Abrams L. and Trachtenberg D. I. (1974) Hemisection: technique and restoration. *Dent. Clin. North Am.* **18**, 415–44.

Basaraba N. (1969) Root amputation and tooth hemisection. *Dent. Clin. North Am.* **13**, 121–32.

Cathey G. M. (1974) Molar endodontics. *Dent. Clin. North Am.* **18**, 345–66.

Stanley H. R. (1968) The cracked tooth syndrome. *J. Am. Acad. Gold Foil Operators* **11**, 36.

Chapter 13

Root canal treatment of incompletely developed teeth

Teeth with incompletely formed root apices often present special difficulties in treatment. When the pulp is vital these difficulties can be avoided by pulpotomy (Chapter 2). Even though pulpal necrosis may eventually follow on such treatment, the pulp usually survives long enough for apex formation to proceed to the stage where root filling is relatively straightforward. This is true even where the coronal part of the pulp is necrotic, provided the level of pulpotomy is such that the wound passes through vital pulp tissue.

It is where the pulp is to all intents and purposes totally necrotic that difficulties occur. These difficulties arise from the anatomy of the root canal, and typically involve the incisor teeth.

1. Root canal anatomy (*Fig.* 231)

On the basis of radiographic appearance, incompletely formed teeth may be divided into three groups according to the stage of root formation that has been reached, namely teeth with root canal walls that diverge gingivo-apically, teeth with parallel root canal walls and finally those with convergent walls. However, such a classification is indicative only of the state of root formation in the mesiodistal plane. In the buccolingual plane root formation proceeds more slowly, so that the buccolingual width of the apical part of the canal, which cannot be assessed radiographically, is rather greater than the mesiodistal width. Thus, Friend (1967) has demonstrated that a canal which, radiographically, is parallel-sided, in fact diverges buccolingually, whilst a radiographically convergent canal is commonly parallel-sided in the buccolingual plane.

It was pointed out in Chapter 3 that in treating a tooth with a necrotic pulp, preparation and filling of the entire canal as far as the vicinity of the apical foramen are necessary for a favourable prognosis. Where the root canal diverges bucco-lingually, or mesiodistally and buccolingually, satisfactory preparation and filling of the flared apical part of the canal are obviously not possible. Even with the convergent type of case, if the root canal is still parallel-sided buccolingually, treatment is difficult, since the presence of a wide apical foramen precludes the formation of an effective apical 'stop' during preparation, so hindering the insertion of a well-condensed filling. It is hardly surprising that Friend (1967) concluded that in most incisor teeth root growth was not sufficiently advanced to enable adequate preparation and filling until considerably more than 3 years after eruption of the tooth.

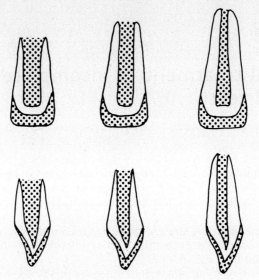

Fig. 231. Mesiodistal and buccolingual root formation in incompletely developed teeth.
Above, In mesiodistal plane. *Left*, divergent root canal; *Centre*, parallel-sided root canal; *Right*, convergent root canal.
Below, Corresponding states in buccolingual plane, in which root formation proceeds more slowly.

2. Inducing root-end closure

It has been realized for some years that although the pulp of an incompletely formed tooth may be necrotic, calcific closure of the apical foramen was possible, even though the extreme apical part of the canal may not have been effectively cleaned or filled (*Fig.* 232). Reports of such closure indicate that it may occur following filling of the root canal with a variety of preparations, including a paste of zinc oxide and various antiseptics (Cooke and Rowbotham, 1960), polyanti-biotic paste (Ball, 1964), iodoform paste (Bouchon, 1966), calcium hydroxide preparations (Crabb, 1965; Frank, 1966), as well as after the insertion of conventional root-filling materials (Rule and Winter, 1966; Friend,1967). Occasionally, an apparent attempt at calcific closure of a pulpless root may even be seen in the complete absence of treatment, as illustrated in Fig. 233; Barker and Mayne (1975) report a similar case. Continued root formation has even been reported following avulsion and loss of an incompletely formed tooth (Gibson, 1969; Burley and Reece, 1976), as well as after replantation of a root-filled tooth (Oliet, 1974).

It is apparent, therefore, that a considerable potential exists for calcific closure of the root-end, and numerous studies have been carried out into methods of encouraging such closure or 'apexification'. Nygaard-Ostby (1961) suggested that, immediately before root filling, the periapical tissues be deliberately traumatized with instruments to promote bleeding, so that the apical end of the canal was occupied by blood clot rather than root-filling material; favourable histological results were reported. Studies by Koenigs et al. (1975) and Roberts and Brilliant (1975), on

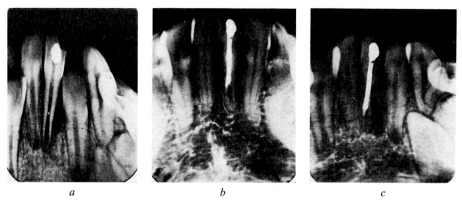

Fig. 232. ⌐⌐. a, After the root canal had been opened for drainage of an acute periapical abscess; b, Following root filling with gutta percha and cement; c, Over 13 years later, root-end closure and periapical repair have occurred, despite the inaccurate root filling.

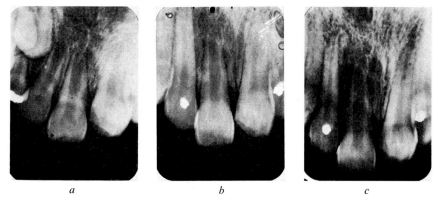

Fig. 233. 1|. a, Shortly after trauma, there is evidence of periapical bone destruction; b, Six months later, bone destruction is apparent mesially, as well as periapically; c, Nine months later, when the patient was referred for treatment. Continued root-end closure is apparent, even though root canal treatment has not yet been instituted.

monkey and human teeth respectively, indicate that good results may be obtained by the use of calcium phosphate ceramic to dress the root canal. However, the most popular method of inducing 'apexification', and that for which there is the greatest evidence, entails the use of calcium hydroxide as a root canal dressing.

3. 'Apexification' treatment with calcium hydroxide (*Fig.* 234)

Although the principles of obtaining access to the pulp cavity of an incompletely formed tooth are the same as with a fully formed tooth, the considerably larger size of both the pulp chamber and the root canal makes it necessary to prepare a significantly larger cavity in the crown. To facilitate access to the lingual wall of the canal, the cavity is made rather closer to the incisal edge than usual.

Although the pulp is necrotic, the apical part of the root canal is sometimes found to contain a plug of vital tissue from which there is haemorrhage; if this occurs, the canal is prepared as far as the level of this tissue. Where the canal is

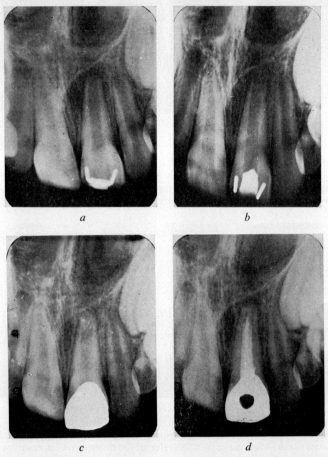

a   *b*

c   *d*

Fig. 234. |1. 'Apexification' treatment; *a*, Prior to treatment; *b*, After root canal preparation and the insertion of a calcium hydroxide-CMCP dressing; in opening the root canal, a large access cavity close to the incisal edge was prepared; *c*, Three months later, when the patient was next seen, calcific closure of the apical end of the root canal is apparent and periapical repair is proceeding; *d*, After root filling with gutta percha and cement.

completely devoid of vital tissue, it is prepared for its entire length. To avoid unnecessarily injuring the soft tissues at the root apex, reamers and files whose pointed ends have been ground flat, or alternatively Batt-ended instruments, are used. Although gross necrotic tissue may be removed with reamers, the bulk of root canal preparation is performed with files. These are inclined from one side of the root to the other during use in an attempt to reach all parts of the canal. The use of measuring devices is advisable to avoid trauma to the apical tissues. The canal is irrigated copiously with hypochlorite solution during and after instrumentation to remove residual necrotic tissue.

Following drying of the root canal, an antiseptic dressing is sealed in the pulp chamber and the patient seen again in 24–36 hours. At this second visit exudate is absorbed and the root canal dressed with calcium hydroxide. This may be used in powder form or as a paste with CMCP, cresatin, or sterile water or saline. Alternatively, a suspension of calcium hydroxide in methyl cellulose or hydroxyethyl cellulose solution may be employed; this form of preparation may be injected from a preloaded syringe employing either a wide-bore needle, or a narrow calibre needle and a screw-type of plunger (*Fig.* 235). A paste preparation, usually with CMCP, is probably employed most commonly.

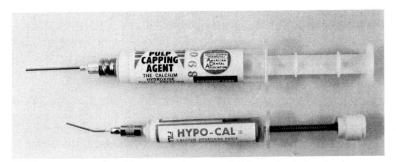

Fig. 235. Calcium hydroxide preparations supplied in preloaded syringes. *Above*, Syringe with conventional plunger action and wide-bore needle. *Below*, Syringe with screw-type of plunger and narrow calibre needle.

To ensure that calcium hydroxide reaches the apical region, the entire root canal is filled with the preparation. Calcium hydroxide powder may be introduced with an amalgam gun and then pushed apically with a large root canal plugger. Pastes are propelled apically with a spiral root filler. Syringe preparations are introduced by inserting the needle of the syringe as far as the apical region of the canal and then slowly withdrawing it whilst the preparation is being injected. Whatever preparation is used, it should not be deliberately forced into the periapical region. Surplus paste is removed from the crown and a pledget of wool placed in the pulp chamber prior to sealing the tooth.

Subsequently the patient is seen every 2 or 3 months when the tooth is examined radiographically for evidence of calcific closure and, if necessary, redressed with calcium hydroxide. Where radiographic evidence of a calcific barrier is not apparent after 6 months, the apical end of the canal may be gently probed with a fine root canal file, since radiographic interpretation of apical closure may be unreliable (Roberts and Brilliant, 1975). As will be discussed presently, the calcific barrier formed at the root-end commonly contains voids, and these could permit renewed periapical irritation from residual necrotic material within the canal. When obvious evidence of closure is apparent, therefore, the residual calcium hydroxide is removed and the canal obliterated with some form of conventional root filling (*Fig.* 234).

4. Repair and prognosis after calcium hydroxide treatment

The nature of the tissue which forms at the apical end of the root following calcium hydroxide treatment has been investigated by a number of workers. Reports based on the histological examination of human teeth have described the tissue as consisting of cementum [*](Klein and Levy, 1974), cementum with connective tissue inclusions [*](Cvek and Sundstrom, 1974) and cementum, dentine and pulp [°](Heithersay, 1970). Investigations following the experimental treatment of monkey teeth have reported the presence of osteodentine (Dylewski, 1971), cementum (Steiner and Van Hassel, 1971), cementum and bone (Ham et al. 1972) and cementum, bone and dentine (Torneck et al., 1973c). In many of these studies it was found that complete closure of the apical foramen did not occur, a conclusion also reached by Roberts and Brilliant (1975). Both Ham et al. (1972) and Torneck et al. (1973c) state that despite necrosis of the pulp and periapical disease, residual vital pulp sometimes persisted; however, whilst dentine deposition and further root development did not occur in the former study, in the latter there was some degree of apex formation postoperatively. It was also found by Torneck et al. (1973c) that moderate to severe periapical inflammation persisted despite substantial apical closure, presumably due to residual necrotic tissue both in the canal and within the spaces of the newly formed barrier.

The available evidence indicates a good prognosis following calcium hydroxide treatment and root filling. The most extensive study into this aspect is probably that of Cvek (1972), who found that of 55 teeth with necrotic pulps and periapical lesions, 50 were successful, with radiographic evidence of both complete periapical repair and apical closure. A later report evidently involving the same group of teeth states that further observation indicated the number of successful teeth to have increased to 52 (Cvek, 1973). There was no correlation between the time needed for apical closure, which was from 3 to 22 months, and that necessary for periapical repair, nor did further growth in root length occur. In a similar investigation of 21 teeth, Heithersay (1970) found that 19 showed some degree of apical closure, whilst complete periapical repair occurred in 20 teeth. In a histological study following the experimental treatment of monkey teeth, Steiner and Van Hassel (1971) observed apical calcification in 9 out of 10 teeth.

The reports of Van Hassel and Natkin (1970) and Roberts and Brilliant (1975) indicate that apical closure of an incompletely formed root may occur in adults as well as young persons.

5. Calcium hydroxide versus other techniques for apexification

Reference has already been made to the fact that apical closure can occur with a variety of materials, and sometimes in the absence of treatment. This aspect has been the subject of a number of comparative studies on experimental animals.

In a series of experiments, Torneck et al. (1973a, b, c) found that although the extent of foraminal closure was actually less when the root canal was cleaned and dressed with CMCP than where it was left untreated and open to the mouth, the greatest degree of closure occurred where the canal was cleaned and dressed with a paste of calcium hydroxide and CMCP. Ham et al. (1972) concluded that apical calcification occurred more often and in greater amounts after the insertion of a calcium hydroxide paste than after inducing the formation of a blood clot in the apical part of the canal, whilst Binnie and Rowe (1973) state that far more teeth showed continued root formation following the use of calcium hydroxide preparations than after filling with Grossman's root canal sealer. Vojinovic and Srnic (1975) report that whilst apical closure occurred with both a calcium hydroxide and an iodoform paste, it was faster and more complete with the former. Although perhaps of more relevance to periapical repair than to apical closure, Spangberg (1969) found that of various root filling materials implanted into the mandibles of experimental animals, only calcium hydroxide was replaced by bone.

It would therefore seem that the use of calcium hydroxide as a root canal dressing is the method of choice for inducing root-end closure in incompletely formed teeth with necrotic pulps. However, this is not to say that more effective methods or materials will not be discovered. Thus, the recent report by Roberts and Brilliant (1975) suggests that just as good results can be obtained using calcium phosphate ceramic, so indicating that it is not necessary to use a material with a highly alkaline pH. Nevins et al. (1976) describe good results with a collagen–calcium phosphate gel, claiming 'revitalization' and ingrowth of connective tissue into the root canals of immature pulpless teeth.

6. Conventional root canal treatment

Although the use of calcium hydroxide to promote apical closure, followed by root filling, has largely superseded other forms of treatment for incompletely formed pulpless teeth, on occasions it is still necessary to employ a conventional form of treatment. For example, where it is necessary to crown the tooth following root filling and the patient is moving to an area with no adequate dental facilities, there may be insufficient time for treatment with calcium hydroxide to be effective. Under these circumstances the canal is prepared in the manner described and conventional root canal dressings inserted preparatory to filling with gutta percha.

Where the canal apparently tapers in a gingivo-apical direction, it is usually possible to obtain a tight fit apically with a large gutta percha point, although the apical end of the latter may have to be shortened. The gutta percha should bind 0·5–1·0 mm short of the apical limit; the lubricant action of the root canal cement and the pressure used in condensation of the filling will result in complete seating of the point. To provide a check on its position during root filling the point is marked or shortened to correspond to the working length of the tooth. The walls of the canal and the point itself are now lightly coated with cement, the point inserted and the remainder of the canal filled using the lateral condensation technique (*Fig.* 236).

Teeth with radiographically parallel or divergent root canal walls are also filled by a lateral condensation technique. However, to obtain as tight a fit as possible in the apical part of the canal, the master gutta percha point has to be fitted coronal end foremost (*Fig.* 237); this has the added advantage of providing extra room in the coronal part of the canal for the introduction of additional points. The latter are inserted into the wider buccal and lingual parts of the canal first, where it may prove possible to introduce some of the points butt end foremost. During filling care has to be taken not to thrust any of the points beyond the apical limit, and to this end each point is marked or shortened beforehand to correspond to the working length. The master point should be firmly grasped to prevent it being forced beyond the apical limit as each additional point is inserted.

The absence of an apical stop in a parallel-sided or divergent canal can sometimes lead to extrusion of filling material into the periapical tissues with resultant haemorrhage into the apical part of the canal before the completion of root filling. To prevent this complication as well as to facilitate condensation of the filling,

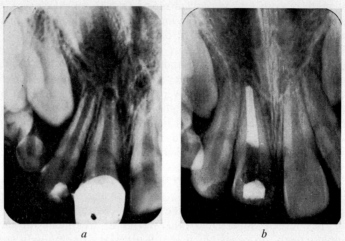

a   *b*

Fig. 236. 1|. *a*, 'Convergent' canal, prior to treatment; *b*, After root filling with gutta percha and cement. Space is available in the coronal part of the canal for the retention of a temporary post crown.

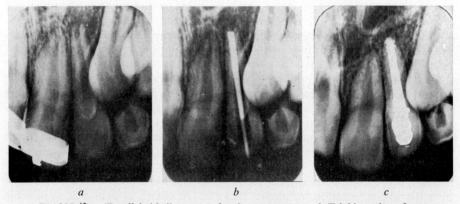

a   *b*   *c*

Fig. 237. |2. *a*, 'Parallel-sided' root canal, prior to treatment; *b*, Trial insertion of gutta percha point, coronal end foremost; *c*, After root filling with gutta percha and cement.

Dimashkieh (1975) suggests that the extreme apical end of the canal and the immediately adjoining periapical region first be occluded with sterile oxidized cellulose, packed apically with root canal pluggers. After surplus cellulose has been removed from the sides of the canal, the root filling is inserted; if preferred, amalgam can be used to fill just the apical part of the canal (Chapter 8). The oxidized cellulose left in the periapical region is absorbed.

7. Surgical treatment

Occasionally calcium hydroxide treatment fails and surgical treatment of an incompletely formed tooth becomes necessary. Such a tooth often has a parallel-sided or divergent canal, and therefore relatively thin root canal walls. Also, being

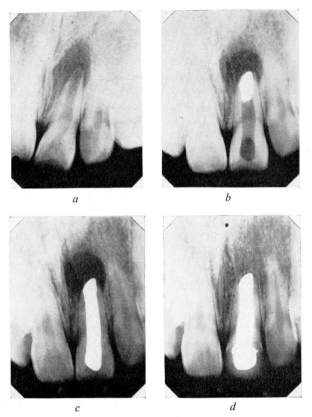

Fig. 238. |1. *a*, Fairly large periapical lesion present; *b*, After reverse filling of the apical part of the canal with amalgam; *c*, The completed root filling; *d*, Complete periapical repair 12 months later. (*Figs.* 238*a, b* and *c* from Nicholls E. (1962) *Oral Surg.* **15**, 463. Missouri, C. V. Mosby Co.)

incompletely formed, the root is likely to be relatively short. In consequence it is inadvisable to treat the tooth simply by performing apicectomy at such a level as to pass through an adequately filled part of the root. Apicectomy with reverse apical filling is often preferable, and as little root structure as possible is removed compatible with producing a smooth rim to the apical end of the root and obtaining enough access for the insertion of a filling. In obtaining access to the root-end, bone is penetrated beyond the apex. If a root filling is already present, filling material is removed to give a root-end cavity about 2 mm deep. Any necrotic tissue on the side walls of the cavity is carefully removed with round burs. Because of the thinness of the walls of the canal, only a slight undercut at the base of the cavity is generally possible; the mesial and distal walls are chosen for this purpose, since they are thicker.

Where the tooth is not already root filled, the canal is first cleaned by way of the pulp chamber as far as the level of divergence, following which a wool pledget moistened with CMCP is placed in the pulp chamber to prevent gross recontamination of the canal by salivary organisms. The region is then anaesthetized, diseased periapical tissue is removed, and the root apex is trimmed to allow preparation of the root-end cavity. It is sometimes advocated that at this stage, instead of inserting a separate apical filling, the entire canal be filled through the pulp chamber by introducing multiple gutta percha points and condensing these against the divergent canal walls by counter-pressure from the apical end of the root. A disadvantage of this method is that if a post crown becomes necessary later, the absence of an apical stop may lead to disruption of the apical seal should one of the points be disturbed when preparing the post hole. To obviate this risk it is better to fill the apical and coronal parts of the canal separately (*Fig.* 238). After the root-end cavity has been prepared, the largest reamer or file which will reach the level of the 'base' of the cavity is trimmed so as to flatten its apical end. The instrument is inserted to the appropriate level and is wedged firmly in position by packing gutta percha or absorbent points alongside it, so forming a suitable base on which to condense amalgam. After filling the root-end cavity and removing the instrument and points, the coronal part of the canal may be obliterated with gutta percha and cement.

An alternative method which can be used where the tooth is not already root filled is described by Messing (1960). A stainless-steel device with a matrix covering the apical end of the root and an adjustable platform engaging the incisal edge is fitted to the tooth. Amalgam is condensed against the apical matrix by way of the pulp chamber.

REFERENCES

Ball J. S. (1964) Apical root formation in a non-vital immature permanent incisor: report of a case. *Br. Dent. J.* **116**, 166.

Barker B. C. W. and Mayne J. R. (1975) Some unusual cases of apexification subsequent to trauma. *Oral Surg.* **39**, 144.

Binnie W. H. and Rowe A. H. R. (1973) A histological study of the periapical tissues of incompletely formed pulpless teeth filled with calcium hydroxide. *J. Dent. Res.* **52**, 1110.

Bouchon F. (1966) Apex formation following treatment of necrotized immature permanent incisor. *J. Dent. Child.* **33**, 378.

Burley M. A. and Reece R. D. (1976) Root formation following traumatic loss of an immature incisor: a case report. *Br. Dent. J.* **141**, 315.

Cooke C. and Rowbotham T. C. (1960) Root canal therapy in non-vital teeth with open apices. *Br. Dent. J.* **108**, 147.

Crabb H. S. M. (1965) The basis of root-canal therapy. *Dent. Practnr. Dent. Rec.* **15**, 397.

Cvek M. (1972) Treatment of nonvital permanent incisors with calcium hydroxide. I, Follow-up of periapical repair and apical closure of immature roots. *Odontol. Revy* **23**, 27.

Cvek M. (1973) Clinical procedures promoting apical closure and arrest of external root resorption in non-vital permanent incisors. In: Grossman L. I. (ed.), *Transactions of the 5th International Conference on Endodontics*. Philadelphia, University of Pennsylvania, pp. 30–41.

Cvek M. and Sundstrom B. (1974) Treatment of non-vital permanent incisors with calcium hydroxide. V, Histologic appearance of roentgenographically demonstrable apical closure of immature roots. *Odontol. Revy* **25**, 379.

Dimashkieh M. R. (1975) A method of using silver amalgam in routine endodontics, and its use in open apices. *Br. Dent. J.* **138**, 298.

Dylewski J. J. (1971) Apical closure of nonvital teeth. *Oral Surg.* **32**, 82.

Frank A. L. (1966) Therapy for the divergent pulpless tooth by continued apical formation. *J. Am. Dent. Assoc.* **72**, 87.

Friend L. A. (1967) The treatment of immature teeth with non-vital pulps. *J. Br. Endodontic Soc.* **1**, 28.

Gibson A. C. L. (1969) Continued root development after traumatic avulsion of partly formed permanent incisor. *Br. Dent. J.* **126**, 356.

Ham J. W., Patterson S. S. and Mitchell D. F. (1972) Induced apical closure of immature pulpless teeth in monkeys. *Oral Surg.* **33**, 438.

Heithersay G. S. (1970) Stimulation of root formation in incompletely developed pulpless teeth. *Oral Surg.* **29**, 620.

Klein S. H. and Levy B. A. (1974) Histological evaluation of induced apical closure of a human pulpless tooth: report of a case. *Oral Surg.* **38**, 954.

Koenigs J. F., Heller A. L., Brilliant J. D., Mefi R. C. and Driskell T. D. (1975) Induced apical closure of permanent teeth in adult primates using a resorbable form of tricalcium phosphate ceramic. *J. Endodontol.* **1**, 102.

Messing J. J. (1960) An adjustable apical matrix for condensation of amalgam in root canals. *Br. Dent. J.* **109**, 456.

Nevins A. J., Finkelstein F., Borden B. G. and Laporta R. (1976) Revitalization of pulpless open apex teeth in Rhesus monkeys, using collagen–calcium phosphate gel. *J. Endodontol.* **2**, 159.

Nygaard-Ostby B. (1961) The role of the blood clot in endodontic therapy: an experimental histologic study. *Acta Odontol. Scand.* **19**, 323.

Oliet S. (1974) Apexogenesis associated with replantation: a case history. *Dent. Clin. North Am.* **18**, 457–64.

Roberts S. C. and Brilliant J. D. (1975) Tricalcium phosphate as an adjunct to apical closure in pulpless permanent teeth. *J. Endodontol.* **1**, 263.

Rule D. C. and Winter G. B. (1966) Root growth and apical repair subsequent to pulpal necrosis in children. *Br. Dent. J.* **120**, 586.

Spangberg L. (1969) Biological effects of root canal filling materials. 7, Reaction of bony tissue to implanted root canal filling material in guineapigs. *Odontol. Tidskr.* **77**, 133.

Steiner J. C. and Van Hassel H. J. (1971) Experimental root apexification in primates. *Oral Surg.* **31**, 409.

Torneck C. D., Smith J. S. and Grindall P. (1973a) Biologic effects of endodontic procedures on developing incisor teeth. II, Effect of pulp injury and oral contamination. *Oral Surg.* **35**, 377.

Torneck C. D., Smith J. S. and Grindall P. (1973b) Biologic effects of endodontic procedures on developing incisor teeth. III, Effect of débridement and disinfection procedures in the treatment of experimentally induced pulp and periapical disease. *Oral Surg.* **35**, 532.

Torneck C. D., Smith J. S. and Grindall P. (1973c) Biologic effects of endodontic procedures on developing incisor teeth. IV, Effect of débridement procedures and calcium hydroxide camphorated parachlorphenol paste in the treatment of experimentally induced pulp and periapical disease. *Oral Surg.* **35**, 541.

Van Hassel H. J. and Natkin E. (1970) Induction of foraminal closure. *J. Dent. Assoc. S. Afr.* **25**, 305.

Vojinovic O. and Srnie E. (1975) Induction of apical formation by the use of calcium hydroxide and iodoform-Chlumsky paste in the endodontic treatment of immature teeth. *J. Br. Endodontic Soc.* **8**, 16.

FURTHER READING

Heithersay G. S. (1975) Calcium hydroxide in the treatment of pulpless teeth with associated pathology. *J. Br. Endodontic Soc.* **8**, 74.

Chapter 14

Treatment of special cases

PERFORATIONS

Perforation of the base of the pulp chamber or of the root of a tooth may result from operative trauma during dental treatment, resorption, or occasionally from caries, and leads to irritation of the adjoining periodontium. Adequate treatment of such a defect is as essential to the health of the supporting tissues as treatment of the root canal, and should be performed as soon as the perforation is detected and with the same regard to asepsis as in root canal treatment.

1. Classification

In discussing treatment, it is useful to classify perforations according to aetiology, time of occurrence and position. The following classification is a modification of that proposed by Nicholls (1962):
  1. Perforations due to resorption.
  2. Perforations due to trauma (or caries).
      a. Perforations diagnosed during root canal treatment.
          i. Perforations of the pulp chamber floor.
          ii. Perforations of the root side.
              α. Perforations of the coronal one-third of the root.
              β. Perforations of the middle one-third of the root.
              Mesial and distal perforations.
              Buccal and lingual perforations.
              γ. Perforations of the apical one-third of the root.
      b. Perforations diagnosed after root filling.

2. Treatment

The treatment of each of these classes of perforation will be considered in turn. A separate account of the surgical treatment of root perforations will be given subsequently.

1. *Perforations due to resorption*

In the past, perforations due to resorption have usually been treated by way of a surgical approach in order to eliminate the tissue associated with the resorptive process. Recently, however, reports by Frank and Weine (1973) and Heithersay (1975) suggest that applications of calcium hydroxide paste can be followed by arrest of the process and the deposition of hard tissue at the site of the perforation, so enabling the insertion of a conventional root filling. As much soft tissue as

264

possible within the pulp cavity in the vicinity of the perforation is removed during root canal preparation. Dressings of calcium hydroxide paste are then packed into the region of the perforation and allowed to remain for some weeks at a time. When there is no more than slight haemorrhage from the region, the tooth is root filled with gutta percha. A vertical condensation technique of filling is used to obtain a close adaptation of gutta percha to the walls of the defect (*Fig.* 239).

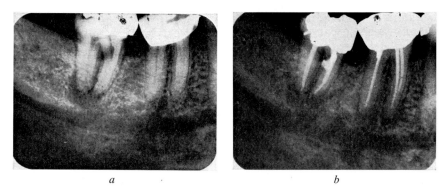

a   *b*

Fig. 239. ⁊̄. *a*, Prior to treatment, resorption and perforation of the distal aspect of the coronal part of the mesial root are apparent; *b*, After root filling with gutta percha and cement by vertical condensation. During root canal treatment, calcium hydroxide dressings were applied to the mesial root.

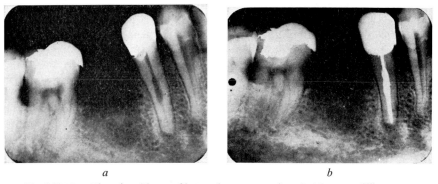

a   *b*

Fig. 240. 5̄|. *a*, There is evidence of internal root resorption; *b*, After root filling.

Occasionally, early evidence of internal resorption is seen during routine radiographic examination. In such a case, root filling should be performed as soon as possible before perforation occurs (*Fig.* 240).

2. *Perforations due to trauma*

Most perforations of the root are traumatic in origin, occurring during root canal treatment or subsequent restoration of the crown.

a. PERFORATIONS DIAGNOSED DURING ROOT CANAL TREATMENT

There is both clinical and histological evidence that where a traumatic perforation has occurred under aseptic conditions, immediate filling of the defect is associated with the most favourable prognosis, whilst deferring the time of filling is followed by destruction of the adjoining bone (Lantz and Persson, 1965, 1967), so eliminating the 'matrix' against which filling material may be condensed and making sealing of the defect more difficult. Where perforation occurs during the treatment of a tooth with a vital pulp with no clinical evidence of infection and bone has not been penetrated, immediate filling of the defect is therefore indicated. If there is evidence of pulpal necrosis, or if cutting instruments have penetrated the supporting bone rather than merely nicking the periodontal membrane, however, the application of dressings to the region of the perforation is indicated prior to filling. In an attempt to encourage the formation of a barrier of hard tissue, a paste of calcium hydroxide may be used. Where this is unsuccessful and the perforation involves a significant area of the root, sterile oxidized cellulose may be packed into the bony defect to form a base for the condensation of filling material (Dimashkieh, 1975a).

i. *Perforations of the pulp chamber floor*: By definition, perforations of the floor of the pulp chamber occur only in multi-rooted teeth. Although occasionally arising during restoration of a tooth, they usually result from incorrect opening of the pulp chamber during root canal treatment. Typically the pulp chamber is shallow and a small instead of a large round bur, run at high speed, has been used to open it. It is easy under these circumstances for the operator to be unaware that the bur has penetrated not only the roof of the pulp chamber but also the chamber itself (Chapter 12).

Experimental studies by Lantz and Persson (1967) and Seltzer et al. (1970) have demonstrated that perforation of the base of the pulp chamber is commonly followed by severe inflammation of the adjoining periodontium with loss of the supporting bone and the development of a periodontal pocket in the region of the defect. This finding is substantiated by clinical experience. Thus, Stromberg et al. (1972) report that of 10 perforations of the floor of the pulp chamber that were treated only 4 were successful.

Perforations in this position are best treated by radisectomy or hemisection; with mandibular molars it is occasionally possible to retain both roots (Chapter 12). If filling is attempted, the defect should be small and amenable to immediate obliteration according to the criteria previously described; in view of the significant risk of failure, treatment should not be performed if a complex restoration will be needed for the crown of the tooth. Immediately the perforation is diagnosed, root canal treatment is discontinued. The exposed periodontal membrane is cleaned by irrigation, gently dried and then covered with a calcium hydroxide cement. If the perforation is actually at the base of a cylindrical cavity in the pulp chamber floor, a filling of gutta percha or amalgam may be inserted over this. Root canal treatment is then resumed. Postoperative observation of such a tooth should include periodic checks on the periodontal condition.

ii. *Perforations of the root side*: A perforation of the side of the root during the course of root canal treatment usually arises from the use of an engine reamer, or from the use of excessive pressures with a hand instrument, especially after failing to employ the previous size of instrument. Occasionally it is caused by a bur. Provided it is not in close proximity to the alveolar crest, treatment of this type of perforation has a good prognosis, as indicated by the study of Stromberg et al. (1972).

Treatment depends on which part of the root is involved.

α. *Perforations of the coronal one-third of the root*: A perforation of the coronal one-third of the root is generally visible and accessible through the pulp chamber, although both the chamber and the coronal part of the canal may have to be judiciously widened.

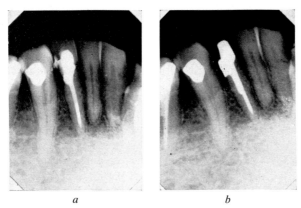

a   *b*

Fig. 241. 2͞]. *a*, Perforation of coronal one-third of root distally, temporarily sealed with zinc oxide–eugenol cement; *b*, Perforated region of root included in metal core for post crown.

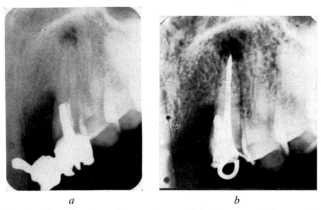

a   *b*

Fig. 242. [3. *a*, Small perforation of coronal one-third of root mesially, resulting from inaccurate post hole preparation; *b*, After obliteration of perforation with zinc oxide–eugenol cement followed by condensation of gutta percha through coronal opening into canal.

The treatment of a perforation in this part of the root depends on its relation to the alveolar crest. Where it is close to the latter, periodontal pocket formation is likely following treatment (Lantz and Persson, 1965, 1967). In these cases surgical exposure with recontouring of the alveolar crest is indicated, either to permit the insertion of a separate filling in the perforation (*see Fig.* 252) or to facilitate inclusion of the latter within a larger coronal restoration (*Fig.* 241). In either case the defect is temporarily sealed with cement until the root canal has been filled.

Where the perforation is rather further from the gingival crevice, it may be obliterated in the same way as a perforation of the floor of the pulp chamber. With this type of case, Harris (1976) recommends obliterating the perforation with Cavit (Espe), claiming a favourable response in 89 per cent of cases. If the defect is of long standing, granulation tissue from the exposed periodontal membrane may have grown into the pulp cavity; such tissue should be removed during root canal preparation and the wound dressed with a calcium hydroxide paste.

In the event of access to the perforation being restricted, the apical section of the canal is filled first. The perforation and the remainder of the canal may then be obliterated without danger of obstructing access to the apical end of the canal (*Fig*. 242).

β. *Perforations of the middle one-third of the root*: Since a perforation of the middle one-third of the root cannot normally be seen by way of the pulp chamber,

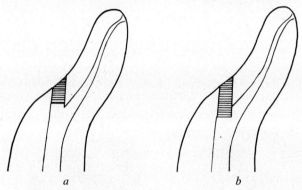

a   *b*

Fig. 243. It is often difficult to treat effectively through the pulp chamber a perforation of the middle one-third of the root if the perforation is in line with the coronal part of the canal. In filling the perforation, either a ledge is left in the root canal wall (*a*) or excess filling material projects into the canal (*b*).

it is necessary to estimate from a radiograph its distance from some occlusal point if it is to be accurately prepared and filled through the pulp chamber. The possibility of using the knowledge so gained depends on the relation of the perforation to the general long axis of the canal, whilst the possibility of obtaining it depends on which aspect of the root is involved.

Where the root canal is curved apically and the perforation is in line with the coronal part of the canal, accurate filling through the pulp chamber of both the perforation and the apical part of the canal is often difficult. If the perforation is filled first, the passage of instruments to the apical part of the canal will be hindered either by excess filling from the perforation or by a ledge in the wall of the canal at this site (*Fig*. 243). This ledge also impedes filling the apical part of the canal before the perforation. This type of perforation generally involves the mesial or distal aspect of the root and is associated with curvature of the canal. Although it usually occurs in the apical part of the root, it is occasionally seen in the middle one-third, often in a molar tooth. Whilst some of these cases may be adequately treated by way of the pulp chamber, in many instances a surgical approach is necessary. With an anterior tooth this may comprise apicectomy at the level of perforation and the insertion of an endodontic stabilizer, as described later in this Chapter. With multi-rooted teeth radisectomy or hemisection may be indicated.

Typically, though, the perforation is not in line with the long axis of the coronal part of the canal. Treatment then depends on which aspect of the root is involved. Usually this may be determined quite easily by comparing the buccolingual inclination of a reamer inserted into the defect with that of one inserted to the vicinity of the apical foramen. Similar inclinations indicate the defect is mesial or distal, whilst divergence of the instruments denotes it is buccal or lingual. The latter conclusion may be confirmed by radiographic examination, when the position of the tip of the instrument placed in the perforation will vary considerably with relatively small changes in horizontal angulation of the X-ray tube (*Fig.* 244).

Mesial and distal perforations: With mesial and distal perforations the distance between the root surface at the site of perforation and a suitable occlusal measuring point is assessed by radiographic examination in exactly the same way that the

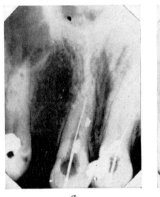 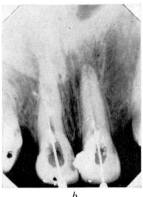

a   b

Fig. 244. 1|1. *a*, The instrument in the buccal perforation in 1| is apparently in line with the root canal, whilst that in the buccal perforation in |1 projects distally; *b*, With a small change in horizontal angulation to the tube, the instrument in 1| apparently projects distally, whilst that in |1 is in line with the root canal.

working length of the tooth is assessed. Since the long axes of the perforation and the coronal part of the canal do not coincide, adequate treatment of both should be possible, especially where, as is typically the case, the perforation has resulted from the injudicious use of an engine reamer or hand instrument and is consequently small. Where due to a bur, however, the perforation tends to be large and ragged in outline; unless a hard tissue barrier can be induced by calcium hydroxide treatment, so allowing obliteration of the defect by the vertical condensation of gutta percha, a surgical approach is necessary in this type of case.

Assuming that treatment by way of the pulp chamber is indicated, the root canal and the perforation are treated concurrently. Reamers, whose pointed ends have been ground flat, are used to widen the artificially created channel, but not the perforation itself, until it is large enough to fill. After irrigation, dressings are applied to both the perforation and the root canal proper. When the tooth is ready to root fill, the perforation, which is not visible through the pulp chamber, is filled before the root canal proper, otherwise access to it may be impeded by excess material. To avoid obstruction of the root canal by excess material from the perforation, a sectional technique is used; because of the difficulty of access, it is usually necessary to employ silver. The 'coronal' end of the sectioned point should not project into the canal in case post crown construction is necessary later (*Fig.* 245).

Buccal and lingual perforations: A buccal or lingual perforation cannot be accurately located by radiographic examination, since its image is superimposed upon that of the root (*Fig.* 246). If the defect is to be filled by way of the pulp chamber,

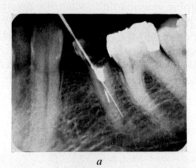 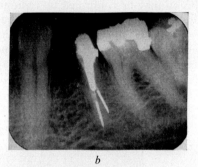

a   *b*

Fig. 245. |5. *a*, Perforation of distal aspect of root, with a broken instrument halfway down the canal; *b*, After filling the perforation and root canal proper through the coronal opening into the canal. The broken instrument was bypassed.

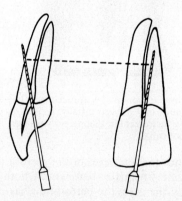

Fig. 246. The site of a buccal, or lingual, perforation cannot be accurately assessed by radiographic examination.
Left, Level of perforation in bucco-lingual plane (broken line).
Right, 'Radiographic' appearance in mesiodistal plane.

therefore, the use of calcium hydroxide treatment is indicated in order to induce the formation of a hard tissue barrier against which the filling may be condensed; alternatively, the bony cavity may be packed with sterile oxidized cellulose. If this is unsuccessful and the perforation is situated buccally, treatment by way of a surgical approach is necessary (*see Fig.* 251). Where the perforation is on the lingual aspect of the root, however, access even by a surgical approach is not usually satisfactory. In such cases, apicectomy at the level of the perforation and the insertion of an endodontic stabilizer may be possible. Alternatively, with a multi-rooted tooth, radisectomy or hemisection may be performed.

γ. *Perforations of the apical one-third of the root*: A perforation of the apical one-third of a root is invariably associated with curvature of the root canal and is therefore in line with the coronal part of the canal. Where the perforation is fairly close to the apical foramen it is often possible to fill both the extreme apical part of the canal and the defect itself, especially if chloropercha or a vertical conden- sation technique is used (*Fig.* 247).

Where the perforation is further coronally this may not be possible. In such a case the absence of a root filling in the apical end of the canal should result in a prognosis little worse than in an uncomplicated case deficient of root filling by the same distance. The treatment of this type of case therefore depends on the level

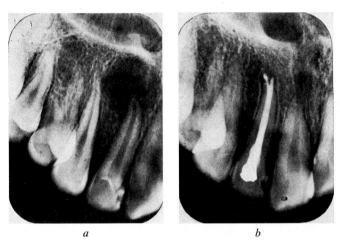

a   *b*

Fig. 247. 2|. *a*, Prior to treatment; *b*, Twenty months after filling of root canal and perforation with chloropercha, there is virtually complete periapical repair.

of the perforation and the state of the pulp. If the pulp is necrotic and the distance between the root apex and the perforation is more than 2·5–3 mm, root filling and apicectomy coronal to the defect are indicated. If the pulp in the apical part of the canal is vital, or if the perforation is within 2·5–3 mm of the root apex, the tooth is root-filled as far as the level of the perforation and observed clinically and radio- graphically afterwards. Often, a successful result is achieved (*Fig.* 248). Should failure occur, apicectomy may still be performed.

b. PERFORATIONS DIAGNOSED AFTER ROOT FILLING

Perforations diagnosed after root filling may be classified according to position in the same way as those diagnosed during root canal treatment. However, the decision whether to perform treatment through the pulp chamber or by way of a surgical approach may be influenced considerably by the nature of the root filling or of the coronal restoration, especially if this is a post crown.

Assuming that only a simple coronal restoration is present, the removal of a poorly condensed root filling, or of one consisting of a resorbable paste, should present little difficulty. Thus, provided surgery is not indicated by virtue of the size or position of the perforation, there is no reason why such a case should not be treated through the pulp chamber. However, the presence of a well-condensed root filling may complicate the problem considerably. Diagnosis of the position of the perforation may not be possible until the root filling has been removed, and this may be difficult and entail a risk of driving material into the supporting tissues in the region of the perforation. If there is an extensive coronal restoration the problem is complicated even further, since much or even all of the restoration may

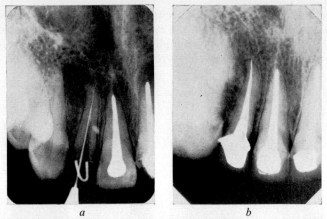

a   *b*

Fig. 248. 2|. *a*, Perforation of apical one-third of root during cleansing, about 2 mm from apical foramen; *b*, Almost complete periapical repair 6 years later, even though the extreme apical part of the canal was not filled.

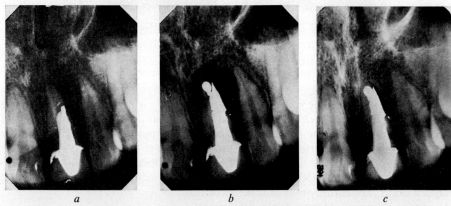

a   *b*   *c*

Fig. 249. |1. *a*, The distal aspect of the root has been perforated by post hole preparation and the apical part of the canal is unfilled. Surgical treatment is indicated due to the presence of a long post and a relatively weak root; *b*, After surgical treatment, with reverse apical filling and obliteration of the perforation with amalgam. Surgical exposure revealed that the root surface had been gouged apical to the perforation, and extension of the amalgam filling in an apical direction was therefore necessary; *c*, Two years after treatment, there is advanced repair.

have to be removed to obtain sufficient access. Such cases are generally treated by way of a surgical approach, therefore (*Fig.* 249).

Perforation of a root during post crown preparation arises from failure to inspect periodically the progress made in preparing the post hole. When such a perforation is diagnosed before cementation of the crown, and is suitable for non-surgical treatment, it is filled by way of the post hole in the same way as a perforation occurring during root canal treatment. The fact that the apical end of the canal is already filled simplifies the problem. Where surgical treatment is indicated, the post is cemented beforehand so as to provide a firm base during filling of the perforation. Should a post crown already be present, treatment depends on whether the crown is adequate. If it is well constructed with a post of adequate length, treatment is invariably surgical. However, should the crown be unsatisfactory and in need of replacement, treatment by way of the pulp chamber may be indicated (*see Fig.* 242).

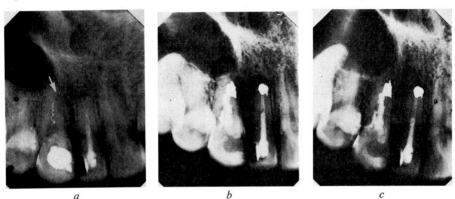

a   *b*   *c*

Fig. 250. 3|. *a*, There is resorption of the mesial aspect of the root. The presence of a perforation is indicated by a small section of broken broach (*arrowed*) projecting into the supporting tissues in the apical part of the resorbed region. There is also a broken rotary paste filler in the root canal. The maxillary antrum is in close proximity. *b*, Immediately after surgical treatment. The root apex was removed at a steep angle so that the amalgam filling used to obliterate the perforation also sealed the apical part of the root canal. *c*, Twenty-seven months later, there is complete repair.

3. Surgical treatment of root perforations

The possible indications for surgery in the treatment of root perforations have already been mentioned. They may be summarized as follows: perforations due to resorption; perforations involving a large area of the root surface, especially those which are ragged in outline; and perforations of the middle one-third of the root which are in line with the coronal part of the canal or which are on the buccal surface of the root. Also, surgical treatment is usually indicated where the tooth is already adequately root filled, especially if an extensive coronal restoration is present and does not need to be replaced. The elimination of a perforation by apicectomy at the level of the defect, with or without the insertion of an endodontic stabilizer, or of an entire root by radisectomy or hemisection, will not be considered here.

The tooth is normally root filled prior to surgery. The position and extent of the flap which is reflected depend on the position of the perforation. Where this is in the middle one-third of the root, the incision is made fairly close to the gingival margins, so avoiding inconvenience due to haemorrhage from the line of incision. Where the coronal part of the root is perforated, however, it is necessary to reflect the flap from the gingival crevices to provide adequate access.

The perforation and the adjoining area of the root are exposed, and any diseased alveolar tissue removed. If perforation has resulted from resorption (*Fig.* 250), softened tissue must be removed in its entirety and the adjoining bone thoroughly curetted. The perforation is now enlarged with suitable burs to form a well-defined cavity, undercut at its base. This is easily done when the buccal aspect of the root is involved (*Fig.* 251). With mesial and distal perforations, access is more difficult, but may be enhanced considerably by working from the same side of the root as

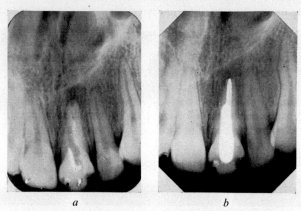

a   b

Fig. 251. |1. *a*, Preoperative view. The root had been perforated buccally; *b*, Postoperative view. The perforation was filled with amalgam by a surgical approach (from Nicholls E. (1962) *Oral Surg.* **15**, 603, Missouri, C. V. Mosby Co.).

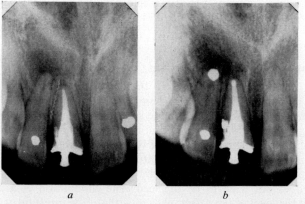

a   b

Fig. 252. 1|. *a*, The distal surface of the coronal one-third of the root has been perforated, and a spiral root filler has been broken in the periodontal membrane, presumably after being passed through the perforation in the root; *b*, After removing the spiral root filler and obliterating the perforation with amalgam, using a surgical approach. The root apices of 21| were also filled.

the perforation. If necessary for adequate access and vision, 'overhanging' cortical bone buccally is removed. Should access still be inadequate, the perforation is enlarged and extended in a buccal direction. In the same way, mesiolingual or distolingual perforations are extended farther on to the mesial or distal aspect of the root (*Fig.* 250).

The bony cavity is now packed with gauze and the cavity in the root dried and filled with amalgam in the same manner as in reverse apical filling. If filling of the perforation should precede filling of the root canal, a silver point of appropriate width is inserted in the canal to ensure it does not become obstructed by excess material. The point should be coated with varnish to prevent amalgamation with the overlying filling.

If the perforation is close to the alveolar crest (*Fig.* 252), surgical treatment is commonly followed by loss of the supporting bone in the vicinity and the development of a periodontal pocket (Lantz and Persson, 1970). Treatment should therefore include appropriate recontouring of the alveolar crest.

Where perforation occurs during root canal treatment and it is known that adequate preparation and filling of a cavity to include the defect will not be possible at the time of surgery, a different approach can sometimes be used. The root is filled with gutta percha, and material deliberately condensed into and beyond the perforation. Immediately afterwards the region is exposed surgically and the excess filling material removed.

BROKEN INSTRUMENTS

The vast majority of instances in which an instrument is broken in a root canal occur unnecessarily and may be avoided by following the simple guidelines suggested by Grossman (1969). Instruments should never be flamed. They should be examined for evidence of weakening each time they are withdrawn from the canal, and should be replaced as necessary. With a broach, weakening takes the form of loss of flexibility; with a reamer, the flute becomes wider or narrower (Chapter 6). Heavy pressure should not be used when a canal proves difficult to negotiate. Reamers and files should be used in the presence of an irrigating solution or other lubricant and in strict numerical sequence, with frequent removal of debris from the flute of the instrument. Reamers should not be used with more than a 180° turn. Stainless-steel instruments are less likely to break than carbon-steel instruments, which corrode in hypochlorite solutions. Fine instruments should not be used on more than one or two teeth before being replaced; larger instruments may be used three or four times. An additional silicone rubber marker may be placed on the instrument each time it is used; alternatively, one side of the existing marker may be cut following use on a tooth. Particular care should be taken in older patients, especially when treating molar teeth since, not surprisingly, instrument breakage is more common in such cases (Grossman, 1968).

On the rare occasions when despite these precautions an instrument is broken, a radiograph is taken immediately to localize it. Usually it is fairly close to the root-end, since it is in the narrow apical part of the canal that the instrument will be gripped tightly.

Either chemical or mechanical methods, or both, may be tried in an attempt to remove a broken instrument. The chemical usually advocated is a concentrated iodine–potassium iodide solution. The action of this preparation when introduced into the canal is to corrode the instrument, leading in favourable cases to its loosening. However, in most instances this successful outcome is not achieved, owing no doubt to the fact that the part of the instrument actually gripped by the root canal walls is not exposed to the solution.

More success is generally achieved by mechanical means. If the broken instrument is a barbed broach or a fine reamer or file, it is sometimes possible to insinuate a fine file alongside to engage it and then to pull it from the canal. A chelating agent may be used to soften the adjoining dentine, but should not be employed if the instrument is broken in a curved part of the canal, since under these circumstances each successive instrument tends to follow a straight path, leading eventually to root perforation. This technique is usually successful with a spiral root filler, since the construction of this instrument prevents it biting into the walls of the canal. If a broken instrument is in the coronal or middle part of the canal, it may be possible to work reamers and files past it and insert a satisfactory root filling to seal it from the periapical region (*Fig.* 253). A broken broach, provided it is not

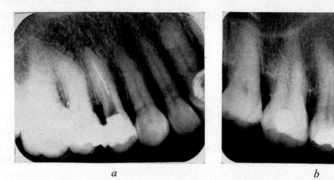

a   b

Fig. 253. 4|. *a*, Broken reamer in canal. Only one root canal could be found in this tooth; *b*, Broken instrument bypassed and root filling inserted.

tightly embedded, may sometimes be removed by engaging it upon a wisp of cotton wool wound round another barbed broach. A large reamer or file wedged in the apical part of a root is difficult to remove. If the coronal end of the instrument is visible it may be possible to widen the adjacent part of the canal with longshank burs, so obtaining sufficient room to insert a longshank excavator and prise out the broken fragment.

Special kits of instruments have been devised by Masserann (1971) and Dimashkieh (1975b) for the removal of root canal obstructions, including broken instruments. In both techniques a tubular end-cutting instrument is used to make a trench around the coronal end of the fragment, so enabling the insertion of a smaller tube to grip and remove it. In the Masserann kit, a special extractor is also provided. Each of these techniques entails drilling a hole 1 mm or larger in diameter to the coronal end of the fragment, and obtaining straight-line access to the latter. They are not readily applicable to slender or curved roots, therefore, especially in the molar region. In an anterior tooth, access through the incisal edge may be needed.

If a broken instrument has not been removed or bypassed within 20–30 minutes, the attempt should be abandoned. The study of Grossman (1968) shows that provided there is no evidence of periapical disease, the prognosis following retention of a broken instrument is still good. Where the periapical condition is normal and the broken fragment is in the apical part of the root, therefore, the remainder of the pulp cavity is filled and the patient informed of the accident. Such a tooth should be periodically checked following treatment. However, where periapical bone destruction is present, or if the fragment is in the coronal or middle part of the canal or projects into the periapical region, the tooth should be treated surgically. This form of treatment is also advisable where a complex restoration will be necessary coronally.

PLANNED REPLANTATION

Replantation is the replacement of a tooth in the socket it originally occupied with the object of obtaining reattachment of the periodontal membrane. The tooth

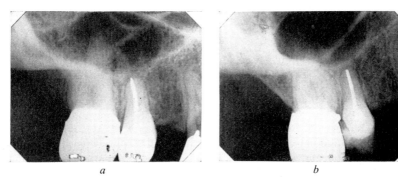

a   *b*

Fig. 254. 5|. *a*, Periapical lesion resulting from failure of previous root canal treatment; *b*, Appearance 1 year after extraction and replantation. Periapical surgery was not performed because of proximity of maxillary antrum. Following extraction the periapical lesion was curetted and the root filling trimmed flush with the apex. The restoration is in the process of being replaced.

may have been displaced from its socket by a blow or, on rare occasions, may have been deliberately extracted. When the tooth is deliberately extracted and replanted, the operation is known as 'planned', or 'intentional', replantation. The procedure is performed to facilitate root filling of a tooth which because of technical difficulties could not otherwise be treated, or the treatment of periapical disease associated with a root-filled tooth (*Fig.* 254).

The following account, although applicable in part to accidentally dislocated teeth also, is concerned only with planned replantation. A description of the replantation of accidentally dislocated teeth is given in Chapter 16.

1. Selection of teeth

Because replantation is commonly followed by root resorption, it is performed only under favourable circumstances and where no other form of treatment will give a reasonably favourable prognosis. Thus, it is normally confined to premolar and molar teeth.

The crown of the tooth must be strong enough to withstand extraction. If there is a large cavity present and a risk of breakage, the tooth should be restored with amalgam 24 hours or more before extraction. The anatomy of the roots must be such that extraction and replantation are possible without dividing the tooth. The tooth should not be involved by periodontal disease.

2. Technique

The available clinical and histological evidence indicates that for a favourable prognosis the periodontal membrane must be maintained in a vital state (Bielas et al., 1959; Löe and Waerhaug, 1961; Hamner et al., 1970), and the tooth must be replanted as quickly as possible after extraction (Flanagan and Myers, 1958). All equipment and materials needed for the operation must be ready to hand, therefore; with proper organization, it should be possible to replace the tooth in its socket within 20 minutes. The roots of the tooth must not be allowed to become dehydrated pending replantation, and the operation must be performed as aseptically as possible. The tooth is scaled and its root canals filled as completely as possible prior to extraction. An acrylic splint is made before the tooth is extracted.

After gaining anaesthesia, the tooth is extracted with as little trauma to the periodontal membrane as possible, following which the opening of the socket is covered with gauze. The tooth is wrapped in gauze soaked in sterile normal saline. It is gripped only by its crown. A slow-running disk is used to section the apical end of each root, which is kept moist with normal saline. This is done partly to facilitate replacement of the tooth in its socket, and partly to ensure that the apical end of each root canal is effectively sealed by filling material. Each root must therefore be sectioned through an adequately filled part of the canal. If, however, a canal has been filled for only a short distance, only the apical part of the root is removed; an undercut cavity is then prepared in the apical end of the remaining portion of the root and filled with amalgam. Neither irritant solutions, such as hydrogen peroxide and sodium hypochlorite, nor filling materials must be allowed to contact the sides of the roots. Periodontal membrane adhering to the roots should not be removed.

When the tooth is ready to be replaced, the blood clot formed after extraction is removed from the socket. Any periapical lesion is curetted, but not the side walls of the socket. Following replantation, the buccal and lingual walls of the socket are squeezed against the tooth and the occlusion checked to ensure the latter is completely seated. The splint is now cemented and left in position for 4–5 weeks. In this connection it should be pointed out that some workers, for example Hammer (1955), contend that splinting of a molar tooth is not necessary, whilst others merely apply a periodontal pack wedged into the interdental regions, or wire the tooth to its neighbour on either side and then apply a pack or acrylic resin to the wire. If this course of action is followed, the occlusal surface of the tooth should be ground out of occlusion before extraction. It is noteworthy that the study of Andreasen (1975) the frequency and extent of ankylosis following planned replantation were significantly less in teeth that were not splinted than in those that were, and further research may show the former approach to be better.

3. Postoperative observation and prognosis

Replanted teeth are re-examined clinically and radiographically 3 months, 6 months and 1 year after treatment, and subsequently at yearly intervals.

Kingsbury and Weisenbaugh (1971) report that of 149 replanted teeth, which were observed for up to 3 years, only 9 showed evidence of root resorption or needed to be extracted. However, most reports indicate that a relatively high proportion of intentionally replanted teeth undergo progressive root resorption or develop periapical disease, or both. Of 29 replanted teeth, Emmertsen (1956) assessed only 41 per cent as successful $3\frac{1}{2}$ years later. In a later study of 100 teeth observed for up to 13 years, Emmertsen and Andreasen (1966) state that only 34 per cent were successful. Deeb (1968) reported that of 117 intentionally replanted teeth, 33 per cent showed resorption after 2 years, whilst Grossman and Chacker (1968) found that of 61 teeth followed for up to 11 years, 57 per cent showed evidence of root resorption or periapical disease. In a large-scale study involving 943 posterior teeth, Bielas et al. (1959) report a success rate of 59 per cent after 5 years.

INTERRELATIONSHIP OF PULPAL AND PERIODONTAL DISEASE

In recent years there has developed a growing realization that pulpal disease can sometimes have an adverse effect on the periodontal state of a tooth. Conversely, evidence has been presented that periodontal disease may give rise to pathological changes in the pulp. These effects are mediated by way of accessory canals, in the form of lateral branches of the coronal part of the main root canal and, with multi-rooted teeth, canals running from the base of the pulp chamber to the region of the furcation.

1. Pulp cavity morphology in furcation region

Bender and Seltzer (1972) have shown in both humans and experimental animals that accessory canals opening in the region of the furcation are common, whilst Kramer (1960) reported that it was not unusual to find major blood vessels entering and leaving posterior teeth in this region. In a later report, Kramer (1968) stated that sometimes the main venous drainage from the pulp chamber emerges in the furcation region. Vertucci and Williams (1974) found that 23 per cent of mandibular first molars had a lateral canal opening into the furcation, whilst 13 per cent possessed a canal leading from the pulp chamber to this region.

Thus, although relatively seldom seen in the anterior part of the mouth, connecting pathways between the coronal part of the pulp cavity and the supporting periodontium are not uncommon in multi-rooted teeth. On occasions they may be filled during the course of root canal treatment (*Fig.* 255).

2. Effect of periodontal disease and procedures on the pulp

Although Mazur and Massler (1964) could find no correlation between pulpal pathology and periodontal state, other workers have shown that where periodontal pocketing has exposed accessory canals in the coronal part of the root or furcation, zones of pulpal inflammation and necrosis may result (Seltzer et al., 1963; Rubach and Mitchell, 1965; Langeland et al., 1974). Also, it is feasible that pulpal damage may occur if chemicals applied to desensitize cervical dentine penetrate such canals, or if blood vessels entering the latter are severed during periodontal procedures such as deep scaling and curettage. It has been demonstrated in experimental animals that stripping of the gingivae to the level of the alveolar crest leads to irritation of the associated part of the pulp (Stahl, 1963).

Seltzer (1971) points out that exposure of accessory canals to saliva has a twofold effect. First, the entry of toxins and perhaps micro-organisms into the pulp cavity becomes possible, with resultant inflammation of the pulp. Secondly, the blood supply to the pulp by way of these canals is eliminated, so reducing the nutritional supply to the pulp and leading to atrophic changes. The toxic products formed from the pulpal damage so created may diffuse back into the supporting structures, so perpetuating the periodontal lesion.

Where periodontal disease has advanced to the root apex (*see Fig.* 261), irritation of the pulp by way of the apical foramen may occur, leading to what is sometimes

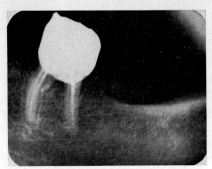

Fig. 255. ⌐6. Extrusion of filling material through a lateral canal in the distal aspect of the coronal part of the mesial root.

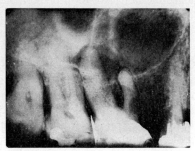

Fig. 256. 6⌐. Resorption of mesial aspect of mesiobuccal root, with pulpal exposure. Periodontal surgery had previously been performed.

called a 'retrograde' pulpitis. Although this may be followed by necrosis of the pulp, the latter may retain its vitality for a long time.

Occasionally, periodontal surgery is followed by a progressive resorption of the root and so leads indirectly to pulpal involvement (*Fig.* 256).

3. Effect of pulpal disease and root canal treatment on the periodontium

Just as toxins from an inflamed or necrotic pulp may pass through the apical foramen and lead to periapical bone destruction, so there is evidence that in both humans and experimental animals they may diffuse from the pulp cavity coronally into the supporting structures and give rise to periodontal inflammation (Winter and Kramer, 1965; Bender and Seltzer, 1972). Periodontitis and resorption of the alveolar crest have been demonstrated following pulp extirpation and root canal treatment (Seltzer et al., 1967), whilst the tendency for crestal bone destruction and periodontal pocket formation to occur following perforation of the pulp chamber floor or the coronal part of the root was discussed earlier in this Chapter.

Sometimes periapical irritation resulting from pulpal disease extends in a coronal direction, leading to a so-called 'retrograde' periodontitis, with the formation of a discharging sinus opening into the gingival crevice (*see Fig.* 23, Chapter 1). This may occur with both acute and chronic periapical lesions.

4. Differential diagnosis and treatment

Thus, although periodontal disease typically is of purely periodontal causation and periapical disease of solely pulpal origin, there are cases where this is not so. These cases may be divided into four categories.

a. Periodontal lesions entirely pulpal in origin
In these cases pulpal disease leads to irritation of the supporting periodontium by way of the apical foramen or accessory canals coronally, and a sinus running along the side of the root and discharging into the gingival sulcus is formed.

Vitality tests will indicate the pulp of the tooth to be largely or completely necrotic, and some cause for pulpal disease, such as a deep restoration or coronal fracture, will be apparent. Where the lesion has resulted from drainage of an acute periapical abscess, as opposed to an acute periodontal abscess, there will be a history of intense pain, usually with swelling in the buccal sulcus and extraorally.

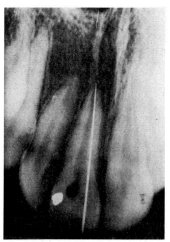

Fig. 257. 1|. A sinus leading from the periapical region to the gingival crevice following the drainage of an acute periapical abscess allowed the insertion of only a fine silver point.

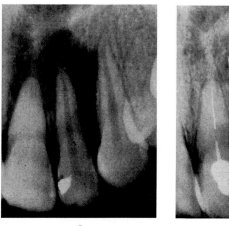
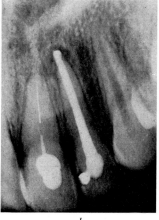

a   *b*

Fig. 258. |2. *a,* An extensive periapical lesion which was associated with drainage into the gingival crevice distally; *b,* Five months after root canal treatment, repair is virtually complete, despite the inaccurate root filling. An instrument has been broken in the root of |1.

10

Probing the sinus will fail to reveal calculus. The sinus is narrow and normally allows the introduction of only a fine silver point (*Fig.* 257). Elsewhere in the mouth and probably elsewhere around the involved tooth also, the periodontal condition is often satisfactory.

Root canal treatment of these teeth is usually followed by closure of the sinus and healing of the lesion (*Fig.* 258), and no periodontal treatment is called for.

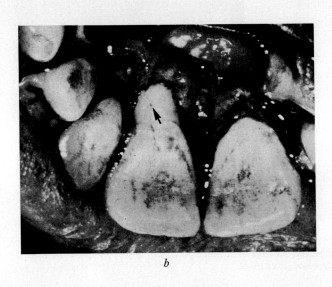

b

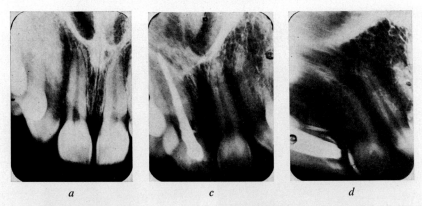

a   *c*   *d*

Fig. 259. 1|. *a*, No apparent cause existed for the acute pulpal pain associated with the tooth, although there was a periodontal pocket palatally; *b*, Surgical exposure revealed a small bleeding point (*arrowed*) on the palatal aspect of the root; *c*, After root filling, a radiograph taken with a slight mesial angulation to the X-ray tube suggests the presence of a lateral canal (*arrowed*); *d*, A different view using a pronounced mesial angulation to the X-ray tube, although leading to distortion of the image, shows the filled lateral canal (*arrowed*) on the palatal aspect of 1| and supports the diagnosis of pulpitis arising from exposure of a lateral canal by periodontal disease.

b. Periodontal lesions of pulpal origin, with secondary periodontal involvement

If the type of case just described remains untreated, plaque will tend to form on the root face along the sinus tract, with the apical migration of epithelium and the formation of a true periodontal pocket. As Bender and Seltzer (1972) point out, when this has occurred it is often possible to insert a large point, or even multiple points, into the pocket and along the length of the root. Probing the pocket will reveal calculus.

When this stage has been reached, both root canal treatment and periodontal treatment with curettage and planing of the root surface are indicated. The reports of Hiatt (1959, 1963) indicate that the prognosis following this treatment is good.

c. Pulpal lesions of periodontal origin, contributing to periodontal disease

Where periodontal treatment is followed by only partial resolution of a periodontal lesion and plaque control is satisfactory, exposure of accessory canals with

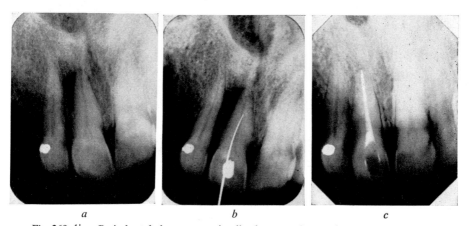

a	*b*	*c*

Fig. 260. 1|. *a,* Periodontal abscess opposite distal aspect of root, close to root apex;
b, Silver point inserted into sinus leading from abscess and opening into gingival crevice;
c, Six years after curettage of the bone lesion and the sinus. During curettage, the neurovascular bundle to 1| was severed, and the tooth was therefore root filled immediately. There has been no recurrence of the sinus.

resultant pulpal disease and continued irritation of the supporting periodontium may have occurred. Although the pulp may initially be vital, vitality tests will eventually indicate necrosis. Often there may be no evidence of a deep cavity or other cause of pulpal disease. Sometimes acute pulpal pain may develop (*Fig.* 259). If allowed to progress, periapical bone destruction may occur, at which stage it will not be possible to determine whether the periapical and periodontal lesions are interrelated or totally unrelated; eventually the lesions may become confluent.

In these cases root canal treatment must obviously be used to supplement periodontal treatment. Root canal treatment may also prove necessary where periodontal pocketing extends as far as the middle part of the root, even though initially the pulp may apparently still be vital and healthy, since periodontal treatment in such a case may subsequently lead to pulpal disease. Where splinting by means of a fixed appliance is planned for such teeth, the advisability of root canal treatment beforehand should be considered, since restorative procedures may cause further pulpal irritation.

d. Periapical disease of periodontal origin

Sometimes a periapical lesion is caused by direct extension of a periodontal pocket in an apical direction, with no obvious loss of crestal bone. The lesion may take the form of an acute periodontal abscess (*Fig.* 260) or it may be chronic in nature (*Fig.* 261). Unless there happens to be concomitant pulpal disease, the pulp may retain its vitality for a considerable time.

Root canal treatment of such cases will obviously be ineffective. If the tooth is to be retained the treatment is essentially periodontal, although root canal treatment

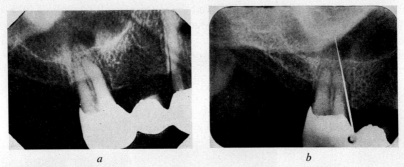

a   *b*

Fig. 261. 7]. *a*, A lesion situated periapically, with no obvious loss of crestal bone; *b*, The lesion was caused by a narrow periodontal pocket, demonstrated by the insertion of a silver point; the pulp of the tooth was vital.

is often necessary to facilitate radisectomy or hemisection of a multi-rooted tooth, or because periodontal treatment jeopardizes the vitality of the pulp.

It is important, therefore, to assess pulpal vitality where an isolated periodontal lesion occurs and the remaining teeth are largely free of periodontal disease, or where plaque control is satisfactory but there is incomplete resolution following periodontal treatment. Root canal treatment of multi-rooted teeth should include thorough obliteration of the coronal part of the root and the pulp chamber with sealing of the pulpal aspect of accessory canals to ensure that the adjoining periodontium is not subject to irritation from any residual necrotic material within the pulp cavity. Where a tooth is associated with pulpal pain or with a periapical lesion and there is no apparent cause for pulpal disease, the periodontal condition should be examined carefully to ensure that there is no periodontal causation.

ENDODONTIC ENDOSSEOUS IMPLANTS

Endodontic endosseous implants, also known as 'diodontic' implants or 'endodontic stabilizers', are used to stabilize loose teeth. Although previously employed by other workers, it was Orlay (1960, 1964) who popularized the use of these appliances, and Frank (1967) who developed a standardized technique for their use.

Endodontic stabilizers take the form of tapered rods of chrome–cobalt or titanium (*see Fig.* 263). They may have smooth or threaded sides, and may be polymer-coated (Hodosh et al., 1974). Stabilizers are available in sizes 40–140, matching the corresponding sizes of root canal instruments. Treatment consists of cementing a stabilizer into the root canal so as to extend beyond the root-end into periapical bone. By artificially lengthening the root in this way, the fulcrum for tooth movement is placed further apically, so reducing tooth mobility.

1. Periapical response to stabilizers

Histological studies on the periapical response to endodontic stabilizers have shown considerable differences in their findings. Frank and Abrams (1969), reporting on 2 implants, state that although the cementing agents used evoked an inflammatory response, the implants themselves were well tolerated with no evidence of inflammation. Scopp et al. (1971), using experimental animals, also noted a favourable response after the use of implants in intact teeth with vital pulps, but chronic inflammatory changes following their use in teeth originally associated with periapical lesions. The latter finding, however, may have been associated with the method of root treatment, since the implants were evidently inserted immediately after root canal preparation, with presumably no form of antiseptic medication to the pulp cavity. Langeland et al. (1971) report a severe inflammatory response to an implant, whilst Seltzer et al. (1973) found evidence of corrosion and an accompanying inflammation following the insertion of 8 Vitallium implants in a dog. Seltzer et al. (1976) also report an inflammatory response to titanium implants, which they consider was probably due to corrosion.

Histological reports on the tissue response to intraosseous implantation of lengths of chrome–cobalt alloy have also differed in their findings. Although Bernier and Canby (1943) stated that such alloys were well tolerated, Neuman et al. (1975) found evidence of chronic inflammation.

In view of these conflicting reports, the use of endodontic stabilizers, although common and apparently successful clinically, must still be regarded as experimental.

2. Indications and contraindications

The use of an endodontic stabilizer may be considered where there is undue tooth mobility due to loss of periodontal attachment from root fracture, apical root resorption, or previous apical surgery, or where the elimination by apical surgery of a perforation in the coronal or middle part of the root would lead to undue mobility. Endodontic stabilizers are also commonly advocated as a means of stabilizing a tooth with advanced bone loss from periodontal disease. However, the fact that a fairly wide opening has to be made through the root apex to accommodate the stabilizer leads to irritation of the tissues in the vicinity of the apex and may detract from the prognosis in these cases. The creation of such an opening not only inflicts trauma on the apical periodontium, but also makes the extrusion of cement into the periapical tissues more likely and may result in an inadequate apical seal; thus, further bone loss is possible. If bone destruction from periodontal disease extends to the close vicinity of the apex, therefore, the use of an endodontic stabilizer would seem dubious. Needless to say, if such an appliance is used to stabilize a periodontally diseased tooth, effective periodontal treatment must also be performed.

An endodontic stabilizer is contraindicated where impingement on a major anatomical structure, such as the maxillary antrum or the inferior dental nerve, is likely, or where the buccolingual alignment of the tooth and configuration of the cortical plate are such that the stabilizer would project into soft tissues. In view of the experimental nature of stabilizers, they should not be used in patients with a history of endocardial damage.

3. Technique

To ensure satisfactory retention within the root, the stabilizer should make close contact with the walls of the prepared canal for as great a distance as possible. Preparation is performed entirely with reamers, therefore, so that the prepared canal will be as near circular in cross-section as possible. Anterior teeth should wherever possible be enlarged to at least no. 70. Because of the rigidity of the stabilizer and the degree of root canal widening often necessary, access to the pulp cavity of an anterior tooth has to be through the incisal edge, or close to it.

To avoid unnecessary pressure and irritation and to ensure that it is completely seated within the prepared canal, the apical end of the stabilizer should not press against bone. Following insertion, sufficient room should be left in the coronal part of the root to allow post crown construction should this be necessary later, but at least 5–6 mm of the stabilizer should extend into the root. Where it is not possible to meet the former requirement because of the need to remove the apical part of the root, the stabilizer should extend into the pulp chamber; if crown construction is necessary later, the coronal end of the stabilizer may be serrated and used to assist in retaining a pinned amalgam or composite core.

The stabilizer is used to root-fill the tooth in the same way that a sectional silver filling is performed (Chapter 8). A deep groove is cut around the periphery of the rod at an appropriate level so that, following cementation, the coronal end of the rod may be rotated and removed, leaving the apical part within the tooth.

Depending on the particular indication for its use, the removal of tissue to accommodate the periapical part of the stabilizer may be performed either by a surgical approach or by way of the root canal. Stabilizers may also be used to join two parts of a fractured root and so eliminate tooth mobility. Whichever method is employed, effective sealing of the root canal is essential for success. Where there is still obvious mobility of the tooth immediately following treatment, temporary splinting is indicated.

a. Technique with periapical surgery

This technique is used where surgical removal of the apical part of the root is necessary because of root fracture or perforation, or where an existing root filling can only be removed by a surgical approach (*see Fig.* 262). In such cases the insertion of a stabilizer to the vicinity of the original root apex effectively eliminates tooth mobility and the removal of additional periapical bone is unnecessary.

The root canal is first prepared to a level just short of the root apex. Periapical surgery is then performed and the apical part of the root removed. Where preparation of the entire length of the root canal was not possible prior to surgery, due to misalignment of the apical part of a fractured root or the presence of an existing root filling, preparation is now completed with the introduction of reamers beyond the root face roughly to the original level of the root apex; this ensures that the stabilizer fits closely against the walls of the prepared canal.

The appropriate stabilizer is tried in the tooth and its fit and apical extension checked. Cement is applied to the walls of the prepared canal and to the coronal part of the stabilizer, and the latter seated firmly in position. A fast-setting cement is used to facilitate the removal of surplus material from the bony cavity and the projecting rod. After excess cement has been removed, the wound is closed with sutures.

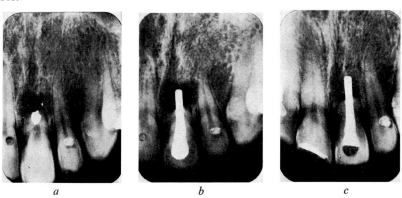

Fig. 262. ⌊1. *a*, Undue shortening of the root from previous periapical surgery had led to pronounced mobility; *b*, After periapical surgery to allow the removal of the existing apical amalgam filling, and the insertion of an endodontic stabilizer; *c*, One year later, periapical repair is in progress.

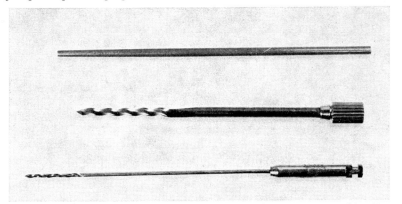

Fig. 263. *Above*, Tapered chrome-cobalt endodontic stabilizer. *Centre*, matching 40 mm hand reamer. *Below*, Engine-driven drill used for apex penetration.

b. Technique without periapical surgery

This technique is used where tooth mobility is the result of periodontal disease. Periapical bone is removed by way of the root canal, using hand reamers 40 mm in length (*Fig.* 263).

Normally the pulp will be vital and both root canal treatment and the insertion of the stabilizer may be performed at the same visit. With an infected or necrotic pulp, root canal preparation and antiseptic medication are first necessary, and perforation of the root apex and insertion of the stabilizer are performed at a subsequent visit. Because of the large size of instruments used for final widening of the root canal, the prepared canal will be straight. Where there is an obvious curvature of the canal, therefore, the latter should first be prepared in a conventional manner and a gutta percha filling inserted prior to further root canal enlargement and perforation of the apex. The removal of periapical bone will necessitate local anaesthesia lingually as well as buccally.

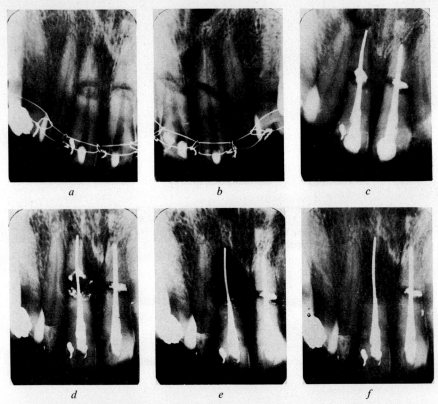

Fig. 264. 1|1. *a* and *b*, Middle-third root fractures; *c*, After root canal filling with endodontic stabilizers and cement; the use of a wider rod in 1| was not possible because the root fragments were slightly out of line; *d*, Nine months later there is obvious bone loss around the fracture site of 1|; *e*, After periapical surgery, with splitting and removal of the apex of 1|, so converting the stabilizing rod into an implant; *f*, Nine months after periapical surgery there is virtually complete periapical repair around 1|. The |1 was still satisfactory both clinically and radiographically. Neither 1| nor |1 showed undue mobility.

The initial preparation of the root canal should extend to the radiographic apex rather than to the normal level of the apical limit, otherwise penetration of the root apex later may prove difficult. Only when the root canal is clean is the apex penetrated. This is done with a reamer two or three sizes smaller than the largest instrument used to prepare the canal. If difficulty is encountered an engine-driven drill may be employed (*Fig.* 263); to avoid breakage, this should be used at a slow speed and should be a loose fit within the canal. Reamers are now used to cut a channel extending about 10 mm into periapical bone. This channel is widened with progressively larger instruments until the root canal preparation and the periapical 'preparation' form a continuous taper, with simultaneous cutting of dentine and bone. To ensure that the cortical plate has not been penetrated, the mucosa overlying the root apex is palpated whilst a reamer is rotated within the periapical preparation.

After the appropriate size of stabilizer has been tried in the tooth, the canal is irrigated; since the irrigating solution may enter periapical tissues, sterile water or saline should be used for this purpose. The root canal is dried and haemorrhage arrested by the insertion of absorbent points of appropriate width to the level of the root apex.

To ensure that complete seating of the stabilizer is not impeded by contact with bone at the end of the periapical preparation, the apical end of the rod is reduced in length by 1 mm. As a check on the depth of insertion, a mark corresponding to the combined working length of the root canal and periapical preparations may be made at the coronal end of the rod. The coronal part of the rod and the walls of the canal are now coated with cement and the stabilizer seated firmly in place. Since the prepared root canal has an open end apically, extrusion of a certain amount of cement into the adjoining tissues is inevitable.

c. Alternative technique for fractured roots
Instead of removing the apical part of a fractured root prior to the insertion of an endodontic implant, the latter may be used to join the apical and coronal parts of the root together, so stabilizing the tooth (*Fig.* 264). It is obviously essential that the two parts of the root are in line, or nearly so, and extrusion of some cement at the line of fracture has to be accepted. Since the stabilizer does not extend into the periapical region, it does not constitute an implant. A conventional sequence of root canal treatment is followed.

Although the potential dead space left at the line of fracture constitutes a disadvantage of this technique, treatment is often successful. Where failure does occur, it is still possible to remove the apical part of the root by splitting it in a vertical direction, so leaving the rod projecting into the periapical tissues and converting it into an implant (*Fig.* 264).

4. Postoperative observation and prognosis

In view of the experimental nature of this form of treatment, postoperative observation is especially important.

Andreasen (1968) states that of 12 teeth in which implants were used following removal of the fractured apical part of the root, 8 were successful 1–3½ years later. Hodosh et al. (1974) report that 10 out of 12 implants were successful for periods ranging up to 3 years.

PATIENTS WITH ENDOCARDIAL DAMAGE

Many dental procedures may cause a bacteraemia and so could conceivably lead to a bacterial endocarditis in patients with existing endocardial damage. Opinion differs as to whether extraction or root canal treatment of a tooth with pulpal disease is preferable in such patients, or indeed whether any natural teeth at all should be retained.

There seems no doubt that root canal instrumentation can on occasions cause a bacteraemia. Thus, Kennedy et al. (1957) were able to produce bacteraemias in experimental animals by deliberately inserting instruments beyond the apical foramen and then sealing known organisms within the root canals of the treated teeth. Bender et al. (1960) also demonstrated bacteraemias by instrumentation beyond the apical foramen, but found that no such bacteraemia resulted when instrumentation was confined to the root canal. Even when instruments were thrust beyond the apical foramen, Bender et al. (1963) found that the likelihood of a bacteraemia was far less than with deep scaling, gingivectomy or extraction of a tooth. The recent investigation of Baumgartner et al. (1976) indicates that provided treatment is carried out with proper regard to asepsis, the risk of a bacteraemia is small; of 20 teeth yielding positive cultures from their pulp chambers, in only one instance was root canal treatment associated with a bacteraemia, and this followed instrumentation beyond the apical foramen. The study of Beechen et al. (1956) indicates that there is little or no risk of a bacteraemia following pulpotomy.

From the viewpoint of the risk of a bacteraemia during treatment, therefore, root canal treatment would seem preferable to extraction. However, in the type of case under discussion it is especially important that the general condition of the mouth be considered. If there is widespread periodontal disease or caries, it is unlikely that the patient will maintain a healthy oral condition following treatment, and in such cases a clearance, although imposing a greater immediate risk, is in the long term in the patient's best interests. Conversely, in a well-cared-for mouth, provided that effective treatment is possible and an accurate result can be obtained, root canal treatment is preferable to extraction. There is a strong case in these patients not only for a thorough clinical examination but also for full mouth radiographs and vitality tests of all suspect teeth.

Antibiotic cover is essential during root canal treatment in patients with existing endocardial damage, such as those with a history of rheumatic or congenital heart disease, valvular disease from other causes, or those who have had cardiac surgery. The position with a patient who has had rheumatic fever but in whom there is no known cardiac complication is uncertain, but in view of the possibility of undiagnosed endocardial damage antibiotic cover would seem desirable. Treatment should be so planned that root canal filling of the tooth is completed within the minimum period of time compatible with obtaining a successful result, so that only one course of antibiotic treatment spanning a 3- to 5-day period is needed.

The antibiotic of choice is penicillin. The American Heart Association (1972) recommends the intramuscular administration of 600 000 units of procaine penicillin plus 200 000 units of crystalline penicillin 1 hour preoperatively and once daily thereafter. Where intramuscular injection is impracticable and oral administration is necessary, 500 mg of phenoxymethyl penicillin (penicillin V) is taken 1 hour before treatment, followed by 250 mg four times daily. For patients who are being maintained on continuous oral penicillin or who are sensitive to this drug, oral erythromycin is used. For adults, 500 mg are given $1\frac{1}{2}$–2 hours preoperatively, followed by 250 mg four times daily.

Although the recommendations of the American Heart Association are widely followed, it should be pointed out that experimental work by Pelletier et al. (1975) suggests that a combination of penicillin and streptomycin is preferable to penicillin alone, and that much larger doses are necessary if oral penicillin is to be relied upon. The same study indicates that erythromycin may be less effective than was previously thought in the prophylaxis of bacterial endocarditis, and that cephazolin (Acephalosporin) is preferable as an alternative to penicillin. However, it should be noted that whilst the cephalosporins are usually without side-effects in patients sensitive to penicillins, there is evidence that cross-sensitivity of the two groups of drugs can occur.

Treatment must be performed aseptically; care should be taken during application of the rubber dam not to inflict trauma on the periodontal tissues. If the pulp is vital, the region of the exposure should be cauterized with a hot instrument. Particular care should be taken in assessing the working length. Whether the pulp is vital or necrotic, instruments must be confined to the root canal. It is highly desirable that treatment be controlled by bacteriological sampling. Following treatment the periapical state should be checked both clinically and radiographically at regular intervals, and the patient should be asked to report any untoward symptoms.

In view of the limitations inherent in pulpal diagnosis, pulp capping would seem contraindicated in patients with endocardial damage. This applies especially to capping agents containing corticosteroids, application of which may well be followed by a symptomless necrosis of the pulp. Steroid capping agents which do not incorporate an antiseptic or antibiotic agent are definitely contraindicated, since there is evidence that their application to exposed contaminated pulps may be followed by a bacteraemia (Klotz et al., 1965).

REFERENCES

American Heart Association (1972) Prevention of bacterial endocarditis. *J. Am. Dent. Assoc.* **85**, 1377.

Andreasen J. O. (1968) Treatment of intra-alveolar root fractures by cobalt-chromium implants. *Br. J. Oral Surg.* **6**, 141.

Andreasen J. O. (1975) The effect of splinting upon periodontal healing after replantation of permanent incisors in monkeys. *Acta Odontol. Scand.* **33**, 313.

Baumgartner J. C., Heggers J. P. and Harrison J. W. (1976) The incidence of bacteremias related to endodontic procedures. I, Nonsurgical endodontics. *J. Endodontol.* **2**, 135.

Beechen I. I., Laston D. J. and Garbarino V. E. (1956) Transitory bacteraemia as related to the operation of vital pulpotomy. *Oral Surg.* **9**, 902.

Bender I. B. and Seltzer S. (1972) The effect of periodontal disease on the pulp. *Oral Surg.* **33**, 458.

Bender I. B., Seltzer S., Tashman S. and Meloff G. (1963) Dental procedures in patients with rheumatic heart disease. *Oral Surg.* **16**, 466.

Bender I. B., Seltzer S. and Yermish M. (1960) The incidence of bacteraemia in endodontic manipulation. Preliminary report. *Oral Surg.* **13**, 353.

Bernier J. L. and Canby C. P. (1943) Histologic studies on the reaction of alveolar bone to vitallium implants (a preliminary report). *J. Am. Dent. Assoc.* **30**, 188.

Bielas I., Fuchs M., Horbal B. and Pankiewicz Z. (1959) Die Bewertung der Replantation der Zahne auf Grund von 1030 Experimentellen Versuchseingriffen. *Schweiz. Monatsschr. Zahnheild.* **69**, 497.

Deeb E. (1968) Intentional replantation of endodontically treated teeth. In: Grossman L. I. (ed.), *Transactions of the 4th International Conference on Endodontics.* Philadelphia, University of Pennsylvania, pp. 147–57.

Dimashkieh M. R. (1975a) A method of using silver amalgam in routine endodontics, and its use in open apices. *Br. Dent. J.* **138**, 298.

Dimashkieh M. R. (1975b) The management of obstructed root canals: the hollow tube technique. *Br. Dent. J.* **138**, 459.

Emmertsen E. (1956) Replantation of extracted molars. *Oral Surg.* **9**, 115.

Emmertsen E. and Andreasen J. O. (1966) Replantation of extracted molars: a radiographic and histological study. *Acta Odontol. Scand.* **24**, 327.

Flanagan V. D. and Myers H. I. (1958) Delayed reimplantation of second molars in the Syrian hamster. *Oral Surg.* **11**, 1179.

Frank A. L. (1967) Improvement of the crown-root ratio by endodontic endosseous implants. *J. Am. Dent. Assoc.* **74**, 451.

Frank A. L. and Abrams A. M. (1969) Histologic evaluation of endodontic implants. *J. Am. Dent. Assoc.* **78**, 520.

Frank A. L. and Weine F. S. (1973) Non-surgical therapy for the perforative defect of internal resorption. *J. Am. Dent. Assoc.* **87**, 863.

Grossman L. I. (1968) Fate of endodontically treated teeth with fractured root canal instruments. *J. Br. Endodontic Soc.* **2**, 35.

Grossman L. I. (1969) Guidelines for the prevention of fracture of root canal instruments. *Oral Surg.* **28**, 746.

Grossman L. I. and Chacker F. M. (1968) Clinical evaluation and histologic study of intentionally replanted teeth. In: Grossman L. I. (ed.), *Transactions of the 4th International Conference on Endodontics*. Philadelphia, University of Pennsylvania, pp. 127–44.

Hammer H. (1955) Replantation and implantation of teeth. *Int. Dent. J., Lond.* **5**, 439.

Hamner J. E., Reed O. M. and Stanley H. R. (1970) Reimplantation of teeth in the baboon. *J. Am. Dent. Assoc.* **81**, 662.

Harris W. E. (1976) A simplified method of treatment for endodontic perforations. *J. Endodontol.* **2**. 126.

Heithersay G. S. (1975) Calcium hydroxide in the treatment of pulpless teeth with associated pathology. *J. Br. Endodontic Soc.* **8**, 74.

Hiatt W. H. (1959) Regeneration of the periodontium after endodontic therapy and flap operation. *Oral Surg.* **12**, 1471.

Hiatt W. H. (1963) Periodontal pocket elimination by combined endodontic-periodontic therapy. *Periodontics* **1**, 152.

Hodosh M., Shklar G. and Povar M. (1974) Polymer-coated metal endodontic stabilizers. *Oral Surg.* **38**, 804.

Kennedy D. R., Hamilton T. R. and Syverton J. T. (1957) Effects on monkeys of introduction of hemolytic streptococci into root canals. *J. Dent. Res.* **36**, 496.

Kingsbury B. C. and Wiesenbaugh J. M. (1971) Intentional replantation of mandibular premolars and molars. *J. Am. Dent. Assoc.* **83**, 1053.

Klotz M. D., Gerstein H. and Bahn A. N. (1965) Bacteremia after topical use of prednisolone in infected pulps. *J. Am. Dent. Assoc.* **71**, 871.

Kramer I. R. H. (1960) The vascular architecture of the human dental pulp. *Arch. Oral Biol.* **2**, 177.

Kramer I. R. H. (1968) The distribution of blood vessels in the human dental pulp. In: Finn S. B. (ed.), *Biology of the Dental Pulp Organ: A Symposium*. Alabama, University of Alabama Press, pp. 369–77.

Langeland K., Dowden W. E., Tronstad L. and Langeland L. K. (1971) Human pulp changes of iatrogenic origin. *Oral Surg.* **32**, 943.

Langeland K., Rodrigues H. and Dowden W. (1974) Periodontal disease, bacteria, and pulpal histopathology. *Oral Surg.* **37**, 257.

Lantz B. and Persson P-A. (1965) Experimental root perforation in dogs' teeth: a roentgen study. *Odontol. Revy.* **16**, 238.

Lantz B. and Persson P-A. (1967) Periodontal tissue reactions after root perforations in dogs' teeth: a histologic study. *Odontol. Tidskr.* **75**, 209.

Lantz B. and Persson P-A. (1970) Periodontal tissue reactions after surgical treatment of root perforations in dogs' teeth: a histologic study. *Odontol. Revy* **21**, 51.

Löe H. and Waerhaug J. (1961) Experimental replantation of teeth in dogs and monkeys. *Arch. Oral Biol.* **3**, 176.

Masserann J. (1971) Entfernen Metallischer Fragmente aus Wurzelkanalen. *J. Br. Endodontic. Soc.* **5**, 55. (Translation).

Mazur B. and Massler M. (1964) Influence of periodontal disease on the dental pulp. *Oral Surg.* **17**, 592.

Neuman G., Spangberg L. and Langeland K. (1975) Methodology and criteria in the evaluation of dental implants. *J. Endodontol.* **1**, 193.

Nicholls E. (1962) Treatment of traumatic perforations of the pulp cavity. *Oral Surg.* **15**, 603.

Orlay H. G. (1960) Endodontic splinting treatment in periodontal disease. *Br. Dent. J.* **108**, 118.

Orlay H. G. (1964) Splinting with endodontic implant stabilizers. *Dent. Practnr Dent. Rec.* **14**, 481.

Pelletier L. L., Durack D. T. and Petersdorf R. G. (1975) Chemotherapy of experimental streptococcal endocarditis. IV, Further observations on prophylaxis. *J. Clin. Invest.* **56**, 319.

Rubach W. C. and Mitchell D. F. (1965) Periodontal disease, accessory canals and pulp pathosis. *J. Periodontol.* **36**, 34.

Scopp I. W., Dictrow R. L., Lichtenstein B. and Blechman H. (1971) Cellular response to endodontic endosseous implants. *J. Periodontol.* **42**, 717.

Seltzer S. (1971) *Endodontology: Biologic Considerations in Endodontic Procedures.* New York, McGraw-Hill, pp. 419–21.

Seltzer S., Bender I. B., Nazimov H. and Sinai I. (1967) Pulpitis-induced interradicular periodontal changes in experimental animals. *J. Periodontol.* **38**, 124.

Seltzer S., Bender I. B. and Ziontz M. (1963) The interrelationship of pulp and periodontal disease. *Oral Surg.* **16**, 1474.

Seltzer S., Green D. B., De La Guardia R., Maggio J. and Barnett A. (1973) Vitallium endodontic implants: a scanning electron microscope, electron microprobe, and histologic study. *Oral Surg.* **35**, 828.

Seltzer S., Maggio J., Wollard R. and Green D. (1976) Titanium endodontic implants: a scanning electron microscope, electron microprobe, and histologic investigation. *J. Endodontol.* **2**, 267.

Seltzer S., Sinai I. and August D. (1970) Periodontal effects of root perforations before and during endodontic procedures. *J. Dent. Res.* **49**, 332.

Stahl S. S. (1963) Pulpal response to gingival injury in adult rats. *Oral Surg.* **16**, 1116.

Stromberg T., Hasselgren G. and Bergstedt H. (1972) Endodontic treatment of traumatic root perforations in man. *Sven. Tandlak. Tidskr.* **65**, 457.

Vertucci F. J. and Williams R. G. (1974) Furcation canals in the human mandibular first molar. *Oral Surg.* **38**, 308.

Winter G. B. and Kramer I. R. H. (1965) Changes in periodontal membrane and bone following experimental pulpal injury in deciduous molar teeth in kittens. *Arch. Oral Biol.* **10**, 279.

FURTHER READING

Myall R. W. T. and Gregory H. S. (1969) Current trends in the prevention of bacterial endocarditis in susceptible patients receiving dental care. *Oral Surg.* **28**, 813.

Seltzer S. (1971) *Endodontology: Biologic Considerations in Endodontic Procedures.* New York, McGraw-Hill, pp. 440–70.

Simon J. H. S., Glick D. H. and Frank A. L. (1972) The relationship of endodontic-periodontic lesions. *J. Periodontol.* **43**, 202.

Chapter 15

Other methods of endodontic treatment

RESORBABLE ROOT-FILLING MATERIALS

Although most root-filling materials may be resorbed if forced into the periapical region, the expression 'resorbable root-filling material' is generally used to denote a paste which does not set after being introduced into the root canal and which is rapidly removed if forced into the periapical region; paste may also be removed from within the root canal. By contrast, the disappearance from the periapical region of a so-called 'non-resorbable' root-filling material is a slow process (*Fig.* 265) and does not normally continue into the root canal. Conventional root-filling materials are of the non-resorbable type and, when in the form of cements, set after insertion into the canal.

Resorbable pastes are of two kinds, namely those consisting largely of iodoform, and those formed mainly of calcium hydroxide.

1. Iodoform pastes

Iodoform, alone or in combination with other substances, has been used as a root-filling material for a considerable time, as shown by the publication of Röse (1894).

Walkhoff's method of root canal treatment

The best-known resorbable iodoform paste, at least in Europe, is that devised by Walkhoff (1928).

Walkhoff's root-filling paste consists of 60 parts of iodoform and 40 parts of a solution containing 45 per cent parachlorphenol, 49 per cent camphor and 6 per cent menthol (Castagnola and Orlay, 1956). An equivalent commercial preparation is known as 'Kri' paste. In the Walkhoff method of treatment, as described by Castagnola and Orlay (1952, 1956), the parachlorphenol-camphor-menthol solution is used for antiseptic medication of the canal prior to filling. When treating a tooth with a vital pulp, the canal is prepared and filled with iodoform paste as far as the apical foramen. When the pulp is necrotic, the apical foramen is intentionally widened during preparation and paste is deliberately driven with a spiral root filler into the periapical region during filling. This is done whatever the state of the periapex. If a sinus is present, paste is propelled beyond the canal until it exudes through the opening of the sinus. Where there is no sinus present and it is thought that the excess filling will cause pain, a bur is used to make an opening in the buccal cortical plate over the root apex. With very large periapical lesions the paste may be used not only to root fill the tooth but also as the antiseptic dressing beforehand. It is unnecessary to insert a gutta percha or silver point as part of the root filling; if one is used, it should not reach the apex.

Assessment of iodoform paste fillings

Various advantages are claimed for the use of Walkhoff's paste and other iodoform pastes by the technique described. One is that it is unnecessary to estimate the level of the apical foramen, so saving time and eliminating one of the difficult

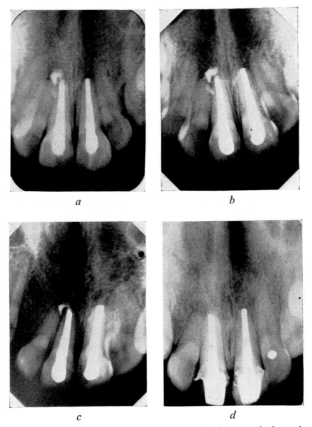

Fig. 265. 1|. *a*, Excess cement at time of root filling; *b*, Twelve months later the excess is disappearing; *c*, Two and a half years later the excess has almost disappeared; *d*, Seven and a half years later the excess has completely disappeared.

stages of treatment. However, most workers would contend that this estimation presents little difficulty, and that treatment may be so arranged that little time need be spent in making it. In any event, if iodoform paste is used by the technique described, such an estimation would seem essential for filling a canal to the apical foramen, or for widening the foramen without also inflicting severe and unnecessary trauma on the periapical tissues.

Although the rapid removal of filling material inadvertently forced into the periapex is no doubt an advantage, it is doubtful if the deliberate introduction of excess material is beneficial from either the bacteriological or histological stand-point. If the periapex is normal before filling, it would certainly seem pointless deliberately to drive a material into it merely to have that material resorbed. Also, quite apart from periapical irritation and pain due to the pressure exerted by the paste, some degree of chemical irritation would seem inevitable. This is also true if a periapical lesion is present, and in such a case it is doubtful if the antiseptic effect

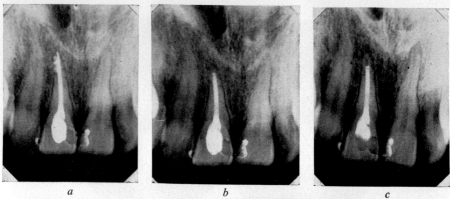

| *a* | *b* | *c* |

Fig. 266. 1]. *a*, At time of root filling. Resorbable paste has been extruded into the periapical region; *b*, Eight days later the paste has disappeared from the periapical region and the extreme apical part of the canal; *c*, One month later, further paste has disappeared from the apical part of the canal.

of an iodoform paste on the lesion constitutes any real advantage, since Hedman (1951) has shown that the periapical region is without evidence of infection follow-ing adequate treatment of the root canal. Although some workers contend that iodoform paste stimulates the periapical tissues and may even accelerate bone regeneration, there seems no evidence to support their view. Indeed, Bell (1969) concluded that Kri paste actually retarded connective tissue and new bone forma-tion, and that successful treatment occurred in spite of, rather than because of, the use of Kri paste.

Friend and Browne (1968) concluded that the initial tissue response to Kri paste was marked inflammation and necrosis followed by fibrous tissue formation. Although Castagnola (1950) believes that removal of paste occurs only by the action of tissue cells, Barker and Lockett (1971) concluded from animal experiments that it was due to a combination of leaching, phagocytosis and direct drainage to the associated lymph nodes.

Paste may disappear not only from the periapical region but also from the root canal itself (*Fig.* 266), with the ingrowth of tissue into the latter (Honegger, 1932; Engel, 1950; Erausquin and Muruzabal, 1969; Barker and Lockett, 1971). Occasionally this process may take place for the entire length of the canal. However, both Honegger (1932) and Erausquin and Muruzabal (1969) found that disappearance of paste from the canal was not synonymous with a successful result, since the tissue which invaded the canal was sometimes inflamed. Also, Barker and Lockett (1971) noted that the tissue ingrowth was limited in extent and did not always reach the level of the residual paste. Thus, a space devoid of both root-filling material and vital tissue may result. Apart from the report of Hyakusoku (1959), there seems no evidence that deposition of cementum in the apical part of the canal is more likely after filling with iodoform paste than with other materials.

Data on the prognosis following root filling with iodoform paste are difficult to evaluate, since factors related to the techniques used as well as the filling material itself may affect the prognosis. The best known clinical study is that of Castagnola (1950), who quoted success rates of 73–80 per cent, according to the type of case.

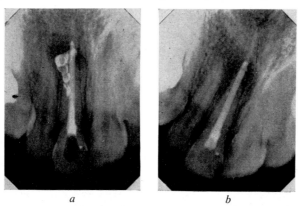

a   *b*

Fig. 267. 1|. *a*, Immediately after root filling. Resorbable paste has been driven into the periapical region. The root canal has been cleared of paste and filled with gutta percha and cement; *b*, Two months later the excess paste has disappeared from the periapical region.

Whilst these results are not so impressive as those of studies in which non-resorbable fillings were used, it should be pointed out that they were based on students' work.

A distinct disadvantage of iodoform pastes is the hazard of periapical irritation during construction of a post crown should the apical part of the canal no longer contain filling material. The insertion of a gutta percha point during root filling does not eliminate this hazard, since there is nothing other than friction against the paste to prevent movement of the point. Also, gutta percha is to some degree soluble in the chlorphenol component of the paste.

It is to avoid this hazard, but at the same time to exploit any beneficial action the paste may have on a periapical lesion, that some workers have advocated that the canal be cleared of paste and filled with a non-resorbable material after paste has been forced periapically (*Fig.* 267). Another technique described by Laws (1959) is to fill the apical one-quarter of the canal with a section of gutta percha and paste, and the remainder of the canal with non-resorbable materials. However, the presence of a gutta percha point apically does not necessarily prevent loss of the adjoining paste (*Fig.* 268). If an iodoform paste is used for root filling, excess material should be eliminated from the pulp chamber and the coronal part of the root canal, otherwise the crown of the tooth may discolour. The introduction of iodoform into a root canal may lead to a rise in the blood level of iodine (Goransson, 1957); iodoform pastes should therefore not be used in patients sensitive to iodine.

2. Calcium hydroxide pastes

Pastes of calcium hydroxide have also been used as resorbable root-filling materials, but would seem to suffer from many of the disadvantages of iodoform pastes.

However, such pastes are undoubtedly useful when used as temporary root 'fillings' in incompletely formed pulpless teeth (Chapter 13) and in teeth with root perforations (Chapter 14).

3. Iodoform paste fillings versus conventional root fillings

As Juge (1959) points out, filling materials that are non-resorbable and effectively seal the root canal retard healing if extruded into the periapical region, whilst

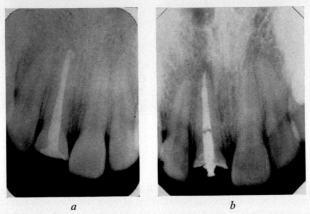

a   *b*

Fig. 268. 1|. *a*, Appearance at time of root filling. The radiograph was supplied by the dentist who referred the patient; *b*, Disappearance of paste from the apical part of the canal with the development of a periapical lesion which gave symptoms. The interval of time since root filling was not known.

materials that are rapidly removed from this region and leave it free to repair fail to give a durable seal. Since the extrusion of significant amounts of filling material into the periapical region is easily avoided in the vast majority of cases, most authorities agree that non-resorbable materials should be used for root filling.

BIOCALEX

Bernard (1952) claimed that following the introduction of a paste of calcium oxide and alcohol into the pulp cavity, the calcium oxide reacted with water in the root canal to form calcium hydroxide. A resultant expansion of more than 250 per cent occurred, so leading to penetration of paste into accessory canals.

Hendra (1970), quoting the work of Bernard (1967), states that since the absorption of water and expansion occur simultaneously, there is no danger of pressure developing and forcing necrotic pulpal tissue into the periapical region. Also, following the formation of calcium hydroxide, it is claimed that the latter reacts with carbon dioxide formed from pulpal decomposition to produce calcium carbonate and water. This leads to a 'chemical incineration' of micro-organisms and to the complete sealing of dentinal tubules and accessory canals, whilst the water that is formed reacts with further calcium oxide. It is stated that the reaction ceases when vital tissue is reached and that periapical bone regeneration can occur within 5–6 weeks.

This method of treatment is known as the 'Biocalex' technique and is recommended mainly for the treatment of teeth with necrotic pulps. It is not necessary to prepare more than the coronal two-thirds of the canal, which is then moistened with distilled water. A paste of Biocalex liquid and powder is inserted into the canal and the pulp cavity sealed. The root canal is subsequently redressed with paste as necessary, prior to the insertion of a conventional root filling.

There is a paucity of independent reports on the efficacy of this method of treatment. Frajlich and Goldberg (1975) assessed the effects of Biocalex paste on extracted teeth and concluded that sealing of neither the accessory canals nor the main root canal occurred. Furthermore, extraction and histological examination of 6 teeth which had been treated with Biocalex paste failed to substantiate the claims made for the technique.

Any beneficial effect associated with the Biocalex technique may be due at least in part to the antibacterial effect of calcium hydroxide, and a comparison of the results of treatment with Biocalex and calcium hydroxide could well prove instructive. Frajlich and Goldberg (1975) found that Biocalex liquid contained approximately 17 per cent water, and concluded that prior to insertion into the canal a considerable proportion of the mixed paste consisted of calcium hydroxide.

PULP MUMMIFICATION

Pulp mummification, also known as 'mortal amputation' and 'non-vital pulpotomy', consists of removing the coronal part of the pulp but retaining the radicular part(s) in a devitalized, fixed state. The pulp must be vital beforehand.

This method of treatment was advocated as long ago as 1866 by Chase. Its main advantage is that instrumentation and filling of the root canal(s) are avoided. Thus, its greatest use, by those who practise it, is in the treatment of molar teeth.

1. Technique

One of two techniques may be followed. Formerly the pulp was first devitalized by applying an arsenical preparation to the base of the cavity. After 3–7 days the coronal part of the pulp was removed and a mummifying agent applied to the base of the pulp chamber to fix the radicular pulp. A layer of cement was then inserted and the cavity restored. Since the advent of effective local anaesthetics, preliminary devitalization has become unnecessary. Thus, treatment consists of a conventional pulpotomy, followed by the application of a mummifying agent to the vital pulp stumps and restoration of the tooth.

The active agent of mummifying compounds is paraformaldehyde; in an attempt to maintain the remaining radicular pulp in a sterile condition, as well as to fix it, other antiseptics are also included in these compounds. Two popular preparations are Gysi's Triopaste, which contains paraformaldehyde, tricresol, creolin, glycerine and zinc oxide, and a variation of Buckley's Formocresol, comprising formaldehyde, cresol and glycerine.

2. Apical reaction to mummification

The account of Hess (1929) of the apical reaction to pulp mummification has been confirmed by various workers, including Rzeszotarski (1939) and Inskipp and Markee (1941). In successful cases there is an ingrowth of periodontal tissue into the apical part of the canal, with a distinct line of demarcation between this tissue and the devitalized pulp farther coronally. The apical part of the canal is first widened by resorption and then becomes progressively narrower as cementum is deposited over the resorbed areas.

3. Assessment of mummification: indications

Although pulp mummification was popular for many years, by 1930 it had largely fallen into disrepute as a method of treating permanent teeth. Whilst this may seem rather surprising in view of the apparently favourable histological reports which have been quoted, there are various factors to account for it. The strongest objection to pulp mummification is the deliberate retention in the body of non-vital tissue, and this objection must have weighed very heavily in an era when the Theory of Focal Infection was so widely held. Even if the compound used to mummify a pulp does succeed in sterilizing it, it is by no means certain that the pulp will remain sterile indefinitely. Thus, s'Gravenmade (1975) states that most actions of formaldehyde on the pulp are reversible, and that penetration of formaldehyde into the periapical tissues is possible, so leading to irritation. The view that reinfection occurred, or that infection persisted, was supported by the experience of many workers, who found that although a tooth might remain symptomless for some time, periapical disease often eventually developed. Partly for these reasons, and partly because acute periapical inflammation not uncommonly followed application of the arsenical devitalizing agents then used, many of those who had formerly practised pulp mummification discontinued its use.

Even those who still use the method generally state that in the permanent dentition it is applicable to only a small minority of teeth, and should be used only where root canal treatment is not possible and where there is no evidence of infection or inflammation of the radicular parts of the pulp. Even under these circumstances it is debatable whether mummification is preferable to pulpotomy.

THE N2 METHOD

The term 'N2' describes both a method of root canal treatment and the materials used in this method. Sargenti and Richter (1961), who introduced N2, state that the term is meant to denote the 'second nerve' of the tooth.

1. Materials

Two N2 preparations exist, each in the form of a powder and liquid which are mixed to form a cement. One is known as 'N2 Permanent', or 'N2 Normal', and is used for root filling. The other is known as 'N2 Temporary', 'N2 Medical' or 'N2 Apical', and is used for antiseptic medication of the canal. The materials are banned in certain countries, except for experimental use.

Various formulas have been given for the N2 preparations, no doubt due in part to periodic changes in composition. With both N2 Permanent and N2 Temporary, the essential constituent of the liquid is eugenol, whilst the powder consists chiefly of zinc oxide, paraformaldehyde and compounds of lead and other metals. The recent formula given by Sargenti (1973) for N2 Permanent was referred to in Chapter 8. In the same publication, Sargenti recommends the use of N2 Temporary in conjunction with an ophthalmic preparation containing oxytetracycline, polymyxin and hydrocortisone.

2. Technique

The following account gives the salient features of the N2 method, as described by Sargenti and Richter (1961).

Treatment of a tooth with a vital pulp consists essentially of partial pulpectomy and immediate root filling. The pulp is removed as far as the apical one-third of the canal, or alternatively to a level where the diameter of the pulpal wound is less than 0·5 mm. Thus, with the finer canals of molar teeth the levels to which the radicular parts of the pulp are removed may be virtually the same as in pulpotomy (*Fig.* 269). In root filling a tooth with N2 Permanent, the insertion of gutta percha or silver points is unnecessary.

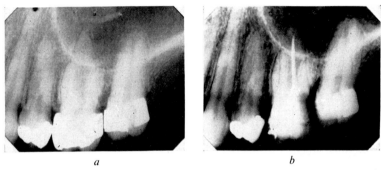

a   *b*

Fig. 269. |6. *a*, Preoperative appearance; *b*, Appearance after root filling with N2. The levels worked to in the mesiobuccal and distobuccal canals are virtually the same as would be used in pulpotomy.

Recently (Sargenti, 1973) the technique has apparently been modified in that it is recommended that a vital pulp should be removed as completely as possible.

In treating a tooth with a necrotic pulp, the canal is prepared for its entire length and N2 Temporary is used as the antiseptic dressing. The tooth is filled with N2 Permanent at the second or third visit.

3. Tissue response to N2 Permanent

The technique advocated for the treatment of pulpless teeth by the N2 method corresponds closely to that of other methods. For this reason, most of the research on N2 has been concerned with the treatment of teeth with vital pulps with N2 Permanent.

Numerous investigations into the effect of N2 Permanent on the non-dental tissues of experimental animals have been performed. Spangberg (1969, 1974) found that implantation into bone led to necrosis. Both Guttuso (1963) and Rappaport et al. (1964) noted a severe inflammatory response following implantation into connective tissue, but Friend and Browne (1968) reported that this response rapidly resolved. Overdiek (1960a) obtained a favourable reaction following implantation into muscle.

Several studies on the response of pulpal and periapical tissues of experimental animals have also been reported. Barker and Lockett (1972a) found that the application of N2 Permanent to pulpotomy wounds was followed by pulpal necrosis. However, when used as a root filling, relatively favourable responses have been reported by Rowe (1967) and Barker and Lockett (1972b). Whilst noting pulpal necrosis and periapical inflammation following partial pulpectomy and filling with N2 Permanent, Snyder et al. (1966) state that the latter was less irritant than a silver-containing cement. Engstrom and Spangberg (1969) and Muruzabal and Erausquin (1973), on the other hand, reported marked periapical inflammation and necrosis respectively.

The results of histological studies on the responses of human pulpal and periapical tissues are less conflicting. Overdiek (1960b) and Hannah and Rowe (1971) found that the application of N2 Permanent to pulpotomy wounds in permanent and primary teeth respectively was followed by pulpal necrosis. Although Rowe (1964) and Schonherr and Brauer (1964) reported the presence of uninflamed pulp and hard tissue formation in the apical part of the canal following partial pulpectomy and root filling with N2 Permanent, the majority of studies report necrosis or fixation of the remaining pulp, sometimes with periapical inflammation (Iten, 1958; Klock, 1959; Nicholls, 1963; Langeland et al., 1969).

Both Nicholls (1965) and Snyder et al. (1966) point out that the level to which the pulp is removed may influence the response of the residual pulp apically. It is noteworthy that whilst Sargenti and Richter (1961) claim that the residual pulp is not devitalized, Sargenti (1973) states that the pulp adjacent to the root filling is fixed.

4. Toxicological studies

Recent investigations have shown that lead from N2 Permanent may enter the systemic circulation. Harndt and Kaul (1973) demonstrated the presence of lead in the organs of experimental animals following implantation of N2 Permanent. Shapiro et al. (1975) found that the insertion of root fillings of N2 Permanent in monkey teeth was followed by a rise in the blood-lead level. Extrapolating their results to humans, the latter authors conclude that although the increase observed would be insufficient to cause overt or subclinical symptoms of lead poisoning, accidental extrusion of the material periapically or root resorption following filling with N2 Permanent could lead to a greater rise in the blood-lead level.

5. Other properties of N2 Permanent

The use of N2 Permanent, in conjunction with a root-filling point, has been shown by Grieve and Parkholm (1973) to provide an effective seal to the root canal.

6. Assessment of N2 Permanent

The use of the N2 method for the treatment of a tooth with a vital pulp is followed by devitalization if an appreciable part of the pulp is left, and under these circumstances is a form of mummification. Sargenti (1973) now states it is wrong to leave a large part of the pulp, although this has been common practice in the past.

The removal of a vital pulp to a level close to the root apex, as has been recently suggested (Sargenti, 1973), corresponds to the level to which the canal is normally prepared. The choice of a root-filling material under these circumstances is to some degree a matter of personal preference. However, in view of the possibility of periapical irritation and absorption of lead from N2 Permanent, especially if the material is extruded into the periapical tissues, the use of some other material is indicated.

REFERENCES

Barker B. C. W. and Lockett B. C. (1971) Endodontic experiments with resorbable paste. *Aust. Dent. J.* **16**, 364.

Barker B. C. W. and Lockett B. C. (1972a) The effect of N2 and other paraformaldehyde preparations on dog pulp. *Dent. Practnr Dent. Rec.* **22**, 329.

Barker B. C. W. and Lockett B. C. (1972b) Periapical response to N2 and other paraformaldehyde compounds confined within or extruded beyond the apices of dog root canals. *Dent. Practnr Dent. Rec.* **22**, 370.

Bell J. W. (1969) Kri 1 paste. *N.Z. Dent. J.* **65**, 96.

Bernard P. D. (1952) Technique complémentaire de l'ionophorèse: le remplissage intégral des canaux aberrants par obturation expansive au moyen d'un échange moléculaire. *L'Odontologie* **73**, 277.

Bernard P. D. (1967) Thérapie Ocalexique. S.A. Paris: Librairie Maloine. Quoted by Hendra L. P. (1970) *J. Br. Endodontic Soc.* **4**, 37.

Castagnola L. (1959) 1000 Fälle von Gangränbehandlung nach der Walkhoffschen Methode aus dem statistischen Material der konservierenden Abteilung. *Schweiz. Monatsschr. Zahnheilkd.* **60**, 1033.

Castagnola L. and Orlay H. G. (1952) Treatment of gangrene of the pulp by the Walkhoff method. *Br. Dent. J.* **93**, 93.

Castagnola L. and Orlay H. G. (1956) *A System of Endodontia for the General Dental Practitioner.* London, Pitman, Chs. 3, 8, 9 and p. 131.

Chase H. S. (1866) Results of pulp treatment. *Dent. Cosmos* **8**, 517.

Engel H. (1950) Die Behandlung infizierter Wurzelkanäle und Granulome nach der Methode von Walkhoff. *Schweiz. Monatsschr. Zahnheilkd.* **60**, 1077.

Engstrom B. and Spangberg L. (1969) Effect of root canal filling material N2 when used for filling after partial pulpectomy. *Sven. Tandlak. Tidskr.* **62**, 815.

Erausquin J. and Muruzabal M. (1969) Tissue reactions to root canal fillings with absorbable pastes. *Oral Surg.* **28**, 567.

Frajlich S. R. and Goldberg F. (1975) Estudio 'in vitro' de las propiedades del Biocalex en el tratamiento endodontico. *Rev. de la odont. Argentina* **62**, 189.

Friend L. A. and Browne R. M. (1968) Tissue reactions to some root filling materials. *Br. Dent. J.* **125**, 291.

Göransson K. (1957) Über die Resorptions-Möglichkeiten aus der Pulpa. *Neues. Zahnk.* **3**, 277. Quoted in *Dent. Abstr., Chicago* **3**, 277, 1958.

Grieve A. R. and Parkholm J. D. O. (1973) The sealing properties of root filling cements: further studies. *Br. Dent. J.* **135**, 327.

Guttuso J. (1963) Histopathologic study of rat connective tissue responses to endodontic materials. *Oral Surg.* **16**, 713.

Hannah D. R. and Rowe A. H. R. (1971) Vital pulpotomy of deciduous molars using N2 and other materials. *Br. Dent. J.* **130**, 99.

Harndt V. R. and Kaul A. (1973) Untersuchungen über den verbleib des bleies im Wurzelkanalfullmaterial N2. *Dtsch. Zahnaerztl. Z.* **28**, 580.

Hedman W. J. (1951) An investigation into residual periapical infection after pulp canal therapy. *Oral Surg.* **4**, 1173.

Hendra L. P. (1970) Biocalex: a new approach to endodontia dependent upon biological principles and chemical action only. *J. Br. Endodont. Soc.* **4**, 37.

Hess W. (1929) Pulp amputation as a method of treating root canals. *Dent. Items* **51**, 596.

Honegger I. (1932) Histologische Untersuchungen über die apikalen Heilungsvorgänge entpulpter Zähne nach Einwirkung von Chlorphenolkampfermenthollösung und Chlorphenolkampfermenthol-jodoformpaste (Methode Walkhoff) auf das gesunde Periodontium. *Schweiz. Monatsschr. Zahnheilkd.* **42**, 761.

Hyakusoku H. (1959) Effect of filling material on healing of periapical tissues in treatment of human infected root canal. *Tokyo Dent. Coll. Bull. Oral Path.* **4**, 51.

Inskipp E. F. and Markee J. E. (1941) Experimental and clinical study of pulp amputation. *J. Dent. Res.* **20**, 277.

Iten J. (1958) Klinische und histologische Untersuchungen mit dem Wurzelfüellmaterial N2. Inaugural Dissertation. Basle, Arnaud Druck Bern.

Juge H. (1959) Resorbable pastes for root canal fillings. *Int. Dent. J., Lond.* **9**, 461.

Klock F. (1959) Experimentelle und klinische Erfahrungen mit der N2-Wurzelbehandlung. Inaugural Dissertation. Bonn, Rheinische Friedrich-Wilhelms-Universität.

Langeland K., Guttuso J., Langeland L., K., and Tobon G. (1969) Methods in the study of biologic responses to endodontic materials. Tissue response to N 2. *Oral Surg.* **27**, 522.

Laws A. J. (1959) Kri-1 for root fillings. *N.Z. Dent. J.* **55**, 131.

Muruzabal M. and Erausquin J. (1973) The process of healing following endodontic treatment in the molar of the rat. In: Grossman L. I. (ed.), *Transactions of the 5th International Conference on Endodontics.* Philadelphia, University of Pennsylvania, pp. 126–54.

Nicholls E. (1963) Resorbable canal fillings, including N2. In: Grossman L. I. (ed.), *Transactions of the 3rd International Conference on Endodontics.* Philadelphia, University of Pennsylvania, pp. 144–57.

Nicholls E. (1965) Research and clinical practice in endodontics. *Dent. Practnr Dent. Rec.* **16**, 81.

Overdiek H. F. (1960a) Zur Gewebsreaktion auf implantierte Wurzelfullmaterialien im Vergleich zum N2. *Zahnarztl. Rsdch.* **69**, 402.

Overdiek H. F. (1960b) Pulpenreaction auf N2 im Kurzzeitversuch. *Dtsch. Zahnaeztl. Z.* **15**, 786.

Rappaport H. M., Lilly G. E. and Kapsimalis P. (1964) Toxicity of endodontic filling materials. *Oral Surg.* **18**, 785.

Röse C. (1894) The treatment of teeth with diseased pulps. *Dent. Cosmos* **36**, 358.

Rowe A. H. R. (1964) Treatment with N2 root canal sealer: histological report of three teeth. *Br. Dent. J.* **117**, 27.

Rowe A. H. R. (1967) Effect of root filling materials on the periapical tissues. *Br. Dent. J.* **122**, 98.

Rzeszotarski J. S. (1939) Clinical and histologic studies of partial pulp amputation. *Bur.* **39**, 59.

Sargenti A. (1973) Is N2 an acceptable method of treatment? In: Grossman L. I. (ed.), *Transactions of the 5th International Conference on Endodontics.* Philadelphia, University of Pennsylvania, pp. 176–95.

Sargenti A. and Richter S. L. (1961) *Rationalised Root Canal Treatment*, 2nd ed. New York, AGSA Scientific Publications, pp. 12, 28, 34–54, 78, 104–20, 204.

Schonherr E. and Brauer K. H. (1964) Röntgenologische und histologische Befunde von mit N2 behandelten pulpitischen Zähnen. *Zahnarztl. Praxis* **15**, 161.

s'Gravenmade E. J. (1975) Some biochemical considerations of fixation in endodontics. *J. Endodontol.* **1**, 233.

Shapiro I. M., Iaquinta S., Mitchell G. and Grossman L. I. (1975) Blood-lead levels of monkeys treated with a lead-containing (N2) root canal cement: a preliminary report. *J. Endodontol.* **1**, 294.

Snyder D. E., Seltzer S. and Moodnik R. (1966) Effects of N2 in experimental endodontic therapy. *Oral Surg.* **21**, 635.

Spangberg L. (1969) Biological effects of root canal filling materials. 7, Reaction of bony tissue to implanted root canal filling material in guineapigs. *Odontol. Tidskr.* **77**, 133.

Spangberg L. (1974) Biologic effects of root canal filling materials: the effect on bone tissue of two formaldehyde-containing root canal filling pastes: N2 and Riebler's paste. *Oral Surg.* **38**, 934.

Walkhoff O. (1928) *Mein System der medicamentosen Behandlung schwerer Erkrankungen der Zahnpulpa und des Periodontiums.* Berlin, Meusser. (Quoted by Castagnola L. and Orlay H. G. (1952) *Br. Dent. J.* **93**, 93.)

FURTHER READING

Langeland K. (1973) Debate: is N2 an acceptable method of treatment? In: Grossman L. I. (ed.), *Transactions of the 5th International Conference on Endodontics.* Philadelphia, University of Pennsylvania, pp. 205–38.

Chapter 16

Treatment of traumatized anterior teeth

Injury to the anterior teeth, with or without tooth fracture, is not an uncommon result of a blow or fall on the face. Thus, Grundy (1959) found that 5·1 per cent of the children he examined had had an anterior tooth fractured, quite apart from any other injuries to the teeth, whilst Clarkson et al. (1973) report that 10 per cent of schoolchildren had one or more injured teeth, sometimes with actual loss of a tooth.

In almost all cases it is desirable that the affected teeth be retained. In so far as appropriate therapeutic measures may prevent the development of pulpal or periapical disease, therefore, the immediate treatment of traumatized anterior teeth merits separate consideration.

With permanent teeth most of these injuries occur in the 6–15 years' age group, especially in children aged 8–11 years (Hallett, 1953). The maxillary teeth, particularly the central incisors, are involved far more commonly than the mandibular teeth (Rock et al., 1974) and, as might be expected, significantly more injuries occur in boys than in girls (Ellis, 1960). Proclined maxillary anterior teeth are especially prone to injury (Hallett, 1953). In more than 50 per cent of patients two or more teeth show evidence of injury (Rock et al., 1974).

The role of mouthguards in the prevention of traumatic dental injuries is discussed by Stevens (1972).

CLASSIFICATION

Numerous classifications, mostly variations of that suggested by Ellis (1960), have been used when discussing the treatment of traumatized anterior teeth. In the present account the following classification will be used:

Class 1: a tooth with no fracture of the crown or root, or with a chipped crown with only the enamel involved.

Class 2: a tooth with a fracture of the crown exposing the dentine.

Class 3: a tooth with a fracture of the crown exposing, or very nearly exposing, the pulp.

Class 4: a tooth with a fracture of the root, with or without a fracture of the crown also.

Class 5: a tooth which has been dislocated completely from its socket.

Class 6: a tooth which has been intruded into the supporting bone.

In each of the first four classes, the tooth may be firm or loose in its socket.

EXAMINATION

An account of history taking and examination was given in Chapter 1. The present account deals mainly with features of particular importance in the immediate treatment of traumatized anterior teeth.

1. History

In cases of traumatized anterior teeth, the following facts especially should be elicited: the age of the patient, the interval of time that has elapsed since the accident, the cause of the accident and the features of any pain which is, or has been, experienced. In addition, the patient should be asked whether there has been previous trauma to the anterior teeth, since such an occurrence may affect the prognosis of treatment of the present injury. Estimates of the number of patients with a history of repeated trauma to the teeth range from 4 to 24 per cent (Andreasen, 1972).

2. Examination

a. Visual examination

i. EXTRAORAL

An extraoral examination is first made. Swellings and cuts of the lips and other soft tissues are noted. Wounds are examined visually for contamination by dirt. The facial skeleton is gently palpated for possible fractures.

ii. INTRAORAL

The inner surface of each lip is also examined. Where a wound is present and the crown of a nearby tooth has been fractured, the possibility that the lip was penetrated by the tooth and that a fragment of the latter is embedded in the wound must be considered (Allan, 1961).

Examination of the occlusion will help not only in assessing the orthodontic status but also in establishing a diagnosis when a fractured jaw is suspected. Premature contact between the two arches anteriorly may be indicative of a displaced tooth. Haemorrhage in the region of the gingival crevice is very suggestive of displacement of the entire tooth or, in the event of a fracture involving the root, of the coronal part of the tooth (see Fig. 277, p. 316).

The alignments of the incisal edges and labial surfaces of the teeth are inspected for evidence of tooth displacement. The latter may take the form of extrusion of the tooth from its socket, intrusion into its socket or displacement of the tooth in the labiolingual plane. Each tooth is examined for coronal fracture and loss of translucency or actual discoloration. If a tooth has been fractured, the class of fracture is determined. The probable nature of the eventual restoration is also considered, since this may affect the plan of treatment.

b. Mobility; Percussion; Palpation

Each anterior tooth is tested for mobility and tenderness to percussion. This needs to be done carefully, since the tissues may be very sensitive. Usually, if either of these tests is 'positive', the other is also.

Pronounced mobility may be indicative of displacement of the tooth or fracture of its root, or both. Tenderness of the tissues over the root denotes bruising, perhaps with fracture of the alveolar bone.

c. Vitality tests

Thermal and electrical tests are now carried out on the teeth. With a fractured tooth, a probe may be gently drawn across any exposed dentine to assess its sensitivity, but care should be taken to confine the application of thermal and electrical stimuli to the enamel. Although it is common practice to perform vitality tests only on teeth in the arch obviously affected, it is preferable to test both arches.

The results of vitality tests on traumatized teeth must be interpreted with caution. As was pointed out in Chapter 1, incompletely formed teeth with no evidence of pulpal disease sometimes do not respond to electric pulp tests. Moreover, although a traumatized anterior tooth may respond to these tests some weeks after the accident, it may not do so immediately, presumably because of the shock sustained by the pulp. If these tests are carried out soon after the accident, therefore, care must be taken not to apply too great a stimulus to a tooth which has not responded.

Rock et al. (1974) report that of teeth giving a negative or doubtful response to electric pulp testing when the patient was first seen, approximately 50 per cent subsequently showed evidence of pulpal vitality; of teeth giving a vital response initially, 82 per cent retained pulpal vitality. These findings support the concept of shock or concussion of the pulp from movement of the tooth in its socket and resultant damage to apical blood vessels and nerves. They also indicate that continued vitality of the pulp is more likely in teeth giving a positive response to pulp tests immediately after the accident.

d. Radiographs

Periapical radiographs are taken to show each anterior tooth in the affected arch. These radiographs are used not only to assist in the initial diagnosis, but also to provide a basis for comparison with later ones.

In viewing the films, each tooth is examined for the size of its pulp, the proximity of the pulp to any fractured surface coronally, the state of development of the root apex, the presence of root fractures and the state of the periapical region. Obvious widening of the periodontal membrane space apically suggests extrusion of the tooth from its socket.

If from the radiographic examination or the mobility test a root fracture is suspected, one or two additional films are taken with different vertical angulations to the tube. If there is reason to believe that a fragment of tooth is embedded in one of the lips, a radiograph is taken with the film placed between the lip and teeth, with a reduction in exposure time or voltage; alternatively, an anterior occlusal radiograph may be taken.

If after examining the patient it is decided that extraction is necessary, the problem of whether to maintain the space or to close it by orthodontic treatment, perhaps with crowning of other teeth later, should be considered.

TREATMENT

1. General considerations

a. Soft-tissue injuries

Deep cuts of the lips may need suturing. If the tissues are lacerated and have been contaminated by dirt, antitetanus serum or antitetanus toxoid, in combination

closed cap splint. Stewart (1963) draws attention to the use of clear polystyrene sheet, which after being heated can be moulded to the model by hand and then trimmed. Whichever material is used, holes are made in the splint to leave the centre of the lingual surface of each traumatized tooth uncovered, so facilitating further vitality tests and, if necessary, root canal treatment, before the splint is removed (*see Fig.* 270). Either zinc phosphate or fast-setting zinc oxide–eugenol cement may be used to fix the splint in position. With both acrylic and silver, zinc oxide–eugenol cement is quite satisfactory, and has the advantage that it provides less resistance when the splint is eventually removed. Exposed dentine of fractured teeth is covered with calcium hydroxide cement before applying the splint.

With each of the three materials just mentioned, either the entire arch or just four or six anterior teeth may be splinted. Where there is a large overjet, only the anterior teeth need usually be covered. However, with mandibular teeth, and in cases where some of the teeth are only partly erupted or are unerupted or missing, it is generally necessary to cover the entire arch in order to gain sufficient retention. Coverage of the entire arch is also indicated where splinting the anterior teeth only would result in severe occlusal interference.

Where the degree of eruption of the existing teeth and the number of missing teeth are such that even complete coverage of the arch will not ensure retention, Stewart (1963) suggests the use of a removable appliance of clear acrylic which covers the palate and is retained by cribs in the molar region. The plate is made to overlap the incisal 1–2 mm of the labial surfaces of the anterior teeth. Occlusal coverage of the posterior teeth is necessary if the mandibular incisors make premature contact with the appliance. A similar appliance can be made for traumatized mandibular incisors. Although this form of appliance does not give the rigid fixation provided by a cemented splint, it is far more acceptable aesthetically and, since it is removable, is more conducive to oral hygiene.

Other forms of splint make use of arch wire or similar devices. The teeth are fixed to the arch wire by means of interdental wiring or orthodontic bands cemented to the teeth. A disadvantage of this type of splint is that it is not readily applicable in cases where the exposed dentinal surfaces of fractured crowns have to be covered.

The introduction of acid etching in conjunction with the application of composite materials provides obvious possibilities for the fixation of traumatized teeth by way of their approximal surfaces, and may well supplant many currently used methods where splinting for only a few weeks is necessary.

c. *Protection of exposed dentine*

Although a splint often serves the dual purpose of immobilizing loose teeth and protecting the exposed dentine and the pulps of fractured teeth, in many instances immobilization is not indicated. Under these circumstances the construction of a splint is hardly justified unless three or four teeth in the same arch have coronal fractures. Usually, however, only one or two teeth need treatment. In such cases, a separate covering is applied to each fractured tooth to retain a protective dressing over the exposed dentine.

Although copper or stainless-steel bands may be used, a preformed stainless-steel crown generally provides a more satisfactory form of temporary covering. As far as possible the crown should restore both the length and contact areas of the original crown so as to prevent drifting of the fractured tooth and its neighbours and overeruption of the teeth. Before cementation a protective layer of calcium hydroxide cement is applied to the exposed dentine and a hole cut in the surface of the crown so as to facilitate vitality tests later. The crown is left in position for 3–6 months before restoring the tooth.

A recent report by Scheer (1975) suggests that the restoration of fractured incisors with etch-retained composite material immediately after injury entails little or no risk of pulpal necrosis. Where this form of treatment is employed, a minimal preparation confined to enamel should be used. Exposed dentine should obviously be protected, using calcium hydroxide cement.

The report of Friend (1973) indicates that pulpal necrosis is less likely where the exposed dentine of a fractured tooth is protected than where it is left unprotected.

2. Treatment according to class of injury

a. Class 1

i. PROGNOSIS

The stage of development of the root apex has a considerable influence on the prognosis of Class 1 injuries. Where root formation is incomplete, there is a good chance that the pulp will remain vital, especially if the tooth is still firm in its socket. Where formation of the root apex is well advanced, however, the pulp often becomes necrotic, especially if the tooth has been loosened or extruded (Andreasen, 1970b). Necrosis of the pulp is more likely where the crown is intact than where fracture through the enamel or dentine has occurred (Rock et al., 1974). It is generally held that this is because in the latter type of case, part of the energy of the blow is dissipated in fracturing the tooth, whereas when the latter remains intact the full force of the blow is transmitted to the pulp apically. The fact that loosening of one or more teeth is commoner with Class 1 injuries than with other classes of injury may be explained on the same basis.

The stage reached in root formation may also be related to the frequency of root resorption following trauma. Thus, Skieller (1960) concluded that resorption seemed to occur more commonly in completely formed teeth, although it apparently proceeded at a faster rate in teeth with incompletely formed roots. In some instances the pulp remains vital but resorption of the root apex (*Fig.* 274) or internal resorption of the root (*Fig.* 275) occurs.

The results of Andreasen (1970b) indicate that internal resorption is relatively rare, and that external root resorption occurs much more often, whilst Cvek (1973) found that in teeth with necrotic pulps external root resorption almost always ceased following routine root canal treatment.

Instead of resorption, progressive calcification of the pulp cavity may take place (*Fig.* 272). This response occurs mainly in teeth which are injured before the completion of root formation (Andreasen, 1970b; Friend, 1973) and subsequent pulpal necrosis is uncommon (Andreasen, 1970b). Although the pulp cavity may appear radiographically to be completely obliterated, a remnant of root canal is always present (Andreasen, 1972; Fischer, 1974).

ii. TREATMENT

Many cases of Class 1 injury will need splinting. It is sometimes not possible to reduce completely any tooth displacement present, with the result that the tooth remains slightly extruded. This is of no significance, since it may be corrected by grinding of the incisal edge after the splint is removed. Chipping of the enamel is treated in the same way. Where immobilization of the tooth is not necessary, it is freed from occlusal contact by grinding the opposing teeth. Stoning and polishing of any chipped enamel may be performed straightaway.

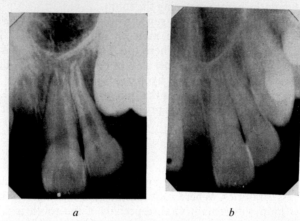

a   *b*

Fig. 272. |12. *a*, Immediately following trauma; *b*, Seven months later, showing very rapid calcification of pulp cavities.

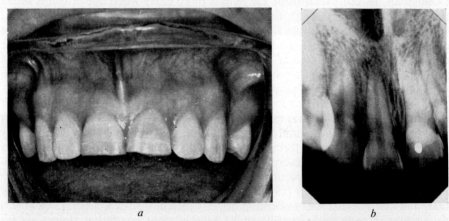

a   *b*

Fig. 273. *a*, Discoloration of 1|1 still apparent some years after trauma; *b*, The pulp of 1| still responds normally to vitality tests. The pulp cavity of |1 is virtually obliterated by calcification and the tooth does not respond to vitality tests. Neither tooth showed definite evidence of periapical disease.

Often, although the crown of the tooth remains intact, cracks in the enamel are apparent. Andreasen (1972) uses the term 'crown infraction' to describe these cases. No special treatment is required for such cracks.

Clinical examination and vitality tests are performed 3–4 weeks after the accident and when the splint is removed, and thereafter every few months for at least 1 year. Radiographs are taken when the splint is removed 6 weeks after the accident, and thereafter two or three times at 6-monthly intervals. Where there is no response to vitality tests immediately after the injury, pulpal recovery, as manifested by reaction to vitality tests, often occurs within 1 or 2 months, but may take up to a year (Skieller, 1960; Friend, 1973). Unless there is pain or radiographic evidence of periapical disease, therefore, root canal treatment should be deferred for at least 1 year in cases showing no evidence of pulpal recovery. On the other hand, teeth which initially respond to vitality tests but subsequently fail to do so should have root canal treatment without delay; pulpal necrosis in such cases is often apparent within 2 months of the injury (Skieller, 1960). It should be noted that although a bluish-grey discoloration of the crown from pulpal haemorrhage usually indicates necrosis of the pulp, the significance of such a change must be assessed in conjunction with the results of vitality tests and radiographic examination, since occasionally the pulp recovers (*Fig.* 273).

Cases in which resorption of the root apex or calcification of the pulp cavity becomes apparent are observed until there is definite evidence of pulpal necrosis. Resorption usually affects only the apical part of the root and does not progress further (*Fig.* 274). However, where resorption of a lateral wall of the root canal becomes apparent (*Fig.* 275), the pulp should be removed immediately and root canal treatment performed before the side of the root is perforated. If resorption is not detected until after the root has been perforated, extraction (*Fig.* 276), or root canal treatment, possibly supplemented by surgery (*see* Chapter 15), is necessary.

b. Class 2

With adequate emergency treatment, vitality of the pulp may be maintained in a high proportion of teeth with Class 2 injuries (Lieban, 1947; Friend, 1973). The teeth are first isolated with wool rolls and the exposed dentine of each fractured tooth cleaned of debris with a wool pledget moistened in warm water. Temporary restorations are then used to cover the exposed dentine, or a splint is applied to the teeth, as described previously. Clinical and radiographic examinations and vitality tests are performed at intervals similar to those used when treating Class 1 injuries.

If after 3–6 months the pulp is still vital, the tooth is restored with an etch-retained composite. When the patient is older and the pulp cavity smaller, a jacket crown may be made, if indicated.

In some instances where a relatively small amount of tooth substance has been lost and the adjacent contact area is intact, it is possible by careful contouring of thefractured surface to obtain a satisfactory appearance. If necessary, the incisal edges of other teeth may also be stoned to improve the appearance still further. Usually this form of treatment is satisfactory only when the fracture has involved the distal part of the crown, since it is this part of the incisal edge which is naturally rounded. If there is any doubt concerning the effectiveness of such treatment or the amount of tissue which would need to be removed, it is useful to trim the teeth on a model beforehand.

c. Class 3

The treatment of a tooth with a Class 3 injury depends largely on the stage of formation of the root apex.

i. INCOMPLETELY FORMED APEX

Where the apical foramen is wide and the radicular part of the pulp is vital, the main aim of treatment is to maintain the vitality of the pulp in the apical part of the

11

root and so enable formation of the root apex to be completed. Pulpotomy is considered to be the form of treatment most likely to accomplish this end. Provided there is no evidence of involvement of the radicular part of the pulp, pulpotomy should be performed even if owing to delay in treatment the pulp has undergone necrosis coronally.

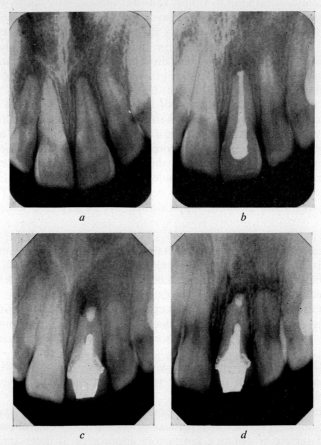

Fig. 274. |12. *a*, Appearance when patient first attended following trauma; *b*, Five months later, |1, which was root-filled, shows obvious apical resorption; *c*, Three years later, |2 shows obvious apical resorption, but its pulp still responds to vitality tests; *d*, Seven years later, |2 still responds to vitality tests and shows no further resorption.

Treatment by pulp capping is generally considered unwise, since the retention of contaminated pulpal tissue is likely to lead to necrosis; however, as was pointed out in Chapter 2, there seem to have been no large-scale studies into the prognosis of capping such teeth. It is also held to be inadvisable to treat a near exposure by applying a protective covering to the exposed dentine, since subsequent necrosis of the pulp is not uncommon, especially if there has been some delay in the patient seeking treatment. However, either of these measures may be useful as an emergency form of treatment if the patient is too distressed or if there is too little time for pulpotomy to be adequately performed when the patient is first seen. By waiting a few days, the operation may be done on a more co-operative patient and in an unhurried manner.

It is unlikely that the exposed tooth itself is mobile and splinting is therefore not indicated unless other teeth need to be immobilized. Following pulpotomy the

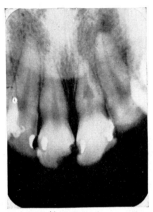

Fig. 275. |1. Internal resorption of lateral walls of root canal following trauma. Root canal treatment should be performed immediately.

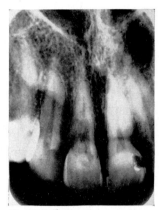

Fig. 276. 1|. Gross resorption of the root makes extraction unavoidable.

tooth is restored with an etch-retained composite filling and observed as described in Chapter 2. Since in most cases a post crown will be needed eventually to restore the tooth, pulpectomy and root canal treatment are carried out directly formation of the root apex has been completed.

Should there be a long delay before the patient seeks treatment and the radicular part of the pulp is necrotic, root canal treatment is indicated (*see* Chapter 13).

ii. 'FULLY' FORMED APEX

Where the walls of the root canal of a tooth with a Class 3 injury show obvious convergence gingivo-apically, root canal treatment is generally indicated, irrespective of the state of the pulp. Even though the latter may be vital and still covered by a very thin layer of dentine, a post crown will usually be needed to restore the tooth eventually. This is invariably so if the fracture has involved both the mesial and the distal aspect of the crown. On the rare occasions when a post crown will not be needed, pulpotomy or simply protection of the exposed dentine— depending on whether or not the pulp is exposed—may be justified, provided the pulp is vital and the tooth is not mobile or tender to percussion.

As with similar injuries involving teeth with incompletely formed apices, pulp capping is contraindicated. However, as a temporary measure pending pulpectomy in a few days' time, capping of an exposure, or coverage of exposed dentine, is often a useful procedure.

Following root canal treatment the tooth is observed in the manner described in Chapter 9. Where hardly any of the natural crown remains, there is little option but to restore the tooth by a post crown. Where a considerable part of the crown is still present, however, post crown construction may be deferred until the patient is older, and the tooth restored with an etch-retained composite filling in the meantime.

Coronal fractures involving periodontal membrane: With a transverse fracture involving both the mesial and the distal aspect to the crown, the line of fracture sometimes extends apical of the epithelial attachment. Thus when the patient is first seen the fractured crown is still held in position, albeit loosely, by attachment to the periodontal membrane. Usually the fracture is oblique in the labiolingual plane, being supragingival labially but subgingival lingually (*Fig.* 277). Although the labial part of the fracture line is visible radiographically, the lingual extent of the fracture is usually not readily apparent (*Fig.* 278).

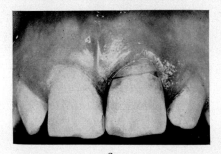 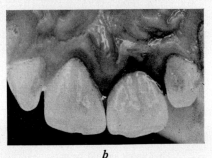

a	*b*

Fig. 277. Coronal fracture ⌊1 involving periodontal membrane. *a*, A labial view shows the fracture; *b*, A mirror view of the palatal surfaces does not show the fracture, but haemorrhage is apparent.

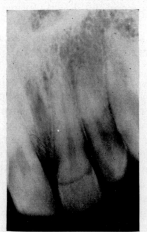 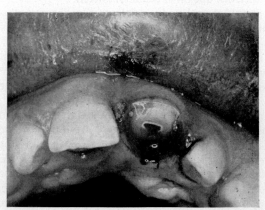

Fig. 278. ⌊1. Radiographic appearance of case shown in *Fig.* 277. The labial part of the fracture line is obvious, but the palatal part is barely discernible.

Fig. 279. ⌊1. Appearance of the case shown in *Fig.* 277 after removing the coronal fragment.

In such cases local anaesthetic injections are given immediately, since even the pressure of an X-ray film against the coronal fragment is likely to disturb the pulp and cause pain. It is necessary first to determine the apical extent of the fracture, and this can only be done by severing the periodontal attachment lingually with a scalpel, and then removing the coronal fragment (*Fig.* 279). Although the fracture may extend some distance apically along the root, a local gingivectomy, sometimes with removal of alveolar bone, will generally make root canal treatment and post crowning of the tooth possible.

An alternative technique makes use of the broken crown itself as the restoration. Ellis (1940), who describes the technique, claims good results from this treatment. After the crown has been removed it is cleaned of all pulpal and periodontal tissue. It is tried back on the tooth to ensure that it fits satisfactorily, and is then stored in normal saline until root canal treatment is completed at a subsequent appointment. Meanwhile, the gingival tissues are prevented from encroaching on the fractured surface of the root by means of a suitable pack. After root filling, the canal is prepared to receive a preformed metal post. This should project a few millimetres beyond the coronal end of the canal into the pulp chamber of the crown. If necessary, the pulp chamber is judiciously enlarged with burs to allow seating of the crown. The pulp chamber and the post hole are now filled with composite or silicophosphate cement and the post and the crown cemented in position simultaneously. After setting, excess cement is removed, particular attention being paid to the lingual aspect of the tooth. Apart from the difficulty in seating the crown in its correct position, disadvantages of this technique are the lack of fit between the preformed gold post and the crown and the possibility of coronal discoloration later.

d. Class 4

Root fractures occur in only a small proportion of patients seeking treatment following trauma to the anterior teeth. Thus, Friend (1973) found that of 801 injured teeth, only 2 per cent had root fractures, whilst in a review of the literature Andreasen (1972) states that they comprised 1–7 per cent of injuries. However, as Lindahl (1958) points out, some root fractures are detected only during routine radiographic examination some time after the accident (*Fig.* 280), and the frequency of the type of injury may therefore be rather greater than the preceding reports suggest.

Most root fractures occur in 'fully' erupted teeth where root formation has been completed (Andreasen and Hjorting-Hansen, 1967), perhaps because the roots of incompletely formed teeth are more elastic and supported less firmly in their sockets. Usually the fracture occurs in the middle one-third of the root and is transverse in the mesiodistal plane (Lindahl, 1958; Andreasen and Hjorting-Hansen, 1967). The fracture is usually oblique to the long axis of the tooth in the labiolingual plane and closer to the root apex labially; this facilitates radiographic diagnosis, since the plane of the fracture is roughly in line with the X-ray beam (Andreasen and Hjorting-Hansen, 1967).

The roots of maxillary central incisor teeth are fractured far more often than those of other teeth (Austin, 1930; Lindahl, 1958). Separate fractures of the crown and the root from the same accident are unusual.

Fractures of the alveolar process, which often occur in conjunction with root fractures (Andreasen, 1970c), usually heal quite uneventfully (Andreasen, 1970a).

i. TEETH WITH VITAL PULPS

α. Prognosis: In the past it was usually held that although the prognosis of a fracture in the apical one-third to the root of a tooth with a vital pulp was good, that of a middle one-third fracture was uncertain, whilst the prognosis of a cervical one-third fracture was hopeless. However, the study of Lindahl (1958) and various case reports by authors such as Hart (1948), Bennett (1959) and Ritchie (1962) indicate that this is probably an unduly pessimistic view. Of 48 root fractures treated by Andreasen and Hjorting-Hansen (1967), pulpal necrosis occurred in

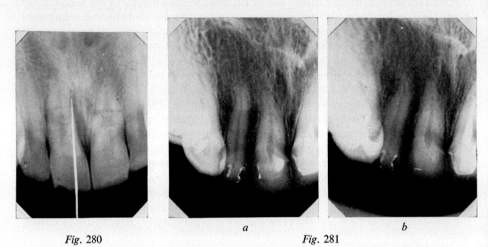

Fig. 280   *a*   *Fig*. 281   *b*

Fig. 280. Fracture of the middle one-third of the roots of 1| and |1, diagnosed some years following the accident. 1| has developed periodontal disease, as shown by the insertion of a silver point by way of the gingival crevice to the vicinity of the fracture line. |1 is still firm and responds normally to vitality tests. Neither tooth had received treatment.

Fig. 281. 2|. *a*, Fracture just visible at junction of apical and middle one-thirds of root. Appearance shortly after accident; *b*, Two years after treatment by splinting, the tooth is still firm. Replacement of the artificial crown showed that the pulp was still vital.

44 per cent; extrusion of the coronal fragment at the time of injury was found to be unfavourable for continued pulpal vitality, whilst splinting reduced the frequency of pulpal necrosis.

Thus, provided certain requirements can be satisfied, it is often possible to maintain the vitality of the pulp and to obtain repair of the fractured root. These requirements are that the fracture line does not extend to the close proximity of the gingival sulcus, that the fragments of the root are close together, and that they remain so by rigid immobilization of the crowns of the teeth.

β. Treatment: In many instances, repair of a fracture of the apical or middle one-third of a root and maintenance of pulpal vitality occur without any form of treatment, the injury only becoming apparent some years after the accident as a result of radiographic examination for some other purpose (*Fig*. 280). However, the fact that this fortunate outcome sometimes occurs in the absence of treatment does not mean that treatment is unnecessary. Even though the tooth seems firm in its socket, it should be splinted as soon as possible, unless of course some weeks have elapsed since the accident. Clinical and radiographic examinations and vitality tests are performed 3–4 weeks afterwards and when the splint is removed, and subsequently two or three times at 6-monthly intervals. Often a successful result is achieved (*Fig.* 281).

γ. *Pattern of repair*: The maintenance of pulpal vitality following root fracture is probably due to the fact that the space between the two fragments allows the escape of inflammatory exudate from the pulp. The report of Miles (1947) suggests that a collateral circulation between the pulp and the periodontal membrane by way of the fracture line may sometimes be formed.

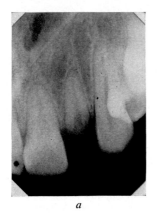 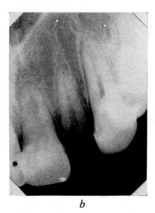

a   *b*

Fig. 282. |1. *a*, Shortly after trauma, showing fracture at junction of apical and middle one-thirds of root; *b*, Seven weeks later there is obvious resorption of the root canal walls in the vicinity of the fracture line.

Andreasen and Hjorting-Hansen (1967) describe three types of repair following successful treatment of root fractures. The two fragments may become united by hard tissue, commonly in the form of dentine on the pulpal aspect of the fracture and cementum laterally. Alternatively, cementum may be deposited over the fractured dentinal surfaces, with the formation of connective tissue between the latter. In some instances there is an ingrowth of bone and connective tissue between the two parts of the root. Where treatment is unsuccessful and pulpal necrosis occurs, the tissues in the vicinity of the fracture line remain inflamed; although the pulp in the coronal fragment is necrotic, that in the apical part of the root almost always retains its vitality where the fracture is apical to the coronal one-third of the root.

Occasionally the dentinal walls of the root canal in the vicinity of the fracture are progressively resorbed (*Fig.* 282). In such cases root canal treatment of the coronal part of the root with the use of calcium hydroxide dressings may lead to cessation of the resorptive process and the formation of a barrier of hard tissue at the fracture site (Heithersay, 1975). If this form of treatment is unsuccessful, periapical surgery with removal of the apical part of the root, and possibly the insertion of an endodontic stabilizer (Chapter 14), is indicated.

ii. TEETH WITH NECROTIC PULPS

Where the pulp is necrotic when the patient is first seen, or becomes necrotic later, root canal treatment is indicated.

Unless there is evidence of pulpal necrosis in the apical fragment, only the coronal part of the root need be treated, but the tooth should be checked radiographically at regular intervals to ensure that periapical bone destruction does not develop.

Where the extent of bone destruction indicates pulpal necrosis in the apical part of the root, a successful result is sometimes achieved by root canal treatment alone (*Fig.* 283), but often surgical removal of the apical fragment proves necessary later.

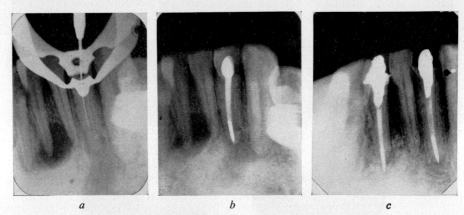

| *a* | *b* | *c* |

Fig. 283. |2̄. *a*, Showing obvious periapical destruction at time of root canal treatment. No root fracture visible; *b*, Fracture of apical one-third of root visible at time of root filling; *c*, Virtually complete periapical repair 8 years later. The apical fracture was not treated.

Where the fracture is in the coronal part of the root and the tooth is mobile, an endodontic stabilizer may be inserted, either to join the two parts of the root or following removal of the apical fragment (Chapter 14).

Vertical root fractures: Compared with transverse fractures, vertical root fractures are rare. The prognosis of such fractures is poor (Michanowicz et al., 1971), and extraction is indicated.

e. Class 5

Complete dislocation of a tooth from its socket is seen less commonly than the other injuries so far described. When it does occur and the tooth is intact, a decision has to be made whether to replant the tooth and accept the fact that it may well be lost in a few years' time as a result of root resorption, or to extract it immediately and either maintain the space or close it by orthodontic treatment. Apart from the orthodontic condition, a major factor to be considered is the length of time that has elapsed since the accident, resorption being more likely the longer the tooth has been out of its socket (Flanagan and Myers, 1958; Andreasen and Hjorting-Hansen, 1966). Replantation more than 2 hours after the accident will almost certainly be followed by root resorption (Andreasen and Hjorting-Hansen, 1966).

Replantation

i. TECHNIQUE

The account of planned replantation given in Chapter 14 applies in large measure to the replantation of accidentally dislocated teeth also. However, certain additional aspects of treatment merit consideration. If the patient or his parent telephones before coming to the surgery, he should be instructed to keep the tooth moist, for example by wrapping it in a clean handkerchief soaked in water. This also keeps the tooth reasonably clean, besides preventing desiccation of its periodontal membrane. If, when the patient attends, there is evidence that the tooth has been on the ground, systemic antibiotic therapy and antitetanus serum or toxoid should be given. Whilst this is being done, the tooth is washed in a solution of normal saline or penicillin to remove extraneous material.

The study of Andreasen and Hjorting-Hansen (1966) indicates that replantation of incompletely formed teeth is followed by revascularization of the pulp in approximately 50 per cent of cases. Provided the patient is seen within 1 or 2 hours of the accident, therefore, such a tooth should be replanted without root filling. Frequent checks should be carried out subsequently, though, and root canal treatment instituted immediately should pulpal necrosis become evident.

With fully formed teeth, on the other hand, revascularization of the pulp rarely takes place, and immediate root canal treatment is therefore indicated. Although it is still common practice among many workers to root fill the tooth before it is replanted, Löe and Waerhaug (1961) reported good results by deferring root filling until after replantation, and this approach, which is favoured by Andreasen and Hjorting-Hansen (1966), is probably preferable.

Blood clot is first removed from the socket by irrigation. The tooth is then replanted and a splint constructed and applied. Root canal treatment is instituted as soon as possible.

A stable tooth following replantation by no means precludes resorption of the root and inflammation of the supporting tissues, as Knight et al. (1964) have shown. The tooth and its supporting structures should be examined clinically and radiographically 3 months, 6 months and 1 year after replantation, and then annually.

ii. PROGNOSIS

The most important factor influencing the prognosis following replantation is probably the time interval that elapses before treatment. Thus, in a study of 110 teeth observed for 2 months to 13 years, Andreasen and Hjorting-Hansen (1966) found that of teeth replanted within 30 minutes of the accident, only 10 per cent showed resorption; of teeth replanted after more than 2 hours, however, 95 per cent underwent resorption.

However, replantation of a tooth within 30 minutes of dislocation is seldom possible, and retention of a replanted tooth for more than 5 years may be considered a very satisfactory result (*Fig.* 284). The studies of Skieller and Lenstrup (1959) and Grossman and Ship (1970) show that the large majority of these teeth are either lost or show radiographic evidence of progressive root resorption within 2 years.

The relatively poor prognosis of replantation emphasizes how unwise it is to extract and replant a tooth which, although severely dislocated and very loose, is still in its socket. Such a tooth should be repositioned and splinted, and later root filled in situ.

f. Class 6

Intrusion of a tooth into the supporting bone, although not uncommon with primary teeth, is relatively uncommon in the permanent dentition. Thus, in the study of Andreasen (1970b), only 23 (12 per cent) of 189 displaced teeth had been intruded.

It is generally agreed that an intruded tooth should be left to re-erupt of its own accord and that no immediate attempt should be made to reposition it.

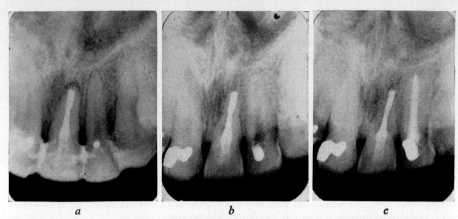

Fig. 284. |1. *a,* Immediately after root filling and replantation; *b,* Two years later, root resorption is apparent; *c,* Five years later, further resorption is apparent. The tooth was eventually extracted about 2 years later.

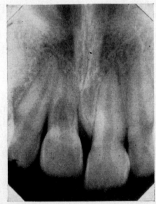

Fig. 285. Gross resorption, probably internal, of root of 1|, following trauma with intrusion of the tooth.

If there is no sign of re-eruption, it may be possible to pull the tooth into position by means of an orthodontic appliance acting on a pin cemented in its crown. After re-eruption, the tooth is observed clinically and radiographically and the pulp periodically tested for vitality.

The long-term prognosis of an intruded tooth is poor. Andreasen (1970b) found that 96 per cent of such teeth underwent pulpal necrosis, whilst 48 per cent showed loss of crestal bone and 52 per cent progressive external root resorption. Occasionally internal resorption occurs (*Fig.* 285).

Chapter 17

Restoration and bleaching of root-filled teeth

PRINCIPLES OF RESTORATION OF ROOT-FILLED TEETH

The retention of a tooth by root canal treatment is of limited value unless the crown of the tooth is satisfactorily restored. The manner in which a root-filled tooth is restored is therefore of considerable importance.

1. Time of restoration

In general, the crown should be restored within a short time of root filling the tooth. Unnecessary deferment of the permanent restoration carries the risk of fracture of the remaining crown. Also, leakage or loss of a temporary filling may lead to discoloration coronally, and so complicate the treatment of an anterior tooth.

Grossman (1974) advises that restoration be deferred for 1 week after root filling, on the assumption that an unfavourable clinical reaction, if it is to occur, will usually take place within 24 hours or so of the completion of root canal treatment. This attitude is certainly advisable where a relatively lengthy procedure, such as that involved in making a gold inlay, is necessary. Where the restoration will take only a little time, on the other hand, there is little to be lost by attending to it immediately after root filling, and this should be done if possible.

Should a relatively complex form of treatment such as a crown be indicated, the possibility of rectifying a later failure of root canal treatment must be considered. Where it would be possible to correct such a failure by periapical surgery, restoration may be carried out a week or so after root filling. Where this is not so, however, it is safer to defer restoration for a few months until radiographs indicate the maintenance of a normal periapex or the regeneration of bone within a periapical lesion. A similar approach is advisable if a root-filled tooth is to be used as an abutment for a bridge or metal denture. Deferring construction of the appliance in these cases may also avoid possible interference with periapical healing from increased stresses on the tooth.

Where restoration is to be deferred for an appreciable time, it is important that the remaining crown is adequately protected against possible fracture. If necessary, a temporary crown is made. Should tissue have been lost mesially, distally, or occlusally from the root-filled tooth, there is a danger of tilting or overeruption of one or more teeth (*Fig.* 286). A well-constructed temporary crown will prevent these complications also.

Before making a temporary crown, the margins of the preparation for the eventual permanent restoration should be considered. Where tooth substance has been lost immediately apical of the gingival crevice, gingival surgery, if not already performed preparatory to root canal treatment, may be indicated. The advantage of performing it at this stage instead of later is that by the time the tooth is ready to be

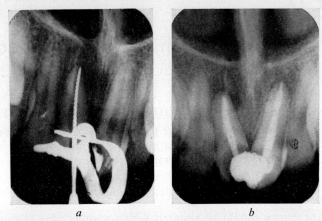

a   *b*

Fig. 286. 1|1. *a*, At time of root canal treatment; *b*, Tilting of 1|1 mesially subsequent to root canal treatment, due to inadequate temporary restorations.

permanently restored the supporting tissues will be in a healthy and 'static' condition.

2. Design of restoration

The design of the restoration is influenced to a considerable degree by the amount of tissue which has been lost. For the same loss of tissue, considerably more of a posterior tooth remains than of an anterior tooth. Also, whilst the restoration must be aesthetically satisfactory in the anterior region of the mouth, this does not necessarily apply to posterior teeth. For these reasons, anterior teeth will be considered separately from posterior teeth. Restorations will be divided, somewhat arbitrarily, into 'simple' and 'complex' types.

a. Simple restorations

i. ANTERIOR TEETH

It was pointed out in Chapter 8 that immediately after filling the canal, surplus filling material should be removed to a level 1–2 mm apical of the cervix of the tooth labially. Besides avoiding discoloration of the coronal dentine from certain constituents, such as the essential oils, of some root-filling cements, this also obviates loss of translucency of the crown due to the opacity of these materials. As a further safeguard against loss of translucency, the dentine of the crown may be treated in the manner described in Chapter 8.

A cavity which comprises only the pulp chamber and the opening into it, or which involves only a small loss of tissue mesially or distally, is best restored, in its entirety, with a composite filling. With a cavity confined to the lingual aspect of the tooth a light shade of material is used, irrespective of the shade of the tooth. This serves to counteract any discoloration of the dentine which may occur later.

For teeth of considerable bulk buccolingually, such as maxillary canines, amalgam may be used provided that discoloration of the coronal dentine is avoided. The major part of the cavity is first filled with composite material, or with silicate or phosphate cement, so that the amalgam used to fill the remainder of the cavity extends no deeper than just 'pulpal' of the amelodentinal junction (*Fig.* 287).

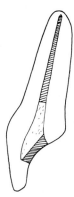

Fig. 287. If amalgam is used to fill the lingual opening into the pulp cavity, it should extend no deeper than just 'pulpal' of the amelodentinal junction. The bulk of the cavity is filled with composite material, or with silicate or phosphate cement.

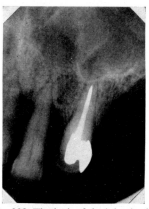

Fig. 288. The lock of the inlay in the root-filled $\underline{3}$ is in the centre of the lingual surface and corresponds to the opening into the pulp cavity.

Since phosphate cement is opaque, it is better to fill the major part of the cavity with composite or silicate.

Where part of the incisal edge is missing, or where there has been an appreciable loss of tissue mesially or distally, an etch-retained composite restoration may be used. Alternatively, where the filling will be largely hidden from view, the tooth may be restored with a gold inlay. If the latter type of restoration is used, the pulp chamber is again filled with composite material or cement; the lock of the preparation is provided by the lingual opening into the pulp chamber, and is therefore somewhat larger and nearer the mesiodistal midline of the crown than in a tooth with a vital pulp (*Fig.* 288).

ii. POSTERIOR TEETH

Vertical fracture of a posterior tooth in a mesiodistal plane is resisted by the roof of the pulp chamber and by the marginal ridges which together serve to join the buccal and lingual aspects of the tooth. Root canal treatment entails removal of the roof of the pulp chamber, so significantly weakening the tooth. Thus, restoration of a root-filled posterior tooth with amalgam is inadvisable unless both marginal ridges are still intact; this is unlikely since pulpal disease is usually the result of advanced caries of an approximal surface.

Where one of the marginal ridges has been lost, a gold restoration with full cuspal coverage is indicated to prevent fracture of the remaining crown. Such a restoration should 'strap' together the buccal and lingual parts of the tooth (*Fig.* 289). Provided the remaining cusps are adequately supported, the same type of restoration is used to restore a tooth in which both marginal ridges have been lost.

b. Complex restorations

The undoubted tendency of root-filled teeth to fracture is due to two factors. First, there is evidence that the calcified tissues of pulpless teeth contain less water than those of teeth with vital pulps (Helfer et al., 1972), and in consequence may be expected to be more brittle. Secondly, a considerable amount of structure has usually been lost from a root-filled tooth, so predisposing to fracture of that which

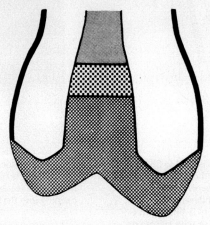

Fig. 289. Where a marginal ridge of a posterior tooth has been lost, the inlay should 'strap' together the weakened buccal and lingual cusps.

remains. Although the relative importance of these two factors is uncertain, there is no doubt that where only a limited amount of the crown remains, special care is needed in restoring it to ensure that it does not fracture subsequently. In general, therefore, the greater the loss of tooth structure the more the restoration has to embrace, and so support, the remaining structure. This implies extension of the restoration to the region of the gingival crevice.

It has already been pointed out that where tooth substance has been lost immediately apical of the gingival crevice, gingival surgery, sometimes with removal of crestal bone, is often necessary. Unless this was done preparatory to root canal treatment, as is usually the case, or before temporarily restoring the tooth following root filling, it is attended to now. The tissues are allowed to heal before the preparation of the crown is completed and impressions taken.

i. ANTERIOR TEETH

When an anterior tooth has lost so much of its structure that complete coverage by an artificial crown is necessary, modification and protection of the remaining natural crown are almost always indicated. A possible exception to this general rule is the maxillary canine tooth, provided it is well formed.

α. *General design of crown*: The stump which remains following jacket crown preparation is invariably weak and therefore has to be reinforced or replaced by a metal core. Retention for this core is gained by extending it into the root canal in the form of a post. Thus, retention of the crown itself is ultimately dependent on the post, and in consequence the eventual restoration is known as a 'post', or 'post-retained', crown.

Post-retained crowns comprise two basic types. Either a 'one-piece' Richmond type of crown, in which the post forms an integral part of the restoration, is constructed, or the core and post and the overlying crown are made as separate entities.

The second type of restoration offers numerous advantages and is generally the more satisfactory. Thus, should caries develop later at the margin of the preparation,

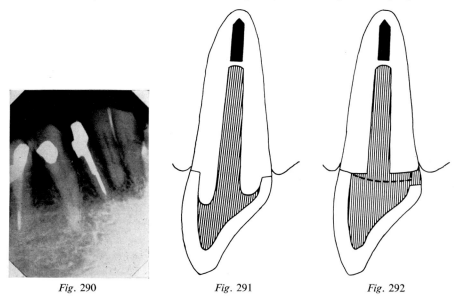

| Fig. 290 | Fig. 291 | Fig. 292 |

Fig. 290. Missing root structure of 2͞| has been replaced by the coronal core, and not by the overlying jacket crown.

Fig. 291. In post crown construction a central stump of dentine resists forces acting on the crown in a labiolingual plane and so prevents their transmission to the opposing surface of the root.

Fig. 292. Where no coronal dentine remains, extension of a post crown preparation gingivally at the periphery of the root face enables the root to be partially encompassed by a collar of gold. In the premolar region, where appearance is less critical, the collar may encircle the entire root face.

only the overlying crown rather than the entire restoration need be removed to permit suitable modification of the preparation. The same procedure is possible should the labial margin of the preparation become visible owing to gingival recession or gingivectomy. Consequently, this type of restoration is particularly indicated where extension of the preparation into the root is necessary in a young adolescent patient, or where there is periodontal disease. Moreover, where there is tilting of the tooth, or of the adjoining teeth, in a mesiodistal direction, the separate paths of insertion of the core and the overlying crown facilitate a better alignment and contour of the latter than when a Richmond type of crown is used. Yet another advantage is that the coronal part of the core, provided it is made of a suitable material, may with little or no modification be used as a bridge abutment should a nearby tooth be lost at a later date. Also, where it is planned beforehand to employ the tooth as an abutment, the use of a separate metal core facilitates alignment of the preparations.

Because of these advantages, the restoration of choice normally consists of a central post and core and a separate overlying crown. The size and shape of the core and the length of the post vary according to the amount of coronal structure which the former has to replace. Sometimes only the incisal tip of the stump is formed by the core, with the result that the post is relatively short. In other cases where little sound coronal dentine remains, the stump is formed entirely, or virtually entirely, by the core, with the result that the post has to be much longer. Missing root structure is replaced by the core rather than by the overlying crown (*Fig.* 290).

Provided it is of adequate strength, a central stump of coronal dentine should be retained wherever possible, since this serves to resist forces acting in a labio-lingual plane and to prevent their transmission to the opposing surface of the root with a consequent risk of root fracture (*Fig.* 291). Where no coronal dentine remains it is advisable to carry the preparation further gingivally around the periphery of the root face; extension of the core in the form of a diaphragm over the root face thus enables the root to be encompassed by a collar of gold (*Fig.* 292). This collar should embrace at least one-half of the periphery of the root, and preferably rather more. Alternatively, if a faced gold crown is to be used, the diaphragm may be omitted and the crown itself so constructed as to achieve the same purpose.

In preparing the post hole, at least 3 mm of root filling should be left apically, otherwise there is a risk of disturbing the apical seal. There should be no radiographic evidence of voids in the apical part of the root filling, which should be of a non-resorbable material. Where the root has been filled by a sectional silver technique, post-hole preparation should not impinge on the silver, the coronal end of which should be covered with a layer of cement (Chapter 8).

It is important that the post is a close fit against the adjacent dentine. The entire root filling, except for the part which remains apically, should therefore be removed (*Fig.* 293). The post should not be located within the original root filling (*Fig.* 294), since this detracts from its value, nor should it be so wide as to cause undue weakening of the root (*Fig.* 295).

To provide sufficient retention it is generally held that the length of the post should be not less than that of the crown which is being restored. A shorter post not only provides less retention but also results in the transmission of forces to a smaller area of the root. Moreover, with a longer post the more are these forces resisted by that part of the root supported by alveolar bone. There is evidence that for optimal distribution of stresses within the root, the post length should approximate to the crown length (Standlee et al., 1972). Where the root is short and a post of effective length cannot be obtained, the core may be extended in the form of a coping over the remaining coronal stump, or an auxiliary pin parallel to the post may be inserted in the root face.

The coronal part of the root canal, and therefore of the root filling, is typically oval in cross-section (Chapter 6). Preparation of the coronal part of the root canal to receive a post of similar oval shape provides resistance to rotational forces acting on the post. Where the shape of the coronal part of the canal is circular in cross-section, or where the post hole is intentionally prepared to receive a post which is circular in cross-section, some form of anti-rotational device is necessary. If a cast core is used, a slot or pin-hole may be cut in the coronal part of one of the walls of the post hole, parallel to the latter and about 2 mm long; normally the lingual wall is selected, since here there is a good bulk of tissue. Alternatively, provided it is strong enough, the entire lingual wall may be cut back so as to produce an oval shape coronally. Where a preformed post and core are used, however,

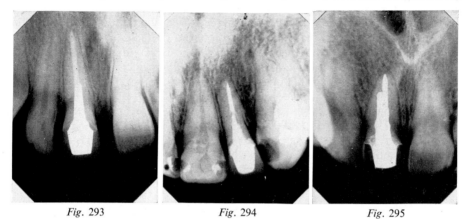

Fig. 293   *Fig.* 294   *Fig.* 295

Fig. 293. A well constructed post in 1|.

Fig. 294. The post in |2 is poorly constructed, since it makes only limited contact with dentine, and is too short.

Fig. 295. Far too much root structure has been removed distally in constructing a post for 1|.

neither of these devices is applicable, and in consequence either the core must be recessed within a slot cut in the root face (*see Fig.* 297) or the uneven height of the shoulder of the preparation for the overlying crown relied upon to resist rotational forces (*see Fig.* 298).

Sharp angles at the coronal opening of the post hole should be avoided, since they produce high levels of stress in the adjacent dentine during loading (Standlee et al., 1972). Also, where a cast core is used, the elimination of such angles facilitates impression taking and construction of the core.

β. *Requirements of post*: The main properties required of a post are that it is retentive, strong, and resistant to rotational forces, but at the same time does not lead to undue weakening of the root.

Tapered posts have been demonstrated not only to be less retentive than parallel-sided posts in the form of right circular cylinders (Colley et al., 1968), but also to have a wedging effect within the root when under load (Standlee et al., 1972), so producing stresses tending to split the root. It might appear, therefore, that ideally a post should be parallel-sided throughout its entire length. As has already been pointed out, though, most root canals not only taper gingivo-apically but are also oval in cross-section coronally, being wider labiolingually than mesiodistally. Thus, unless the apical part of the canal is widened unduly with resultant weakening of the root, preparation of the root for a parallel-sided post will often result in a lack of contact between the coronal part of the post and the adjoining dentine, so leading to loss of retention and a lack of resistance to rotational forces.

In consequence, although it is desirable that the apical part of the post is parallel-sided, or nearly so, coronally the post normally tapers and is often oval in outline. It is desirable that the surface of the post is serrated, or roughened, since this has been shown to give increased retention (Colley et al., 1968). It is also advantageous to 'vent' the post by cutting a groove along its length; by helping the escape of excess cement this should facilitate complete seating of the post, so reducing the thickness of the luting cement and enhancing retention. Venting may also reduce the stresses generated within the apical part of the root (Standlee et al., 1972).

Wrought gold posts are stronger than cast gold posts of corresponding width and are preferable for teeth with narrow roots, such as lower incisors. With the exception of such teeth, however, fracture of a cast post is a rarity, and the choice between a cast or wrought post of no consequence.

There is some evidence that some base metal posts may corrode within the root (Dérand, 1971).

γ. *Methods of post and core construction*: Although many methods of post and core construction are available, they are broadly divisible into five groups, of which three are concerned with the construction of a cast post and core.

'Conventional' cast post and core: The post and core may be cast as an entity, using a conventional direct or indirect impression of both the post hole and root face preparation. Even though some taper on the post hole which is prepared is unavoidable if undercuts are to be precluded, this seems to be of no clinical significance provided the post is of adequate length.

Although the clinical and laboratory procedures are relatively exacting, this method of construction is readily applicable to most teeth. However, in a narrow root not only may a cast post be relatively weak, but also an accurate impression of the post hole may be difficult to obtain.

Preformed metal posts: Both parallel-sided and tapered preformed posts are available. If a tapered post is used, it is desirable that its sides should not converge more than 4°, otherwise retention is markedly reduced (Colley et al., 1968). Preformed metal posts are supplied in a range of sizes and may be used in conjunction with either a direct or indirect impression technique. A gold core is cast onto the preformed post.

Matching reamers or drills are used to prepare a post hole of appropriate depth. As previously pointed out, the coronal part of this hole will not be circular in cross-section, either by virtue of the oval shape of the prepared canal or because of the deliberate use of an antirotational feature in the preparation. In taking an impression with the post in position, therefore, impression material is forced alongside the post into the coronal part of the post hole. Thus, when a core is cast onto the post, metal is also added to the coronal part of the latter.

Examples of tapered posts, in increasing order of convergence, are Endoposts (Kerr), P.D. posts (Produits Dentaires) and Mooser posts (Cendres et Metaux). The difference in convergence between the first- and last-named of these is illustrated in *Fig.* 296. Whilst none of these posts is supplied already vented, P.D. posts are serrated, whilst both smooth and sandblasted Mooser posts are made. Endoposts are smooth. Although formerly available in precious metal, P.D. are now made only in stainless steel.

Paraposts (Whaledent) are parallel-sided and are supplied in a grooved and vented form. If wished they may be employed in conjunction with a paralleling jig to enable the drilling of auxiliary pin-holes in the root face, so providing additional retention and resistance to rotational forces; a direct impression technique is used. Schenker posts (Cendres et Metaux) are also parallel-sided and vented, and are sandblasted; the apical end of this type of post is of narrower cross-section than the coronal part. Instead of using a precious metal post, Harty and Leggett(1972)

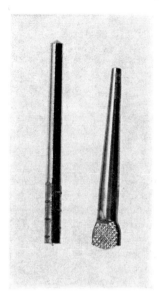

Fig. 296. Preformed metal posts; tapered variety. *Left*, Endopost (Kerr). *Right*, Mooser post (Cendres et Metaux).

advocate the use of a 'post' cut from nickel-chromium clasp wire (Wiptam) of appropriate width; an engineering twist drill of corresponding size is used to prepare the post hole.

Preformed posts can be used in most teeth apart from those with exceptionally wide root canals. Apart from their use in narrow roots, the main advantage of preformed posts in conjunction with cast cores is that an impression of the apical part of the post hole is not needed, since the post fits accurately in this region. In consequence, both clinical and laboratory procedures are simpler than with a cast post and core.

The choice of a preformed metal post is largely a matter of personal preference, but unduly convergent posts are less satisfactory. Endoposts offer the advantage that they are available in a wide range of sizes and have minimal taper. If a parallel-sided post is used, venting is definitely advisable.

Preformed plastic posts: These are also available in a range of sizes and are used in a similar way to preformed metal posts.

Endowels (Star) are vented and are similar to Endoposts in their taper. They are available in a wide range of sizes and may be used with either a direct or indirect impression technique. After investment, the plastic post is burned out together with the waxed core, so resulting in a cast post and core. Tapered P.D. plastic posts are also available.

Although adaptable to a direct impression technique, plastic Paraposts, together with auxiliary pins, are designed for use with an indirect impression technique. The plastic post and pins are withdrawn from the model and replaced with their parallel-sided metal equivalents prior to casting the core.

Preformed plastic posts and cores: One of the advantages of an indirect impression technique is that both the post and core and the overlying crown may be made on the same model, whereas a post and core made from a direct impression has first to be cemented before an indirect impression for the overlying crown can be taken, so entailing an extra visit. However, the former method of construction is open to criticism in that, since both parts of the crown are made on the same model, the position occupied by the post and core after cementation in the tooth is 'proud' relative to that on the model, due to the intervening layer of cement. Thus, when the overlying crown is cemented, the thickness of cement at its margin is, theoretically at any rate, doubled, since the crown cannot be seated as far on the tooth as it could on the model.

The 'KD Gold Post System' is a technique intended to overcome this potential drawback by compensating for the thickness of cement between the post and core and the root. In this technique a plastic core and parallel-sided post are fitted to the root. To ensure close contact between the root face and the core the former is ground flat, following which the post is shortened as necessary. The plastic core may be cut to the shape of a jacket crown preparation either before an indirect impression has been taken or after a model has been cast from the impression. The plastic post and core are now invested and a casting made. A perforated metal disc is slid over the cast post to contact the core, so making the latter stand slightly 'proud' of the model. The overlying crown is then made.

Because of the need for a flat root face, this method is readily applicable only to teeth with little natural crown remaining. The cast post should be vented.

Preformed metal posts and cores: Two types of preformed, one-piece metal post and core are available, each in a small range of sizes.

One of these, introduced by Charlton (1965), is made of stainless steel, and consists of a smooth, parallel-sided post and a partially shaped core blank with flat facets mesially and distally. These facets face the sides of a labiolingual slot which is cut in the root face (*Fig.* 297), so providing resistance to rotational forces. After preliminary widening of the root canal to the necessary depth, a parallel-sided post hole is cut with a flat fissure bur matching in width the selected post. The latter is shortened until the post and core can be fully seated. Before cementation, the core blank is cut to the approximate shape of a jacket crown.

The other type, which is described by Kurer (1967), consists of a threaded stainless-steel post with a staked brass head forming the core blank; the head has a slot 'incisally' to accommodate the end of a screwdriver and projects into a recess countersunk in the root face (*Fig.* 298). After enlargement of the root canal with reamers, a thread is cut along the sides of the post hole with the aid of a hand-tap. The post is shortened as necessary and is then coated with a thin mix of cement and screwed home. After setting of the cement, the brass head is cut to the form of a jacket crown preparation. The uneven height of the shoulder of the preparation is relied upon to resist rotational forces on the crown and their transmission to the post (*Fig.* 298).

As with the K.D. system, both of these methods entail the removal of most or all of the clinical crown. Since it is not possible to cast onto the post, the addition of a diaphragm integral with the post and core is not possible and excessive widening of the apical part of the post hole may be necessary to ensure that the coronal part of the post fits the adjoining root canal walls. Standlee et al., (1972) point out that a threaded post generates considerable stress within the root if the recess which is countersunk is fully engaged by the head or if it is out of line with the long axis of

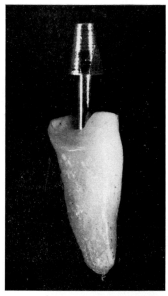

Fig. 297. Preformed stainless steel post and core blank; Charlton type. After insertion, the flat facets on the mesial and distal surfaces of the core face the sides of a labiolingual slot cut in the root face.

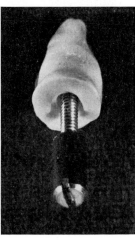
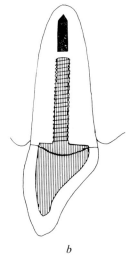

a   *b*

Fig. 298. *a*, Preformed metal post and core blank, Kurer type. The core blank has a 'slot' incisally to accomodate the end of a screwdriver and projects into a circular recess in the root face; *b*, Kurer post and core blank after insertion and jacket crown preparation. The uneven level of the shoulder is relied upon to resist rotational forces acting on the crown being transmitted to the core and post.

the post hole. They also draw attention to the care which is needed to avoid root fracture when using the hand tap.

ii. POSTERIOR TEETH

α. *Some natural crown remaining*: Often, cuspal coverage of a posterior tooth is by itself insufficient to safeguard the remaining crown against fracture. With molar teeth, extending the preparation in the form of a three-quarter or full crown is

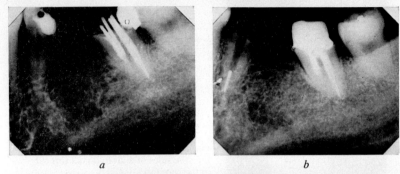

a   *b*

Fig. 299. ⌐7. *a*, Threaded stainless steel pins cemented into mesial and distal canals; *b*, Shaped amalgam core. None of the natural crown remains.

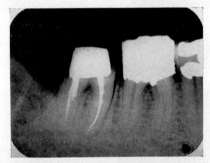

Fig. 300. Amalgam core 7⌐ retained by Dentatus screws in mesial and distal roots.

frequently satisfactory. On other occasions, especially with premolar teeth, the cusps are so severely undermined that there is a risk of horizontal fracture of the tooth at gingival level unless vertical support is given to the remaining crown. This is achieved either by the cementation of a post or screw into one or more root canals, or by the insertion of dentine pins around the periphery of the pulp chamber, or both. These devices are normally used to retain an amalgam or composite core, over which is placed a crown (*see Figs*. 299 and 300).

The choice between peripheral pins and an intra-radicular post or screw, such as a Dentatus screw or a Kurer crown-saver anchor, depends not only on the amount of coronal tissue remaining but also on the amenability of the individual root to periapical surgery should periapical disease develop later. Where the root-end would be accessible to periapical surgery, the choice between peripherally placed dentine pins and a post or screw within the root canal is, from the endodontic viewpoint, immaterial. However, with a root which would be inaccessible, peripheral pins, provided they will adequately support and retain the restoration, are preferable, since unlike a post they would not impede retreatment of the canal by way of the pulp chamber.

β. *Little or no crown remaining*: In teeth with little or none of the natural crown remaining, the insertion of retentive devices into the root canals is unavoidable.

Premolar teeth are normally restored by a conventional post and core and an overlying crown. In the majority of two-rooted premolars, the two canals are parallel coronally, or may safely be made so by the removal of relatively little dentine. In these teeth a post approximately one-half the length of the clinical crown is inserted into each root (*see Fig.* 304).

With two-rooted premolar teeth with widely divergent canals and also with molar teeth, an amalgam core retained by a post or screw in each of the roots is normally satisfactory (*Figs.* 299 and 300); wherever possible the overlying crown should be extended beyond the amalgam in a gingival direction to embrace the remaining tooth substance and so reduce lateral stresses on the posts. If a core of gold is preferred to one of amalgam, one of three techniques may be followed. The simplest of these is to insert a 'master' post at least as long as the clinical crown

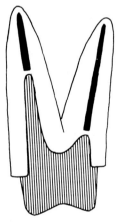

Fig. 301. One type of post and core construction for two-rooted premolars with divergent canals. One root is prepared for a long 'master' post and the other for a short 'accessory' post. A similar construction may be used for multirooted teeth.

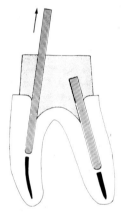

Fig. 302. Alternative post and core construction for teeth with divergent canals. The coronal end of the pre-formed metal post in the 'master' post hole is embedded in an overlying acrylic resin core. The lubricated plastic post in the 'accessory' post hole is withdrawn prior to removal and casting of the core.

into the root canal best suited for this purpose; in a premolar this will be the canal nearer the long axis of the tooth, whereas in a molar it will normally be the wide distal or palatal canal. Into each of the other roots is inserted an 'accessory' post 2–3 mm long; this is in line with the master post and serves as an antirotational device, but provides little retention (*Fig.* 301). Undercuts may need to be eliminated from the pulp chamber.

Alternatively, the accessory post holes may be made of greater depth and in line with their respective canals, and the Parapost technique described by Wearn (1974) used to overcome the undercuts so created. In this technique a preformed metal post is inserted into the master post hole and a lubricated plastic post into each of the other post holes. A core of Duralay is then built up in the mouth, the accessory posts withdrawn, and the core and attached master post removed (*Fig.* 302). After casting, the core and master post are tried in the tooth, with the insertion through the core of the metal equivalent of each accessory plastic post. The master post and core and the accessory posts are cemented simultaneously. A similar technique may be followed using, for example, an Endopost or Endowel as the

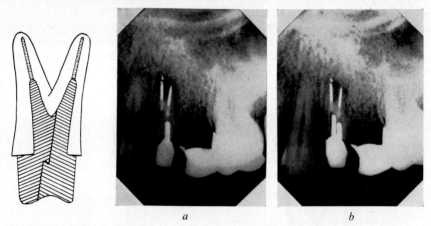

a   *b*

Fig. 303. Two-piece,   *Fig.* 304. |4. *a*, When inserting a split gold core, that part contri-
or split gold core in a   buting less to the occlusal surface is inserted first; *b*, The other
two-rooted premolar.   part of the core is then inserted.

master post and a length of parallel-sided wire such as Wiptam for each accessory post.

The core, instead of forming one piece, may be constructed in two or more separate, interlocking sections, each with a post extending into the preparation within the corresponding root (*Fig.* 303). This technique, described by Rosen (1961), is more complex and uses an elastic, indirect impression technique. The different parts of the core are made to interlock coronally by means of a mortise type of joint or a semi-precision lock. Each section is inserted separately (*Fig.* 304). At the time of cementation the section which contributes least to the occlusal surface is cemented first, and that which contributes most to the occlusal surface last.

Sometimes pulpal disease occurs in a tooth which already has a satisfactory artificial crown, and in consequence root canal treatment is performed through the crown. In such a case there is often some doubt about the amount of coronal dentine which remains to support the restoration after root filling. Under these circumstances the remaining tooth stump is supported by the cementation of a post or screw into the canal most suited for this purpose and amalgam used to obliterate the pulp chamber and access cavity.

BLEACHING OF ROOT-FILLED TEETH

Discoloration of the crown of a root-filled anterior tooth is, unfortunately, not uncommon. In some teeth the discoloration may be eliminated merely by the removal of root-filling material and obviously stained dentine from the interior of the crown. In other teeth this treatment alone is insufficient. Before dealing with the possibility of bleaching such a tooth, a brief account will be given of the causes of discoloration and its prevention.

1. Causes of discoloration

The local causes of discoloration of dentine, other than caries, may be divided into four groups.

a. Decomposition of pulpal tissue or food debris

Decomposition of the pulp is a common cause of discoloration of the dentine. The presence of gas-producing organisms in a necrotic pulp may lead to the formation of black iron sulphide, by the action of hydrogen sulphide on haemoglobin.

Staining of the dentine may also follow upon the accumulation of food debris in the pulp cavity. After drainage of an acute purulent condition, therefore, the pulp cavity should be sealed from the mouth without undue delay.

b. Haemorrhage into pulp cavity

Haemorrhage into the pulp cavity may be caused by trauma, in the form of a blow or fall, by the application of arsenical devitalizing agents to the pulp, or by the extirpation of a vital pulp. Following haemorrhage, the haemoglobin released by lysis of erythrocytes breaks down into products which discolour dentine.

c. Root canal medicaments

Many of the drugs advocated in the past for use in canals, particularly antiseptics, may lead to discoloration. Examples are silver nitrate, concentrated iodine solutions, and the essential oils.

The antibiotics chlortetracycline (Aureomycin) and oxytetracycline (Terramycin) have also been stated to discolour dentine sometimes.

d. Root canal filling materials

Amongst the root-filling materials which can discolour the crown are iodoform and root canal cements which contain silver or essential oils. The presence of silver or copper amalgam in the pulp cavity may cause darkening of the dentine.

2. Prevention of discoloration

Discoloration of a tooth subsequent to root canal treatment can in most instances be prevented by giving proper attention to various aspects of treatment.

It is important that the opening into the pulp chamber is large enough to permit the removal of all pulpal debris in the crown, particularly incisally. After removal of a vital pulp, all traces of blood should be eliminated from the pulp chamber. Haemorrhage should have ceased by the time the pulp cavity is dressed and sealed. Large strands of tissue coronal to the level at which the pulp was severed should not be allowed to remain, since they are likely to bleed later.

Root canal medicaments known to stain dentine are best avoided. After root filling, the pulp chamber and the coronal part of the canal are cleared of material to a level 1–2 mm apical of the cervix of the tooth labially. This is best done immediately after root filling. Should this be impracticable, it should not be deferred for longer than a few days.

As was pointed out earlier in this chapter, in restoring the crown of an incisor tooth the pulp chamber is filled with a translucent material, and not with one which is opaque. Prior to restoration the dentine may be treated with an agent designed to prevent loss of translucency following on dehydration. This aspect has already been dealt with in Chapter 8.

In a minority of cases, despite the utmost care during the root canal treatment and restoration of a tooth, the crown discolours. In certain of these cases the discoloration may be eliminated by bleaching.

3. Bleaching

a. Prognosis; Indications

The factors influencing the prognosis of bleaching the crown of a root-filled tooth are ill-defined. However, it is generally accepted that discoloration from root canal medicaments and filling materials is difficult to eliminate, and that the longer the tooth has been discoloured the less the likelihood of success.

Moreover, even if the crown is successfully bleached, there is a distinct tendency, sometimes manifest within a few months, for discoloration to recur. The reason for this is not clear, but it may be associated with the ingress of pigments from the saliva by way of the enamel, the permeability of which may be increased by the bleaching process. Brown (1965) reports that although some improvement was evident in the majority of teeth treated by bleaching, less than 30 per cent could be counted as completely successful when examined 1–5 years later.

In general a post-retained crown is a far more certain and satisfactory method of treatment for a discoloured tooth than bleaching, especially where discoloration is due to root canal medicaments or materials. However, the construction of an aesthetic crown for a tooth which is thin labiolingually or of an unusual or very light shade may be difficult and under these circumstances bleaching is worth trying.

Bleaching is normally confined to anterior teeth, and obviously is only performed on teeth needing simple restorations. It is desirable that the enamel is free of obvious cracks, since these may contribute to recurrence of discoloration. The uncertainties concerning the procedure should be explained to the patient before treatment is begun.

b. Technique

i. PREPARATORY TREATMENT

The discoloured tooth and the neighbouring teeth are first polished. Since interaction between the bleaching agent and base metals may cause staining of dentine, amalgam fillings in the tooth to be treated are best removed. Silicate and composite restorations, on the other hand, may be left, although it will be necessary to replace the former later, since they become dehydrated during the bleaching process. Any filling surrounded by softened dentine must be removed to allow elimination of the affected dentine.

A rubber dam is used for isolation. Wherever possible, only the tooth under treatment is isolated. Should it be necessary to isolate other teeth as well, any silicate restorations which they contain are coated heavily with varnish to prevent their dehydration. Since the bleaching agent is caustic, it is advisable to protect the labial and lingual gingivae against possible leakage of the agent by coating them with petroleum jelly beforehand.

If the pulp chamber has already been filled, it is re-opened so that all parts of it are freely accessible. All filling material, whether used to restore the crown or to

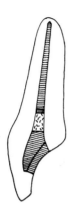

Fig. 305. The bleaching process is continued by sealing a paste of hydrogen peroxide and Bocasan in the pulp cavity. A double seal of gutta percha and fast-setting zinc oxide–eugenol cement is used. When bleaching a tooth, the coronal end of the root filling should be sealed with a layer of cement.

fill the root canal, is removed from the pulp cavity to a level about 3·0 mm apical of the cervix of the tooth labially (see Fig. 305). By working to this level—which takes in the extreme coronal end of the root canal—exposure of a discoloured region of the tooth due to gingival recession later is avoided.

The cavity is now inspected, and as much stained dentine as possible removed without unduly weakening the crown. To prevent the bleaching agent penetrating to the periapical region by way of unsuspected gaps in the root filling, it is advisable to seal the coronal end of the latter with a layer of fast-setting cement, about 1 mm thick (see Fig. 305). This precaution is essential if there is clinical or radiographic evidence of voids in the filling.

In an attempt to eliminate the fatty products of pulpal decomposition, which could prevent penetration of the bleaching agent into the dentinal tubules and thereby interfere with the bleaching process, all accessible dentine is 'scrubbed' with a wool pledget soaked in chloroform. To assist in desiccation of the dentine and penetration of the bleaching agent, the same procedure is repeated with alcohol. Alternatively, instead of using chloroform and alcohol separately, a mixture of two or three parts of alcohol to one of chloroform may be employed.

Drying of the cavity and the adjoining dentine is completed with a stream of warm air.

ii. BLEACHING AGENTS

The principle of bleaching is to convert the compounds causing discoloration into colourless substances. Although this may be done by either oxidation or reduction, an oxidizing agent is usually employed.

The two most popular oxidizing agents which have been used for bleaching teeth are probably a 30 per cent w/v solution of hydrogen peroxide in distilled water

(Concentrated Hydrogen Peroxide Solution, B.P.), which is equivalent to 100 volumes strength, and a 25 per cent solution of hydrogen peroxide in ether. The disadvantages of the second preparation are its nauseating odour and its lack of stability once its container is opened. These drawbacks, which do not apply to the first preparation, outweigh any benefit which the ether confers by encouraging diffusion of the solution into the dentinal tubules. In consequence, Concentrated Hydrogen Peroxide Solution, B.P., is generally favoured, and the following account assumes that this solution is used.

Concentrated Hydrogen Peroxide Solution is provided in dark, glass or plastic stoppered bottles. When not in use it should be kept refrigerated to prevent

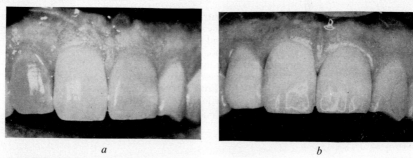

Fig. 306. 2|1. *a*, Before bleaching; *b*, After bleaching.

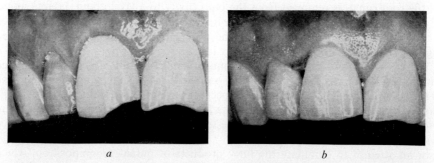

Fig. 307. 2|. *a*, Before bleaching; *b*, After bleaching. The incisal edges of the teeth were recontoured.

decomposition. When required, a little of the solution is transferred to a suitable receptacle, such as a Dappens glass, and the bottle immediately removed from the working area and returned to the refrigerator. Any solution left at the end of each treatment should be discarded from the receptacle. When handling the solution, the operator should take particular care not to splash it over the skin of either the patient or himself. Should such an accident happen, the affected area is immediately washed with water and covered with petroleum jelly. The solution should obviously be kept away from articles of clothing.

iii. BLEACHING PROCESS

Various techniques of bleaching with hydrogen peroxide have been advocated. Each relies upon the release of nascent oxygen from hydrogen peroxide placed within the pulp chamber. Thus, heat may be applied from an infrared lamp, or light from an ultraviolet lamp; alternatively, both heat and light may be employed, using a lamp with a no. 1 photoflood bulb (275 W). However, whilst indicating that the application of heat and light simultaneously is better than the use of either alone, the study of Gray (1964) suggests that forcing peroxide into the dentinal tubules under pressure produces the best results.

A wool pledget is packed into the coronal part of the canal and the pulp chamber and is saturated with hydrogen peroxide. The orifice of the cavity is then sealed with gutta percha and fairly heavy pressure applied to the latter for a few moments with the aid of a ball-ended burnisher or suitably trimmed orange-wood stick. This procedure is repeated two or three times. If it is wished to apply heat and light to the tooth, a fresh pledget of wool saturated with peroxide is inserted into the cavity and the light from a photoflood bulb directed onto the crown from a distance of about 40 cm for 20 minutes; the patient's eyes should be protected with dark glasses and the wool pledget and peroxide replaced every few minutes.

The cavity is now dried and a thick paste of hydrogen peroxide and sodium perborate, or alternatively Bocasan (Knox Laboratories), packed into the coronal part of the canal and adjoining pulp chamber. This paste continues the bleaching process, especially of the thicker cervical part of the tooth which is the slowest to respond, and in fact has been recommended by Nutting and Poe (1967) as a replacement for other methods of applying hydrogen peroxide. The remainder of the cavity is sealed with a layer of gutta percha and then zinc oxide cement in order to prevent disintegration of the latter and consequent leakage (*Fig.* 305).

Since a bleached tooth tends to revert in some degree to its former colour fairly soon after treatment, an attempt should be made to 'overbleach' it to a lighter shade than the adjoining teeth. To this end the patient should be seen again in 3 or 4 days. Provided there has been a significant improvement of the sort shown in *Figs.* 306 and 307, fresh paste should be sealed within the pulp chamber. If no such improvement has occurred, a successful result is unlikely and bleaching should be abandoned.

Directly the necessary colour has been obtained the pulp chamber is cleaned of paste and the tooth restored, otherwise partial or complete loss of the cement seal may lead to fresh discoloration.

iv. MAINTAINING TRANSLUCENCY

In an attempt to restore the translucency of the crown, or to prevent it being lost later, before restoring the tooth the coronal dentine may be treated in the manner described in Chapter 8.

REFERENCES

Brown G. (1965) Factors influencing successful bleaching of the discolored root-filled tooth. *Oral Surg.* **20**, 238.

Charlton G. (1965) A prefabricated post and core for porcelain jacket crowns. *Br. Dent. J.* **119**, 452.

Colley I. T., Hampson E. L. and Lehman M. L. (1968) Retention of post crowns: an assessment of the relative efficiency of posts of different shapes and sizes. *Br. Dent. J.* **124**, 63.

Dérand T. (1971) Corrosion of screwposts. *Odontol. Revy* **22**, 371.

Gray H. S. (1964) The bleaching of artificially stained teeth. *N.Z. Dent. J.* **60**, 93.

Grossman L. I. (1974) *Endodontic Practice*, 8th ed. London, Kimpton, p. 319.

Harty F. J. and Leggett L. J. (1972) A post crown technique using a nickel-cobalt-chromium post. *Br. Dent. J.* **132**, 394.

Helfer A. R., Melnick S. and Schilder H. (1972) Determination of the moisture content of vital and pulpless teeth. *Oral Surg.* **34**, 661.

Kurer P. F. (1967) Retention of post crowns: a solution of the problem. *Br. Dent. J.* **123**, 167.

Nutting E. B. and Poe G. S. (1967) Chemical bleaching of discolored endodontically treated teeth. *Dent. Clin. N. Am.* **11**, 655–62.

Roşen H. (1961) Operative procedures on mutilated endodontically treated teeth. *J. Prosthet. Dent.* **11**, 973.

Standlee J. P., Caputo A. A., Collard E. W. and Pollack M. H. (1972) Analysis of stress distribution by endodontic posts. *Oral Surg.* **33**, 952.

Wearn D. I. (1974) Posts and cores in divergent canals. *Aust. Dent. J.* **19**, 346.

FURTHER READING

Baraban D. J. (1967) The restoration of pulpless teeth. *Dent. Clin. North Am.* **11**, 633–53.

Index